AETCOM

Attitude, EThics and COMmunication

MANUAL

Learning Modules for MBBS Professional Year IV
Competencies for the
Indian Medical Graduate

As Recommended by National Medical Commission

AETCOM

Attitude, EThics and COMmunication

MANUAL

Learning Modules for MBBS Professional Year IV
Competencies for the
Indian Medical Graduate

As Recommended by National Medical Commission

Nitin Ashok John

MBBS MD FRSB (London, UK), FASSOPI (India), FAcad Med Edu (Cardiff, UK 2021), FRSPH (London, UK 2021)
PGDMLE (Medical Law and Ethics, NLSIU Bengaluru), DIH, PGDHA (Hospital Administration)
MA (Public Administration), European Lifestyle Medicine Organization Certified Graduate

Professor and Head
Department of Physiology
All India Institute of Medical Sciences
Bibinagar, Hyderabad

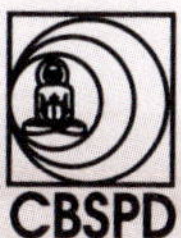

CBS Publishers & Distributors Pvt Ltd

New Delhi • Bengaluru • Chennai • Kochi • Kolkata • Lucknow • Mumbai
Hyderabad • Jharkhand • Nagpur • Patna • Pune • Uttarakhand

Disclaimer

Science and technology are constantly changing fields. New research and experience broaden the scope of information and knowledge. The author has tried his best in giving information available to him while preparing the material for this book. Although all efforts have been made to ensure optimum accuracy of the material, yet it is quite possible some errors might have been left uncorrected. The publisher, the printer and the author will not be held responsible for any inadvertent errors or inaccuracies.

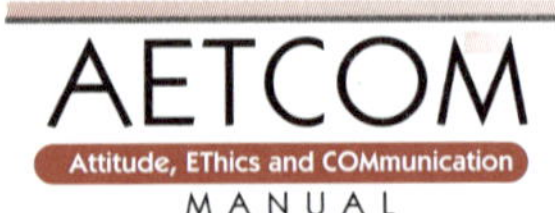

Learning Modules for MBBS Professional Year IV
Competencies for the
Indian Medical Graduate

As Recommended by National Medical Commission

ISBN: 978-93-5466-636-0

First Edition: 2024

Published by **Satish Kumar Jain** and produced by **Varun Jain** for

CBS Publishers & Distributors Pvt Ltd

4819/XI Prahlad Street, 24 Ansari Road, Daryaganj, New Delhi 110 002, India
Ph: 011-23289259, 23266861 Website: www.cbspd.com
e-mail: delhi@cbspd.com

Corporate Office: 204 FIE, Industrial Area, Patparganj, Delhi 110 092, India
Ph: 011-4934 4934 Fax: 011-4934 4935 e-mail: publishing@cbspd.com; publicity@cbspd.com

Branches

- **Bengaluru:** Seema House 2975, 17th Cross, K.R. Road, Banasankari 2nd Stage, Bengaluru 560 070, Karnataka, India
  Ph: +91-80-26771678/79 Fax: +91-80-26771680 e-mail: bangalore@cbspd.com
- **Chennai:** 7, Subbaraya Street, Shenoy Nagar, Chennai 600 030, Tamil Nadu, India
  Ph: +91-44-26680620, 26681266 Fax: +91-44-42032115 e-mail: chennai@cbspd.com
- **Kochi:** 42/1325, 1326, Power House Road, Opposite KSEB, Power House, Ernakulum, Kochi-682 018, Kerala, India
  Ph: +91-484-4059061–67 Fax: +91-484-4059065 e-mail: kochi@cbspd.com
- **Kolkata:** 147, C/o Hind Ceramics Compound,, 1st Floor, Nilgunj Road, Belghoria, Kolkata-700 056, West Bengal, India
  Ph: +91-33-25633055/56 e-mail: kolkata@cbspd.com
- **Lucknow:** Basement, Khushnuma Complex, 7-Meerabai Marg (behind Jawahar Bhawan), Lucknow-226 001, Uttar Pradesh, India.
  Ph: +91-522-4000032 e-mail: tiwari.lucknow@cbspd.com
- **Mumbai:** PWD Shed, Gala No. 25/26, Ramchandra Bhatt Marg, Next to JJ Hospital, Gate No. 2, Opp Union Bank of India, Noorbaug, Mumbai-400009, Maharashtra, India
  Ph: +91-22-66661880, 66661889 e-mail: mumbai@cbspd.com

Representatives

- **Hyderabad** 0-9885175004 • **Jharkhand** 0-9811541605 • **Nagpur** 0-8692091830
- **Patna** 0-9334159340 • **Pune** 0-9664372571 • **Uttarakhand** 0-9716462459

Printed at: Mudrak, Noida, UP, India

Preface

I am happy to share that the *AETCOM Manual* for MBBS fourth year professional is ready to release. The manual has been written with the objective to inculcate high moral principles and ethical values. This manual covers the medical ethics curriculum designed for the students of MBBS as per the recommendation of the National Medical Commission. The book also covers important topics on medical ethics as recommended by the Medical Council of various South Asian countries, UK, the US, Canada, New Zealand, and Australia. The key features of the book are its simplified expression of text, defined learning objectives at the beginning of each chapter, the easy, lucid, and comprehensive language of expression and it includes case scenarios for interactive learning and for better grasping of concepts.

The book also covers important topics on foundations of communication, case studies in medicolegal and ethical situations, case studies in ethics empathy and the doctor–patient relationship, case studies in ethics: The doctor–industry relationship, case studies in ethics and patient autonomy, dealing with death and medical negligence.

Key Features of the Book

- Simplified text for easy reproducibility.
- Well-defined learning objectives.
- Easy, lucid, and comprehensive coverage of all topics.
- Case scenarios for interactive learning and for better grasp of concepts.
- Recommended references for reading for explorative learning.
- Case resolution for a clear understanding of the intricacy of the issue.
- Formative and summative assessment protocol included.
- The manual is so designed that students can note lecture points, resolve case scenarios, write formative and summative assessments, and moreover, after completion of the course,

a record is available to evaluate students' performance and grade them.

I am thankful to Dr Vikas Bhatia, Director, All India Institute of Medical Sciences, Bibinagar, Hyderabad, for his encouragement and support. I am thankful to Mr Satish Jain (CMD), CBS Publishers & Distributors Pvt. Ltd., Mr YN Arjuna (Senior Vice President—Publishing, Editorial and Publicity) and all publishing staff.

I am thankful to my mother Mrs Ujwala Parekh, wife Dr Jyoti and son Joshua for all their support in this endeavor.

I hope that the book will stand immensely helpful to all readers. All efforts have been made to write the script in flawless manner, and mistakes if any due to oversight may be pardoned. Looking forward for your suggestions which i will keep in view when bringing out the next edition of this manual.

Nitin Ashok John

Contents

Index of Competencies

Competency based Undergraduate Curriculum for the Indian Medical Graduate

Module

4.1

The Foundations of Communication

Background: The skills of effective way of communication are being taught from first professional year. The art of communication is important in medical practice for developing rapport with the patient as well as for eliciting proper medical history for right diagnosis as well as for monitoring prognosis and therapy effectively.

Learning Objectives: The student after learning the module must be able to:

1. Demonstrate ability while communicating to an ill person in a patient, respectful, nonthreatening, non-judgmental and empathetic manner.
2. Communicate and inform to patient and family regarding diagnostic and therapeutic options in a simulated environment.

SESSION I

Introductory Small Group Session (1 hour)

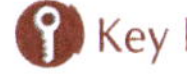

Principles of communication with focus on administering informed consent:

1. The student should learn to communicate with patient respectfully and should never be threatening, judgmental or nonempathic towards patient.
2. While recording patient's medical history he should record each and every problem told by patient regarding the health issues; further, patiently it is necessary to ask questions in relevance to differential diagnosis which the student suspects in order to arrive at an appropriate diagnosis.
3. Informed consent must be obtained from patient for all diagnostic, therapeutic and surgical interventions planned by the doctor.

4. Informed consent should be complete in terms of explaining the patient's health condition, planned management strategies, foreseen complication, prognosis, expected outcome and what is best in patient's health welfare.
5. Written consent is appropriate method for obtaining consent for official records.
6. As consenting for healthcare is patient's fundamental right; the patient should not be pressurized, threatened and bullied for giving consent but it should be by patient's own free will without any pressure or prejudices or under intoxication. The doctor acts as a facilitator for clearing patient's doubt but cannot infringe on patient's right.
7. The patient when coming to doctor is considered to have accepted implied consenting for general physical examination and other routine investigations. But any other management modality, therapeutic, diagnostic and surgical intervention obtaining written consent is a must.
8. A word of caution: Incomplete disclosure may lead to litigation.
9. The students must communicate in simple, lucid and local language and provide complete and adequate information regarding the disease, management, outcome, risks and benefits of treatment, follow-up required and prevention and same be written in easy understandable language for patient.
10. Consent in written be obtained from parent or guardian in case of minor, incapacitated individual or in case if child is having lunacy.
11. The care to be taken to clarify doubts and question of patient / parent/ guardian as applicable.
12. Information revealed should testify prudent patient that is expected of average patient.
13. All consent document should be safely documented.
14. All informed refusal must be entered in recorded and documented.

BIBLIOGRAPHY

1. Etchells E, Sharpe G, Walsh P, Williams JR, Singer PA. Bioethics for clinicians: 1. Consent. *CMAJ*. 1996;155:177–80.
2. Satyanarayana Rao KH. Informed consent: an ethical obligation or legal compulsion? J Cutan Aesthet Surg. 2008 Jan;1(1):33–5.

SESSION II

Focused Small Group Sessions (2 hours)

Note: The students can enact a role play and write their observations as to observe, criticize and discuss common mistakes committed in role play administering informed consent.

Role Play 1:

Dr Raju: **Vinita** you are adult over 18 years and as you are obese we will have procedure of liposuction done as part of management.

Vinita: Yes I am 105 kg, well I want to be slim ... and yes wish to get married in future

Dr Raju: Well you decide and come for admission tomorrow

Vinita's parents are busy businessmen ...

Radhikha Kumari: **Vinita's mother** asks doctor ... whether it is necessary ... Is there any other method for reducing weight?

Dr Raju: **Amma** ... lots of info is available on net ... you can tell Vinita to surf down

Vinita: Please tell me what are risks after the procedure; how much weight will I loose; how will be the follow-up schedule

Dr Raju: Well, I have treated 100 of patients; you can see photo in album in reception ... yes all will be well ... Nurse will explain you all ...

Next patient Nurse..............................

Dr Raju: Ok see you tomorrow... Bring Rs 50000/ as advance deposit

Vinita to Nurse: **Sister** I want to know regarding what are risks after the procedure; how much weight will I loose; how will be the follow-up schedule

Nurse: **Vinita** ... That's all in paper which you will sign tomorrow ... Well one thing...you will look very beautiful after the surgery ...

Next day morning Vinita's mother get her admitted to Dr Raju's hospital ...

Junior Doctor: Get Consent Form signed by Vinita and her mother too.

Without any information and communication the consent is signed.

Observation by

Observe, criticize and discuss common mistakes committed in role-play administering informed consent.

The students shall discuss and record their opinions below:

The group teacher/facilitator to make opinion regarding student's presentation: The students to note important clues and corrective action below—ideal situational modification in such scenario:

Exercise 1: Skills Lab Session: 2 hours

Ask student to comprehend a consent form for 55 years old female patient who needs to be admitted and posted for laparotomy next day. You are attending the patient as junior consultant in OPD:

Exercise 2:

Design and obtain a written consent for management of child reporting for urgent appendectomy with the parent:

Task

1. You have obtained consent for MTP from 16-year-old girl with her mother around. A standard written consent form was handed over to patient for signature.
2. Your friend can be the patient
3. Your teacher is the facilitator
4. Write your observation as self critique, critique by patient and by facilitator

Students Assessment by Faculty Incharge

1. Formative

Assessment of participation of student in session 2 and in session 3 was:

Name of Student: ....

Participation in session 2:
Excellent/Very Good/Good/Satisfactory/Poor

Signature: Faculty Incharge AETCOM ....

Participation in session 3:
Excellent/Very Good/Good/Satisfactory/Poor

Signature: Faculty Incharge AETCOM ....

2. Summative

Administer informed consent provided to patient. Note your designed consent form and obtain patient's signature and record it below:

___

___

___

___

___

___

___

___

___

Disclaimer: All information in **Module 4.1**: The foundations of communication, includes but not limited to, and is for information purpose only. The editor declares that the sincere attempt has been made to give standard accurate information in Module 4.1, but it is not a substitute for any legal or professional advice. The reader should seek advice from legal professional if they seek consultation and advice for any issue associated with fiduciary duty.

Module

4.2

Case Studies in Medicolegal and Ethical Situations

Background: The students are expected to thoroughly grasp and obtain knowledge regarding the medicolegal and ethical aspects of abortion and conflict situation which may arise in adolescent age group. The case is self designed for discussion and is in line with syllabus. The teachers may formulate case study for discussion in their setup.

Learning Objectives: The students after studying the module should be able to discuss and describe the socioeconomical and ethical issues regarding medicolegal and ethical aspects of abortion, medical termination of pregnancy and reproductive health.

ASSIGNMENT I

Introduction to Case: 1 hour

The student should introduce the case and teacher should take a pretest regarding the point of discussion of the case and guide them.

Case: An 18 years old female staying in hostel reach back home and reveals to her mother regarding her state of amenorrhea since 3 months. The mother takes her to gynecologist and after her report of ultrasound which confirmed 12 weeks fetus; the mother was shocked. The daughter cried and confessed her love with classmate. After a lot of hue and cry, the mother revealed to father and later both the parents requested the gynecologist to perform a medical termination of pregnancy (MTP). The daughter refuses to listen to the parents and was firm to continue her pregnancy. She says she is above 18 years old and not minor. Parents considering family reputation feel it is their right over daughter and she cannot refuse it as she is under control till she get married. As a doctor, they would like you to help them to take right decision.

Points for Discussion

1. Who makes healthcare decisions for individuals who are in adolescent's age group?
2. Describe the medical implications of the MTP Act.
3. Enlist the provisions for emancipated minors.
4. Can an adolescent be part of the decision-making process?

BIBLIOGRAPHY

AETCOM for IMG Graduates NMC Syllabus 2019.

Anchoring Lecture: 1 hour

Abortion / Medical Termination of Pregnancy and Medicolegal Framework:

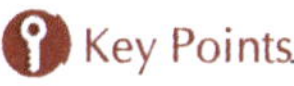

1. As per report of the World Health Organization nearly six of the ten unintended pregnancy ends up in abortion. The unsafe abortion is a leading cause of maternal mortality and can be prevented.
2. **Abortion in Indian Context:** The conduct of abortion got a legal framework after Medical Termination of Pregnancy (MTP) Act, 1971 came into existence. Considering the mortality risk of unsafe abortion, the Medical Termination of Pregnancy Regulations Act 2003 was formed which lead to various provisions for access to safe and legal abortion services by females in India. The further MTP Amendment Act 2021 was enforced vide Government Gazette Notification dated 24 September 2021 which had provision for seeking safe abortion services in cases of contraceptive failure, the gestation limit for abortion was increased to 24 weeks for special categories of women, and the opinion of an abortion service provider was the sufficient requirement for conducting abortion up to 20 weeks of gestation.
   A. **MTP Act 1971 (Act No. 34 of 1971):** The voluntarily termination of a pregnancy was a criminal offence as per the Indian Penal Code, 1860. It was after Medical Termination of Pregnancy Act, 1971 came into existence it allowed doctors having specialized qualification and training to abort pregnancies on certain grounds. As per the Act pregnancy up to 12 weeks could be terminated based on single doctor opinion while pregnancy up to 20 weeks could be terminated based only after the opinion of two doctors.

B. The termination of pregnancy is only permitted when pregnancy if continued involves risk to women's life, or it has chances of causing grave injury to the mental or physical health of the women, or there is evidence of any foetal abnormalities.

C. MTP Amendment Act 2021 has provision which permits that abortion up to 20 weeks can be done on the basis of opinion of single doctor while termination between 20 and 24 weeks in certain categories of women shall require opinion of two doctors. This extension of the gestation period for consideration of MTP up to 24 weeks is given for specially defined category of women such as rape victims, differently-abled women, and minors. Moreover, medical termination of pregnancy up to 20 weeks was permitted in cases of contraceptive failure both in cases of married and unmarried women. It also empowered state level medical board to allow termination of pregnancy after 24 weeks in cases of substantial fetal abnormalities.

3. A woman has reproductive rights under which a woman has a choice for terminating her pregnancy if she feels it is appropriate but the medical practitioner has to adhere to MTP Act and legal bindings as per updated Act. As per Indian Penal Code Section 312 'causing miscarriage' is a punishable criminal offence. Supreme Court of India in July, 2022 held that, a woman's right to reproductive choice the inseparable part of women's personal liberty with the ambit of Article 21 of Constitution.

4. Very important point to be noted by a student is that MTP Act has no provision to allow induced abortions on demand. The medical practitioner should ensure that there is valid legal indication to conduct MTP.

5. Women who is adult and above 18 years of age is a major and she can consent for termination of pregnancy and this shall be a valid consent. Guardian has to consent for MTP if child is minor below 18 years or in case of a lunatic.

6. **Socio-ethical Issues and Abortion**

   A. Any unmarried women getting abortion done in India is a stigma while scenario in cases of married women is different and acceptable in society. With MTP Act being introduced in India the incidences of suicide in unmarried women getting pregnancy is very much reduced.

   B. Rape victims who are also at times stigmatized are benefitted by legal provision of MTP Act.

   C. Unsafe abortion practices especially due to improper sterilization techniques and at times being conducted by unqualified person (which is an offence) may lead to maternal mortality.

7. Economical impact over a women and MTP is marginal as compared to stigma she may face in society and for a lifetime.

8. Legally MTP has to be conducted strictly adhering to MTP Act, any violation amounts to a punishable criminal offence.

9. MTP is to be conducted by a qualified surgeons in registered clinics or hospitals centre only.
10. Legalization of Termination of Pregnancy is the legal laws governing who to conduct, where to conduct, and how to conduct an abortion can be provided and accessed.

Self-directed Learning: 2 hours

The students should read the following and record their findings:

1. **MTP Act 1971**

Read: **"MTP ACT, 1971/Ministry of Health and Family Welfare | GOI"** Ministry of Health and Family Welfare, Government of India. 10 August 1971.

https://www.indiacode.nic.in/bitstream/123456789/1593/1/A1971-34.pdf.

___

___

___

___

___

___

___

___

___

___

___

___

___

___

___

___

___

___

___

___

2. MTP Act 2021

https://ruralindiaonline.org/hi/library/resource/the-medical-termination-of-pregnancy-amendment-act-2021/

3. **Bhavish Gupta and Meenu Gupta. The socio-cultural Aspect of Abortion in India: Law, Ethics and Practise. ILI Law Review. Winter Issue 2016: 140–150.**

4. Shakhatreh HJM, Salih AJ, Aldrou KKAR, Alazzam FAF, Issa MSB. Medicolegal Aspects of Abortion: Updates of the Literature. Med Arch. 2022 Oct;76(5):373–376. doi: 10.5455/medarh.2022.76.373–376.

DISCUSSION AND CLOSURE OF CASE: 1 HOUR

Points for Discussion

1. Who makes healthcare decisions for individuals who are in adolescent's age group?

   In case of minor below 18 years of age and lunatic, its parent/guardian who make decision while adult above 18 years can give valid consent themselves.

2. Describe the indications and medical implications of the MTP Act.

   Indications for MTP are:

   a. If the continuing pregnancy further has risk to the life or likely to cause grave injury to the physical or mental health of a woman.

   b. There are substantial risk of physical or mental fetal abnormalities and this will render the fetus seriously handicapped.

   c. Pregnancy caused due to rape.

   d. Or pregnancy caused due to contraceptive failure.

   e. **Note:** *Pregnant woman's actual or reasonable foreseeable environment must be taken into account before decision regarding conduct of MTP.*

   Implications are that the legal framework under Act governs safe abortion, prevent suicide in unmarried women, prevents occurrence of fetal anomaly and safeguards medical practitioners from conducting any unlawful act.

3. Enlist the provisions for emancipated minors.

   Emancipated minors are minors who before attaining the age of majority are freed from the control of their parents or guardians, and vice versa. An emancipated child may make decisions such as for their marriage, education, carrier and future course of their life. As of now there isn't any legal provision for emancipation in India.

4. Can an adolescent be part of the decision-making process?

   In case of minor below 18 years of age and lunatic, guardian will make decision while adult above 18 years can give valid consent themselves.

Students Assessment by Faculty Incharge

1. Formative

The student may be assessed based on their active participation in the sessions.

Name of Student: ....

Participation in session 2:
Excellent/Very Good/Good/Satisfactory/Poor

Signature: Faculty Incharge AETCOM ....

2. Summative

Short questions on the Medical Termination of Pregnancy Act:

ASSESSMENT

Write short note on Medical Termination of Pregnancy Act 1971.

BIBLIOGRAPHY

1. Abortion. **https://www.who.int/news-room/fact-sheets/detail/abortion. 25th November 2021**.
2. Article 25-A, Reproductive Health Act, New York, **https://legislation.nysenate.gov/pdf/bills/2019/s240;** Frequently Asked Questions, The Reproductive Health Act, New York Senate, **https://www.nysenate.gov/sites/default/files/article/attachment/rha_faqs.pdf.**
3. Bhavish Gupta and Meenu Gupta. The Socio-cultural Aspect of Abortion in India: Law, Ethics and Practise. ILI Law Review. Winter Issue 2016: 140–150.
4. Global Abortion Policies Database: A descriptive analysis of the regulatory and policy environment related to abortion, Best Practice & Research Clinical Obstetrics and Gynaecology, **https://abortion-policies.srhr.org/documents/reference/Regulatory-and-policy-environment-of-abortion.pdf.**
5. **"MTP ACT, 1971 | Ministry of Health and Family Welfare | GOI"** Ministry of Health and Family Welfare, Government of India. 10 August 1971.
6. **"MTP Regulations (Department of Family Welfare) Notification"**. Ministry of Health and Family Welfare, Government of India. New Delhi. 13 June 2003. Archived from the original on 30 September 2022. Retrieved 30 September 2022.
7. RI H5125, The Reproductive Privacy Act, Rhode Island, **https://www.billtrack50.com/BillDetail/1018806.**
8. SB-1301 Reproductive Privacy Act, California, **http://leginfo.legislature.ca.gov/faces/billCompareClient.xhtml?bill_id=200120020SB1301&showamends=false.**
9. Shakhatreh HJM, Salih AJ, Aldrou KKAR, Alazzam FAF and Issa MSB. Medicolegal Aspects of Abortion: Updates of the Literature. Med Arch. 2022 Oct;76(5):373–376. doi: 10.5455/medarh.2022.76.373–376.
10. Tanvi Mathur. Reproductive Rights of Women in India. **https://www.legalserviceindia.com/legal/article-3372-reproductive-rights-for-women-in-india.html**

Disclaimer: All information in **Module 4.2**: Case studies in medicolegal and ethical situations, includes but not limited to, and is for information purpose only. The editor declares that the sincere attempt has been made to give standard accurate information in Module 4.2, but it is not a substitute for any legal or professional advice. The readers should seek advice from legal professionals if they seek consultation and advice for any issue associated with fiduciary duty.

Module

4.3

Case Studies in Medicolegal and Ethical Situations

Background: The student should know the medicolegal and ethical conflicts in organ transplantation. The teachers can self design suitable case to the theme for discussion with students in line with recommendation of the curriculum.

Learning Objectives: The student after studying the module should be able to: Understand and discuss the medicolegal, socioeconomic and ethical issues in reference to organ donation.

Introduction to Case: 1 hour

Naveen Kumar aged 68 years was a chronic alcoholic and been your patient for the last thirty years. You are his family doctor. He was apparently healthy 10 years back but over last 3–4 years he developed alcoholic cirrhosis. He was on treatment with a physician and since two months he was referred to treatment from hepatobiliary surgeon and was advised liver transplant for alcohol cirrhosis with extrahepatic biliary atresia. The doctor advised him to arrange a live donor preferable from/among his relatives if possible and suggested that his 38 years old son can be a donor as only partial liver was required. Naveen kumar was disgusted and dismayed over to ask his only son to donate an organ. Doctor had explained him that liver will regenerate within months and both donor and recipient will have no problem. Formally introduce the case with following question in background for disclosure at the end session.

Points for Discussion

1. Can a liver be bought?
2. Discuss the health economic outcomes of selling a liver.
3. Enlist the medicolegal and ethical implications of the Human Organ Transplantation Act?

Self-directed Learning: 2 hours

The students should read the following research papers and record the summary of the observation and conclusion:

1. **Shroff S. Legal and ethical aspects of organ donation and transplantation. Indian J Urol. 2009 Jul;25(3):348–55.**

2. Government of India. *Transplantation of Human Organs Act, 1994.* https://main.mohfw.gov.in/sites/default/files/Act%20 1994.pdf.

Anchoring Lecture: 1 hour

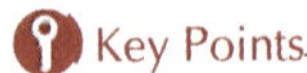

Key Points

1. Organ Donation in India is governed by 'The Transplantation of Human Organs and Tissues Act, 1994'. There were further amendment act Transplantation of Human Organs (amendment) Act 2011 and Transplantation of Human Organs and Tissue Rules 2014.
2. This act was formulated to prevent any commercial and illegal donations of any organ from deceased or live donors. As per the stringent guidelines any unauthorized removal of human organ from deceased or live donor was punishable offence and amounted to imprisonment for the term of three years with a fine of 5 lakh rupees.
3. Transplantation of Human Organs (amendment) Act 2011 includes certain modifications and these were inclusion of grandparents and grandchildren in donors list, brain death certification board simplified with inclusion of more number of experts in the list, national registry of donors and recipient was recommended; provision of retrieval centers among a few other recommendations. This Act provided the regulation of removal, storage and transplantation of human organs for therapeutic purposes and for the prevention of commercial dealings in human organs.
4. Transplantation of Human Organs and Tissue Rules 2014 removed certain impediments in rules interpretation and further curbed down and misuse of the Act. The important issues which were further amended over included authority by living donor for removal of any organ or tissue, duties of registered medical practitioner, composition of authorization committee, scrutiny of applications by Authorisation Committee, Procedure in case of transplant other than near relatives, renewal of registration of hospital or tissue bank, manner of establishing National or regional or state human organs and tissues removal and storage networks and their functions, etc.
5. Many ethical issues are to be safeguarded and adhered to by registered medical practitioner for organ and tissue transplantation. There is acute shortage of organs and demand for organ such as kidney is rising globally. The socio-economical impact of organ donation is many times poor person may opt for selling his organ for acute financial crisis or a middlemen may extract such person and sell kidney for higher price or so on. Incidence of organ selling may become a trade rather than donation.
6. Deceased donation rate is significantly smaller in India.
7. Integrity of medical personnel, proper patient consent and evidence-based successful transplant outcome are key issues associated with ethics in organ transplantation. Ethical issues which need to be addressed are that organ donation should not affect the health of donor, consent given by donor should by his/her own free will and must not be under pressure or coercion; no commercial trade should arise out of this organ donation; healthcare

support is continued for donor if required and benefit to recipient should outweigh the harm to the donor.

8. The ethical issues in organ and tissue occur due to acute shortage in supply.
9. Moral sense of good act of donation may interfere with religious belief and dogmas.
10. Health issues such as transmission of hepatitis B, hepatitis C or HIV may occur if ethics and all procedures laid for safe transplantation are not met with.
11. Cadaver donation and organ donation education program may be arranged in the society to address organ shortage.
12. The government may think of paying financial incentives to the donors in the form of medical health insurance coverage both for the donor and the family.

BIBLIOGRAPHY

1. Delmonico FL, Arnold R, Scheper-Hughes N, Siminoff LA, Kahn J, Youngner SJ. Ethical incentives--not payment--for organ donation. *N Engl J Med*. 2002;346:2002–5.
2. Government of India. *Transplantation of Human Organs Act, 1994*. Central Act 42 of [cited 2007 Mar 9] Available from: **http://wwwmedindianet/tho/thobill1asp.**
3. Ministry of Law, Justice and Company Affairs (Legislative Department) New Delhi, the 28th September, 2011. The following Act of Parliament received the assent of the President on the 27th September, 2011 and is hereby published for general information: The Transplantation of Human Organs (amendment) Act, 2011.
4. Ms. Jayshri P. Khandare. Organ Transplantation: Legal, social and moral issues. https://www.legalservicesindia.com/article/618/Organ-Transplantation-Legal, Social-and-Ethical-issues.html.
5. Shroff S. Working towards ethical organ transplants. *Indian J Med Ethics*. 2007;4:68–9. **[PubMed]** **[Google Scholar]**.
6. Transplantation of Human Organs and Tissue Rules 2014 **(https://main.mohfw.gov.in/sites/default/files/THOA-Rules-2014%20%281%29.pdf.)**

Disclosure of the Case: 2 hours

1. The teacher to discuss prior to discussion of case: The Transplantation of Human Organs and Tissues Act, 1994; Transplantation of Human Organs (amendment) Act 2011 and Transplantation of Human Organs and Tissue Rules 2014.

Write summary of Act

The Transplantation of Human Organs and Tissues Act, 1994.

Transplantation of Human Organs (amendment) Act 2011.

1. **Transplantation of Human Organs and Tissue Rules 2014.**

Points for Discussion

1. Can a liver be bought?

   No, it cannot be bought; you require getting a donor as per the prevailing act.

2. Discuss the health economic outcomes of selling a liver.

   Selling of liver or any organ is illegal and unlawful while, organ donations are legal under the Transplantation of Human Organs Act (THOA), 1994 and amendment in India. Poor person may be lured for financial benefit may sell an organ but such act is not permitted under law. The effect of liver donation on health is that post-surgery patient may complain of pain and discomfort along incision site and this is managed by analgesics. Moreover, liver is an organ which starts regenerating immediately after post-surgery and reverts back to normal size in period of six to eight weeks.

3. Enlist the medicolegal and ethical implications of the Human Organ Transplantation Act.

   Integrity of medical personnel, proper patient consent and evidence-based successful transplant outcome are key issues associated with ethics in organ transplantation. Ethical issues which need to be addressed are that organ donation should not affect the health of donor, consent given by donor should by his/her own free will and must not be under pressure or coercion; no commercial trade should arise out of this organ donation; health care support is continued for donor if required and benefit to recipient should outweigh the harm to the donor.

   Medicolegal issues when any organ donation is not done as per laid law and regulations. Or organ has been sold or traded illegally; health of a forced donor is affected post-donation; transplant is not carried by qualified person at notified authorized centers leading to death of recipient, consent from donor not obtained and/or donor is diseased and still act was conducted as there was organ shortage and so on and this may likely lead to spread of infection like HIV and hepatitis B to recipient, etc.

ASSESSMENT

1. Formative

The student may be assessed based on their active participation in the sessions.

Name of Student: ....

Participation in session 2:
Excellent/Very Good/Good/Satisfactory/Poor

Signature: Faculty Incharge AETCOM ....

2. Summative

Write short notes on Human Organ Transplantation Act.

Disclaimer: All information in **Module 4.3**: Case studies in medicolegal and ethical situations, include but not limited to, and is for information purpose only. The editor declares that the sincere attempt has been made to give standard accurate information in Module 4.3, but it is not a substitute for any legal or professional advice. The readers should seek advice from legal professionals if they seek consultation and advice for any issue associated with fiduciary duty.

Module

4.4

Case Studies in Ethics, Empathy and The Doctor–Patient Relationship

Background: Module 4.4 discusses nuances in the doctor–patient relationship in situation such as failure of therapy, termination of relationships, etc.

Learning Objectives and Competency Addressed: The student after studying the module should be able to:

1. Demonstrate the act of empathy in patient encounters.
2. Discuss and explain care options to patient and family with a terminal illness in a simulated case scenario.

Learning Experience

I. Introduction to case: 1 hour
II. Self-directed learning: 2 hours
III. Anchoring lecture: 1 hour
IV. Discussion and closure of case: 1 hour

BIBIOGRAPHY

AETCOM competencies for IMG, National Medical Commission 2019.

ASSIGNMENT I

Introduction to Case: 1 hour

Patient's Name: Rajesh

Relative: **Suman** (wife)

Suman after expiry of husband writes a letter to the renowned neurosurgeon of the city.

Respected Sir,

I am wife of Rajesh who was under your treatment and expired a fortnight back. I am very much disheartened due to my husband's death. I extend my thanks for all your effort you have taken to treat him. I remember your kind concern and attention you showed to us when we came to you after Rajesh met with a head injury and he was rushed to the hospital as I along with my relatives brought him to your hospital. Rajesh was conscious but wincing in pain. You talk with due care and showed your empathy towards his condition. You even spared some time to explain me regarding emergency measures of getting investigation for CT scan done and if required you agreed to operate him. He was operated by you for hematoma. He was a diabetic and hypertensive and you duly prescribed all medication post-surgery and got him reviewed by the physician too. Unfortunately Rajesh condition deteriorated after three days. I was near Rajesh bed but after his health got bad, neither you, nor attending doctors or nurses spoke to us much. Though Rajesh was conscious at that time, but you never spent time in consoling him. Consent for his management and regarding his deteriorating health and risk thereof was taken. He went into coma, and later was put on ventilator. You came on your rounds everyday but avoided looking at me or any one near him. I approached the nursing staff but none listened to me carefully and at times hushed me away as they were busy and told that ask doctor when he comes on round.

I have written this letter writing not with any vengeance but only to suggest taking a clue from the experience of how Rajesh case was handled after his condition worsened and no empathy and care was shown towards the kilns who were genuinely concerned for complete recovery of Rajesh and this experience may be of help for other patients who in future can receive the compassion and care from you that Rajesh and myself did not receive. Your timely approach of conducting surgery for his head injury made all the difference. I was happy and abundantly thankful to you. But our ill fate that Rajesh slipped into coma. After Rajesh was put on ventilator you did visit him morning and evening on round but paid not so much attention to my queries. You distractedly talk to me and moved to other bed quickly. He succumbed to the injury and was declared dead. As he was being resuscitated only junior doctors were there and you were seen rushing in after much time elapsed. Your junior doctor prepared death certificate and we were discharged. I wanted to meet you but your staff did not allow. It would have been better that would have given a minute of consolation to me and relatives.

We come to hospital with faith that the doctor will help and support us in coping with the illness I feel that you abandoned Rajesh when it was clear that he will not be a case that you can boasted as a success. You abandoned Rajesh and us at the time we needed you most. Please be empathetic to your patient and his relatives and this will count your success irrespective of outcome.

Thanks

Suman

Points for Discussion

1. Discuss the role of a doctor as a healing physician in the case above. What is expected for way he should discharge his duty in treating the patient?
2. Discuss implications of failed treatment on the doctor–patient relationship. What are patient/or relatives feeling if doctor does not pay attention towards them or their patient's misery?
3. Discuss need of empathy and patient care in relevance to the case above.
4. Can doctor–patient relationship be terminated? Can doctor terminate his patient's treatment after the patient's stops recovering or his conditions worsen?
5. Discuss regarding the hospice care in the case above. Hospice is focusing in providing appropriate care, a state of comfort, and quality life to a patient approaching the end of life.

ASSIGNMENT II

Self-directed Learning: 2 hours

The students should read the following papers surfing it from pub med database and understand the importance of topic. They can note important findings as follows:

1. **Hall JA, Stein TS, Roter DL, Rieser N. Inaccuracies in physicians' perceptions of their patients. Med Care. 1999 Nov; 37(11):1164–8.**

2. van Dijk I, Scholten Meilink Lenferink N, Lucassen PL, Mercer SW, van Weel C, Olde Hartman TC, Speckens AE. Reliability and validity of the Dutch version of the Consultation and Relational Empathy Measure in primary care. Fam Pract. 2017 Feb;34(1):119–124.

3. **Wu Q, Jin Z, Wang P. The Relationship Between the Physician–Patient Relationship, Physician Empathy, and Patient Trust. J Gen Intern Med. 2022 May;37(6):1388–1393.**

4. Pellegrini CA. Trust: The Keystone of the Patient–Physician Relationship. J Am Coll Surg. 2017;224:95–102.

ASSIGNMENT III

Anchoring Lecture

Empathy: Doctors responsibilities in the doctor–patient relationship and in care of the terminally ill patient.

Key Points

Empathy

1. Doctor is considered as a person of trust on whom patient looks forward for his healing. The patient expectation includes a standard medical care, reasonable charges for it and a compassionate behavior towards him.
2. Doctors though being considerate are unable to provide ample time for patients to show empathy towards their suffering.
3. The lesser the connection between doctor and physician, the greater the discontent among the patients and their relatives.
4. It may affect their healing too.
5. A good doctor–patient communication helps in patient's satisfaction, his adherence to medical advices, builds patient's trust and hastens recovery.
6. The education level of patients also facilitates better communication of their feelings to doctor and their sufferings; they can understand the empathy being shown by doctor better and so also they develop a better interpersonal relationship with supporting health staff than an health illiterate person.
7. Empathy is governed by the fact that the doctors inherent ability in understanding the patients perspective and their emotional needs. With this approach doctors may put their patients at ease and provide them medical care pertaining to their needs.

Doctor's Responsibilities in the Doctor–Patient Relationship

1. Doctor is expected to provide standard medical care to his patients, maintain the dignity of the profession as well and his patients.
2. He is expected to work in best interest of patient's health in their relationship responding to the calling of the injury and sickness of the patient.
3. He is expected to provide compassionate care to the patients.
4. Doctor is obliged arbitrarily not to refuse treating any patient unless the patient's illness is not under prerogative of his specialty and skill and only then he can refer treatment to other doctor of the specialty concerned.

5. Doctor is expected to maintain confidentiality of patient's illness and secrecy.
6. Doctor must inform regarding the prognosis and condition of his patient to the patient or relatives in best interest of patient's health.
7. Doctor should not neglect the patient regarding the course of treatment.

Doctor's Responsibilities in the Care of the Terminally Ill Patient

1. Doctors are expected to provide standard medical care to their patients, maintain the dignity of the profession as well and their patients.
2. Doctor must in best interest of patient's health rather than on any personal views and interest responding to the timely calling of the terminally ill patients.
3. Doctor should provide compassionate care to the terminally ill patients and should be empathetic towards the sufferings.
4. Doctor should obtain a written consent prior to treatment from patient or from his relatives if patient is critically ill.
5. Doctor must not refuse treating any patient unless the patient's illness is not under prerogative of his specialty and skill and only then he can refer treatment to other doctor of the specialty concerned.
6. Doctor is expected to maintain confidentiality of patient's illness and secrecy.
7. Doctor must inform regarding the prognosis and condition of his patient to the patient or relatives in best interest of patient health.
8. Doctor should not neglect the patient regarding the course of treatment or in case if the patient is not recovering.
9. Doctor should provide necessary information regarding required further line of treatment so that it aids in decision making by patient or relatives and doctor can also plan further intervention. Consent must be sought at all levels of intervention.

The doctor–patient relationship is critical for vulnerable patients as they experience a heightened reliance on the physician's competence, skills, and goodwill. The relationship need not involve a difference in power but usually does, especially to the degree the patient is vulnerable or the physician is autocratic. United States law considers the relationship fiduciary; i.e., physicians are expected and required to act in their patient's interests, even when those interests may conflict with their own.

BIBLIOGRAPHY

1. Dorr Goold S, Lipkin M Jr. The doctor–patient relationship: Challenges, opportunities, and strategies. *J Gen Intern Med*. 1999 Jan;14 Suppl 1(Suppl 1):S26–33.
2. Jenson A, Roter DL, Mkocha H, et al. Patient-centered communication of community treatment assistants in Tanzania predicts coverage of future mass drug administration for trachoma. Patient Educ Couns. 2018;101(6):1075–1081.
3. Krupat E, Bell RA, Kravitz RL, et al. When physicians and patients think alike: Patient-centered beliefs and their impact on satisfaction and trust. *J Fam Pract*. 2001;50(12):1057–63.
4. Riess H, Kelley JM, Bailey RW, et al. Empathy training for resident physicians: a randomized controlled trial of a neuroscience-informed curriculum. *J Gen Intern Med*. 2012;27:1280–1286.
5. Van Den Assem B, Dulewicz V. Physicians' trustworthiness, practice orientation, performance and patient satisfaction. *Int J Health Care Qual Assur 2015*;28(1):82–95.
6. Wu, Q., Jin, Z. and Wang, P. The Relationship Between the Physician–Patient Relationship, Physician Empathy, and Patient Trust. *J Gen Intern Med*. 2022; 37: 1388–1393.

ASSIGNMENT IV

Discussion and Closure of Case: 1 hour

The student after self-reading may further elaborate and note their opinion regarding the case in consultation with teacher incharge.

Points for Discussion

1. **Discuss the role of a doctor as a healing physician in the case above. What is expected for way he should discharge his duty in treating the patient?**

____

____

____

____

____

2. **Discuss implications of failed treatment on the doctor–patient relationship. What are patient or relatives feeling if doctor does not pay attention towards them or their patient's misery?**

3. **Discuss need of empathy and patient care in relevance to the case above.**

4. **Can doctor–patient relationship be terminated? Can doctor terminate his patient's treatment after the patient's stops recovering or his conditions worsen?**

5. **Discuss regarding the hospice care in the case above. Hospice is focusing in providing appropriate care, a state of comfort, and quality life to a patient approaching the end of life.**

ASSESSMENT

1. Formative

Assessment will be based on nature of participation in the various sessions; whether active or passive.

2. Summative

Write short notes on

1. **Empathy**

2. **Doctor's responsibilities in the doctor–patient relationship.**

3. **Doctor's responsibilities in the care of the terminally ill patient.**

Disclaimer: All information in **Module 4.4**: Case studies in ethics empathy and the doctor–patient relationship, includes but not limited to, and is for information purpose only. The editor declares that the sincere attempt has been made to give standard accurate information in Module 4.4, but it is not a substitute for any legal or professional advice. The readers should seek advice from legal professionals if they seek consultation and advice for any issue associated with fiduciary duty.

Module

4.5

Case Studies in Ethics: The Doctor–Industry Relationship

Background: The present module discusses various issues and conflict associated with the doctor–industry relationship.

Learning Objectives: The students after studying the module must be able to:

Understand, recognize, explain and defend medicolegal, socio-cultural, professional and ethical issues in the physician–industry relationships.

Introduction of Case: 1 hour

As a very popular general practitioner, you are always having bunch of medical representatives meeting you daily after OPD and usually load you with many samples of medicine and gifts such as pens, photo frames; diaries; glass sets; crockery, etc. As usual you have summer vacation of your kids and you look forward for happy vacation. The manager of a famous drug company visits you to inform you that tickets for trip abroad has been booked for the family by the company and is inclusive of flight, stay, excursion trips, etc. for grand support of prescribing two of the company's medicine round the years through which the company has made big profits. To make trip more exciting the company has arranged seminar for popularizing the drug at the destination place. They will be paying you Rs two lakhs as compensation of being off the practice.

Points for Discussion

1. Discuss the effect and influence of pharmaceutical industry on doctor's prescription behavior.
2. Limitation of doctor–industry engagement.

Self-directed Learning: 2 hours

The student should read the following research papers from web and write down conclusive summary from the paper.

1. **Keller F, Marczewski K, Pavlović D. The relationship between the physician and pharmaceutical industry: Background ethics and regulation proposals. Croat Med J. 2016 Aug 31;57(4):398–401.**

2. Bes-Rastrollo M, Schulze MB, Ruiz-Canela M, Martinez-Gonzalez MA. Financial conflicts of interest and reporting bias regarding the association between sugar-sweetened beverages and weight gain: A systematic review of systematic reviews *PLoS Med* 201310discussion e1001578 10.1371/journal.pmed.1001578.

3. Elliott C. Relationships between physicians and Pharma: Why physicians should not accept money from the pharmaceutical industry. Neurol Clin Pract. 2014 Apr;4(2):164–167.

4. Rodwin M. Institutional corruption and pharmaceutical policy. *J Law Med Ethics*. 2013;41:544–552.

Anchoring Lecture: 1 hour

Doctors and Industry

1. Doctors to core in general adhere to code of Medical Ethics. Pharmaceutical company also adheres to principle of medical ethics in their clinical trials. A pharmaceutical company influences doctors by luring them financial gains for prescribing company drugs to them. The gift amount may vary depending on sales of the drug. Doctors may prescribe same company drug rather than one which will be most beneficial.
2. Pharmaceutical industry conducting clinical trials in collaboration of prestigious government institute may rig the finding to show that their company's product is better than other company's drug for the same ailment. Doctor may be paid for giving false findings. This is unethical practice at both ends and in routine no doctors or pharmaceutical company indulge in such practices.
3. Pharmaceutical industry may fund money for research to a doctor and may request doctor to give results favorable to them. These are assumption of situations and in general no pharmaceutical company will involve in such an influencing act. Moreover, doctors should refuse such proposal if any and may lodge complain with appropriate body for disciplinary action.
4. Doctors should follow the professional ethics to their core. He needs to be accurate and transparent in all his professional duties and collaborated research. He should never indulge for getting financial gains by compromising his professional judgment and personal integrity.
5. Certain relations in which doctor should be cautious while working with industry and must not get divulge in maintaining code of ethics:
   A. While conducting post-marketing drug surveillance.
   B. Advertising for some products of pharmaceutical company on social media.
   C. Attend industry sponsored meetings or tours in exchange of financial gains.
   D. Should not over demand to give free samples on grounds of more prescription.
   E. Doctors should never utilize their professional expertise for promotion of the interests of industry.

6. A physician may not accept any gifts but may tie up for sponsoring his clinical trials in which the pharmaceutical industry may expect a return favor of findings in their best interest and this may leads to physicians moral and ethical compromises.
7. A physician should rightly refuse favor from industry as this may affect his clinical judgment and he is not pressurized to prescribe the medicine of the same company to patient irrespective of its benefit to patient.
8. Institutional Research and Ethics Committee should stringently ensure that any tie up with industry based clinical trial is screened, scrutinized and then approved after ascertaining that there will no financial foul play between collaborative team and industry. But this has its own limitations.

BIBLIOGRAPHY

1. Blum LA, Hunt DW, Hanks J, Nordberg M, Goldstein SN, Spiro DC, Ludwig GG. Rude awakenings. *Emerg Med Serv*. 1995;24(5):31–34. 73–75, 80–85.
2. Elliott C. Relationships between physicians and Pharma: Why physicians should not accept money from the pharmaceutical industry. Neurol Clin Pract. 2014 Apr;4(2):164–167.
3. Elliott C. White Coat, Black Hat: Adventures on the Dark Side of Medicine. Boston, MA: Beacon Press; 2010:63.
4. Farhud DD, Zokaei S. Conflict of Interest in Medicine and Health. Iran J Public Health. 2022 Jul;51(7):i-ii. doi: 10.18502/ijph.v51i7.10108. PMID: 36248295; PMCID: PMC9529726.
5. Keller F, Marczewski K, Pavlović D. The relationship between the *physician and* pharmaceutical industry: background ethics and regulation proposals. Croat Med J. 2016 Aug 31;57(4):398-401. doi: 10.3325/cmj.2016.57.398. PMID: 27586556; PMCID: PMC5048228.
6. Krumholz SD, Egilman DS, Ross JS. Study of Neurontin: titrate to effect, profile of safety (STEPS) trial: a narrative account of a gabapentin seeding trial. *Arch Intern Med*. 2011;171:1100–1107.
7. Parsa M, Larijani B, Aramesh K, Nedjat S, Fotouhi A, Yekaninejad MS, Ebrahimian N, Kandi MJ. Fee Splitting among General Practitioners: A Cross-Sectional Study in Iran. Arch Iran Med. 2016 Dec;19(12):861–865. PMID: 27998161.
8. Ramsay MA. Conflict in the health care workplace. Proc (Bayl Univ Med Cent). 2001 Apr;14(2):138-9. doi: 10.1080/08998280.2001.11927749. PMID: 16369603; PMCID: PMC1291328.

9. Robinett J, Cruser A, Podawiltz AL. "But doctor, someone has to do something": resolving interpersonal conflicts in the workplace. *J Am Osteopath Assoc*. 1995;95:333–336.
10. Sotile WM, Sotile MO. Part 1, Conflict management. How to shape positive relationships in medical practices and hospitals. *Physician Exec*. 1999;25(4):57–61.

Discussion and Closure of Case: 1 hour

The students should write their opinion in reference to case discussed with them:

1. **The influence of pharmaceutical industry on doctor's prescription behavior.**

____
____
____
____
____
____
____
____
____
____
____
____
____
____
____
____
____
____
____
____
____
____

2. **The limits of doctor–industry engagement.**

ASSESSMENT

1. Formative

The student may be assessed based on their active participation in the sessions.

Name of Student: ....

Participation in session 2:
Excellent/Very Good/Good/Satisfactory/Poor

Signature: Faculty Incharge AETCOM ....

2. Summative

Write short notes on

Can doctors accept gifts from pharmaceutical industry? Explain your choice.

____

____

____

____

____

____

____

____

____

____

____

____

____

____

____

Disclaimer: All information in **Module 4.5**: Case studies in ethics: The doctor–industry relationship, includes but not limited to, and is for information purpose only. The editor declares that the sincere attempt has been made to give standard accurate information in Module 4.5, but it is not a substitute for any legal or professional advice. The reader should seek advice from legal professional if they seek consultation and advice for any issue associated with fiduciary duty. The editor has elaborated ethical issue which may arise in doctor–industry relationship and is editor's personal opinion based on evidence-based research publications and declares no condemnation personally to any profession or industry.

Module

4.6

Case Studies in Ethics and The Doctor–Industry Relationship

Background: The students will be studying the nuances in the professional relationships and conflicts arising thereof.

Learning Objectives and Competency to be Achieved: The student after studying the module should be able to:

1. Identify conflicts of interest in patient care and professional.
2. Discuss the correct response methodology for addressing these conflicts.

Learning Experience Year of Study:
Professional year: 4; Hours: 5

Introduction of Case: 1 hour

Case: A very popular surgeon working in Government Hospital was contacted by a leading private hospital for referring the patient coming to him for treatment to the private hospital. They agreed to give him 15% commission of the total bill per patient, as well as they offered to pay him 25% of all diagnostic lab and radiological investigation of patients referred by him to their hospital instead of getting them investigated in Govt hospital. They offered him to pay off the table one Lakhs per month and operate at least 10 patients in the private hospital. The surgeon was also advice to invest in pharmaceutical company owned by the hospital through which doctor would receive extra dividends. Surgeon bargained for starting a pharmacy in the hospital on sharing basis.

Note: The teacher should introduce the case and discuss points below in the form of relearning test.

Points for Discussion

1. Fee splitting and other practices.
2. Can doctors become entrepreneurs?
3. Can doctors own pharmacies or hold stock in pharmaceutical companies?
4. What comprises professional conflict of interest?

Self-directed Learning: 2 hours

The students should study these papers surfing on web and discussed among the peers.

1. Sotile WM, Sotile MO. Part 2, Conflict management. How to shape positive relationships in medical practices and hospitals. *Physician Exec*. 1999;25(5):51–55.
2. Deng G, Cai W, Yang M, Lio J, Feng C, Ma X, Liang L. Linking doctor–patient relationship to medical residents' work engagement: The influences of role overload and conflict avoidance. BMC Fam Pract. 2021 Sep 24;22(1):191.
3. Norris SL, Holmer HK, Burda BU, Ogden LA, Fu R. Conflict of interest policies for organizations producing a large number of clinical practice guidelines. PLoS One. 2012;7(5):e37413.
4. Elliott C. Relationships between physicians and Pharma: Why physicians should not accept money from the pharmaceutical industry. Neurol Clin Pract.
5. 2 Rodwin M. Institutional corruption and pharmaceutical policy. *J Law Med Ethics*. 2013;41:544–552.
6. Clemens J, Gottlieb JD. Do Physicians' Financial Incentives Affect Medical Treatment and Patient Health? Am Econ Rev. 2014 Apr;104(4):1320–1349. doi: 10.1257/aer.104.4.1320. PMID: 25170174; PMCID: PMC4144420.
7. Fee-Splitting and the Law Br Med J. 1933 Jun 24;1(3781):1112. PMID: 20777618; PMCID: PMC2368872.

1. The student can note the gist of research papers studied below:

____

____

____

____

____

____

____

____

____

____

Anchoring Lecture: 1 hour

Key Points

Conflict of interest in professional medical practice

1. Doctors are working in government and private set up and they should be working towards the goal of the state or organization with whom they are working. All action, planning, decisions and judgment should be in alignment with code of discipline as practiced in their setup. Conflict of Interest arises if the doctor or staff works with any personal interest for any financial or non-financial gain.
2. A doctor may exhibit nepotism in practice by favouring his relatives or friends while on duty rather than being neutral and working under principle of justice by equal care and facilities to all patients.
3. There are concepts pertaining to self-dealing in medical practice; and the doctors usually those in administrative position may indulge in practices such as receiving kickbacks for purchasing drugs or equipments from particular vendor, or doctors may extract money from patients to provide them better medical and surgical care while admitted; or may get their investigations done off the record and do not register them officially or may even provide sample medicines by secretly demanding money, etc. All these practices are unethical and against the Code of Ethics as prescribed by National Medical Commission. Doctor may be punished and disciplinary action can be initiated as per code of ethics.
4. There is concept of **"Excess Compensation"** in which an administrative doctor may make to his employee in the form of financial payments, for example, paying him salary for period when he was absent by adjusting his leave in exchange for personal services which a doctor may extract from the employee.
5. Conflict of interest, examples include that if a doctor prescribes drugs of the pharmaceutical company in which he is holding a share. Or doctor may prescribe drugs of particular pharmaceuticals and asked them personal favour such as financing their medical trip or demanding for gifts, or doctor may collaborate with some pharmaceuticals for newer invention of drugs or intervention secretly not informing authority at his working place and may get financially paid for it unofficially.
6. Personal interest of doctor over his patient's interest or organization goal is unethical. Fee splitting among doctors and hospitals for unnecessary consultation and diagnostic or therapeutics services which were not required is totally unethical.
7. Conflict of interest may occur even due to temperament difference between the doctors and they may show knowledge and skill supremacy by managing

patients by their own will and at the same time may undermine skills of colleagues or junior staff.

8. **Doctors and Industry:** Pharmaceutical company influences doctors by luring them financial gains for prescribing company drugs. The gift amount may vary depending on sales of the drug. Doctors may prescribe same company drug rather than one which will be most beneficial.

   Pharmaceutical industry conducting clinical trials in collaboration of prestigious government institute may rig the finding to show that their company's product is better than other company's drug for the same ailment. Doctor may be paid for giving false findings. This is unethical practice at both ends.

   Pharmaceutical industry may fund money for research to a doctor and may request doctor to give results favourable to them. Doctors should refuse such proposal and may lodge complain with appropriate body for disciplinary action.

   Doctors should follow the professional ethics to the core. He needs to be accurate and transparent in all his professional duties and collaborated research. He should never indulge for getting financial gains by compromising his professional judgment and personal integrity.

   Certain relations in which doctor should be cautious while working with industry and must not get divulge in maintaining code of ethics:

   A. While conducting post-marketing drug surveillance.

   B. Advertising for some product of pharmaceutical company on social media.

   C. Attend industry sponsored meetings or tours in exchange of financial gains

   D. Should not over demand to give free samples on grounds of more prescription

   E. Doctors should never utilize their professional expertise for promotion of the interests of industry.

9. Preventing conflict of interest at working place.

   A. All doctors staff need to abide by Code of Ethics as practiced in the country and a written declaration should be given by all employees while joining.

   B. Any irregularity brought to notice should be immediately addressed; enquired and disciplinary action must be initiated as per Code of Ethics to curb any such events in future.

   C. Every hospital must establish a highly professional environment and teamwork at workplace.

   D. Providing well defined and good pay structure and promotion is likely to prevent conflict of interest in medical services system.

E. All hospital staff should be aware of the gift policy in order to prevent and prohibit the staff from accepting gifts, financial gains and benefits.

BIBLIOGRAPHY

1. Blum LA, Hunt DW, Hanks J, Nordberg M, Goldstein SN, Spiro DC, Ludwig GG. Rude awakenings. *Emerg Med Serv*. 1995;24(5):31–34. 73–75, 80–85.
2. Elliott C. Relationships between physicians and Pharma: Why physicians should not accept money from the pharmaceutical industry. Neurol Clin Pract.
3. Farhud DD, Zokaei S. Conflict of Interest in Medicine and Health. Iran J Public Health. 2022 Jul;51(7):i-ii. doi: 10.18502/ijph.v51i7.10108. PMID: 36248295; PMCID: PMC9529726.
4. Keller F, Marczewski K, Pavlović D. The relationship between the physician and pharmaceutical industry: background ethics and regulation proposals. Croat Med J. 2016 Aug 31;57(4):398-401. doi: 10.3325/cmj.2016.57.398. PMID: 27586556; PMCID: PMC5048228.
5. Parsa M, Larijani B, Aramesh K, Nedjat S, Fotouhi A, Yekaninejad MS, Ebrahimian N, Kandi MJ. Fee Splitting among General Practitioners: A Cross-Sectional Study in Iran. Arch Iran Med. 2016 Dec;19(12):861–865. PMID: 27998161.
6. Ramsay MA. Conflict in the health care workplace. Proc (Bayl Univ Med Cent). 2001 Apr;14(2):138–9. doi: 10.1080/08998280.2001.11927749. PMID: 16369603; PMCID: PMC1291328.
7. Robinett J, Cruser A, Podawiltz AL. "But doctor, someone has to do something": resolving interpersonal conflicts in the workplace. *J Am Osteopath Assoc*. 1995;95:333–336.
8. Sotile WM, Sotile MO. Part 1, Conflict management. How to shape positive relationships in medical practices and hospitals. *Physician Exec*. 1999;25(4):57–61.

The students should know the key findings of the lecture.

Discussion and Closure of Case: 1 hour

Points for Discussion

1. **Fee splitting and other practices.**

2. **Can doctors become entrepreneurs?**

3. **Can doctors own pharmacies or hold stock in pharmaceutical companies?**

4. **What comprises professional conflict of interest?**

ASSESSMENT

1. Formative

The student may be assessed based on their active participation in the sessions.

Name of Student: ....

Participation in session 2:
Excellent/Very Good/Good/Satisfactory/Poor

Signature: Faculty Incharge AETCOM ....

2. Summative

Write short notes on

1. Fee splitting and its implications for patient care.

2. Conflicts in professional relationships.

Disclaimer: All information in **Module 4.6**: Case studies in ethics and the doctor–industry relationship, includes but not limited to, and is for information purpose only. The editor declares that the sincere attempt has been made to give standard accurate information in Module 4.6, but it is not a substitute for any legal or professional advice. The reader should seek advice from legal professional if they seek consultation and advice for any issue associated with fiduciary duty. The editor has elaborated ethical issue which may arise in doctor–industry relationship and is editor's personal opinion based on evidence based research publications and declares no condemnation personally to any profession or industry.

Module

4.7

Case Studies in Ethics and Patient Autonomy

Background: Ethical issues regarding children are discussed in this module.

Learning Objectives: The student after studying the module should be able to:

Recognize conflicts of interest in care of patient and professional relationships thereof and describe the appropriate response to these conflicts.

Introduction of Case: 1 hour

Dilemma of Parent

A 10 years old boy was brought to hospital with history of pain abdomen and difficulty to urinate. The pain was radiating towards groin. The surgeon after careful examination got X-ray KUB and ultrasound done and diagnosed it as case of kidney stones and started treatment with NSAID pain killer and alpha-blocker and informed that he wishes to further conduct extracorporeal shock wave lithotripsy. The patient's parent next morning came to doctor and told him to stop all treatment as they wish to get him treated home with a traditional ritual priest as their family adhered to such practices for generation. Doctor tried to explain the patient but to no avail.

Points for Discussion

Have a formal discussion regarding:

1. Do children have right to decide about their treatment?

2. Will it be right for parents to refuse treatment in life-threatening situations?
3. What if there is a conflict?

Self-directed Learning: 2 hours

The students should explore following papers and note their findings:

1. **Gamble NK, Pruski M. Should parents be asked to consent for life-saving paediatric interventions? J Intensive Care Soc. 2021 Nov;22(4):335–341.**

2. **Diekema DS. Parental refusals of medical treatment: the harm principle as threshold for state intervention.** ***Theor Med Bioeth*** **2004; 25: 243–264.**

3. **Manson NC. Transitional paternalism: how shared normative powers give rise to the asymmetry of adolescent consent and refusal: *Bioethics* 2015; 29: 66–73.**

4. Gamble NK, Pruski M. Should parents be asked to consent for life-saving paediatric interventions? J Intensive Care Soc. 2021 Nov;22(4):335–341.

5. **Frasier LD, Smith N, Crowell K. When Medical Care and Parents Collide—Parents Who Refuse Testing and/or Treatment for Children. J Child Adolesc Trauma. 2019 Aug 2;13(3):277–284.**

Introductory Lecture: 1 hour

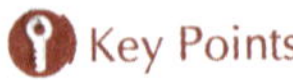

Key Points

1. Consent for medical and/or surgical management requires consent of parent/guardian in cases of all minor individuals below 18 years of age.
2. As much time health issues may be life-threatening its responsibility of parents/guardian to take appropriate decision in reference to their children and not get carried away by any personal, social or religious belief.
3. Parents/guardians should heed to doctors advice as the doctor is bound to give a standard medical care under code of ethics. And if doctors warn the parents/guardian for some foreseen health complications, they should carefully analyze before drawing any hasty conclusion of not following doctor's advice.
4. Doctors while seeking consent should give complete information about the disease, course of management, risk of treatment modality if any, expected outcome and feasible required follow-up.
5. Doctor must give an evidence-based consultation to parents/guardian who have doubts or queries to gain their confidence.
6. Parents caring attitude, literacy and capacity to understand harm and benefits of health are all contributory factors in making right decision for their child's health.
7. Doctor can also arrange for counseling with staff involved in health education about the disease so patient/guardian can further understand the intricacy of disease manifestation and management.
8. Doctor and the state have obligation for protecting children from malevolent or incompetent parent in terms of literacy as far as health of children are concerned.
9. Doctors need to make all measures to minimize parental conflict and build rapport and confidence of parent/guardian and patient too.
10. The situation is tricky as balance is to be achieved between parents authority to accept or refuse treatment and states obligation to safeguard child's health and vetoing act by physician in child's health best interest may be challenged in court if parents have refused for any treatment option.
11. Doctors must recognize the social, moral, religious and ethical barriers of patient/guardian in decision making and attempt should be made to overcome these barriers, by empathetic communication with family members so that they cooperate with and accept medical recommendations.
12. Doctor must ensure that child is neither a case of medical neglect nor a battered child. The family history needs to be carefully drawn to analyze whether the child is cared with love and affection. Many a times poor

economic condition with drunkard father/parent/guardian might affect overall social and mental development of child.

13. To conclude minor patients parental/guardian right of decision making regarding child health is absolute may be challenging and doctors need to have patience and perseverance to convince parents/guardian to opine for treatment in best interest of child's health rather than parents/guardian refusing treatment for want of their dogma and belief.

BIBLIOGRAPHY

1. Boos SC, Fortin K. Medical neglect. *Pediatric Annals*. 2014;43(11):e253–e259. doi: 10.3928/00904481-20141022-08.
2. Brown J, Cohen P, Johnson JG, Salzinger S. A longitudinal analysis of risk factors for child maltreatment: Findings of a 17-year prospective study of officially recorded and self-reported child abuse and neglect. *Child Abuse & Neglect*. 1998;22:1065–1078.
3. Frasier LD, Smith N, Crowell K. When Medical Care and Parents Collide—Parents Who Refuse Testing and/or Treatment for Children. J Child Adolesc Trauma. 2019 Aug 2;13(3):277–284.
4. Gamble NK, Pruski M. Should parents be asked to consent for life-saving paediatric interventions? J Intensive Care Soc. 2021 Nov;22(4):335–341.
5. Satyanarayana Rao KH. Informed consent: an ethical obligation or legal compulsion? J Cutan Aesthet Surg. 2008 Jan;1(1):33–5.

Discussion and Closure of Case: 1 hour

The teachers should discuss the researcher papers read by students in reference to questions for interactive discussion.

1. Do children have right to decide about their treatment?
2. As child is considered to be minor; the parents/guardians are rested with rights to make decision about the child's treatment. The child if understanding usually may assent for doctor advices during course of discussion.
3. Will it be right for parents to refuse treatment in life-threatening situations?
   No it will not be right for parents to refuse treatment in life-threatening situations
4. What if there is a conflict?
   Doctors must recognize the social, moral, religious and ethical barriers of patient/guardian in decision making and attempt should be made to overcome these barriers, by empathetic communication with family members so that they cooperate with and accept medical recommendations.

ASSESSMENT

1. Formative

The student may be assessed based on their active participation in the sessions.

Name of Student: ....

Participation in session 2:
Excellent/Very Good/Good/Satisfactory/Poor

Signature: Faculty Incharge AETCOM ....

2. Summative

Write a note on parental consent.

___

___

___

___

___

___

___

___

___

___

___

___

___

___

___

___

___

Disclaimer: All information in **Module 4.7**: Case studies in ethics and patient autonomy, includes but not limited to, and is for information purpose only. The editor declares that the sincere attempt has been made to give standard accurate information in Module 4.7, but it is not a substitute for any legal or professional advice. The reader should seek advice from legal professional if they seek consultation and advice for any issue associated with fiduciary duty.

Module

4.8

Dealing with Death

Background: The study of science of death is known as Thanatology. All doctors may have to prepare and report death of their patient during course of duty. Dealing with death empathetically is one of the most important skills for doctors to develop in the course of their carrier. Case for discussion can be self-designed as recommended in curriculum for AETCOM from live incidences in your setup.

Learning Objectives: The students after studying the module must be:

1. Understand, recognize and discuss the conflicts of interest in patient care and professional relationships and how accurately one can respond to these conflicts.
2. Demonstrate and express empathy to patient and family with a terminal illness in a simulated environment.

Introduction of Case: 1 hour

Case I

As a Senior Resident of General Medicine, you along with consultant attended a medical emergency in which a women aged 74 years was admitted with dyspnoea, high BP, edema feet and she was restless and complained of generalized weakness. Her ECG and ECHO were done and she was diagnosed as case of mild diastolic failure. The necessary medical management was done and patient appeared restful by the time the 8-hour shift of yours ended. But throughout your duty you were called for smaller complains by patient and accompanying relatives. As she was known patient of hypertension and you had been treating her for last two years your emotion towards patient was motherly and you responded assertively to her repeated check request. During her monthly visit she would wait for you and get treated by you only. Presently she was having some family tension which she did not reveal but told that she was upset from recent past. As you left your duty by meeting her, you anticipated she will be well. But next morning you came you found the bed empty; you enquired from nurse on duty and she told that patient expired last night at 12 pm due to cardiac arrest. You were bit shocked ...

Points for Discussion

1. As a doctor how should you deal with the emotions of patients and family facing death?
2. Can you comprehend the patient experience when he/she is dying?
3. As a doctor can you make the process of death comfortable?
4. Describe the emotions which a doctor is likely to face on confronting death of patients.
5. Will you consider death of your patient as a defeat? Is it right for a doctor be emotionally detached from a dying patient?
6. Describe the cultural aspects of dying.

Case II

You are a family physician and treating a patient of hypertension and diabetes for last 40 years. You are treating the entire family, his children and grandchildren too. Your patient developed albinism six months back. He once a jovial person in spite of being hypertensive is now depressed and meets to tell you and also developed nephropathy. That he is 68 years now; he has got his children married and settled; he does not want to live any more due to stigma, due to the changing skin colour and impending illness; he wants to die ... he wants to know how he can get peaceful death ...

Points for Discussion

1. Can patients have a choice for deciding to die? Do you think you as a doctor have a role in the death of patients? Will as doctor you assist death?
2. Describe your role as a doctor while dealing with the emotions of patients and family facing death.

3. Describe the patient experience at the time of death. Can you as a doctor make the process of death comfortable?
4. Describe your emotions as doctors when confronting death of patients.
5. Whether death is a defeat for the doctor?
6. Will it be appropriate to emotionally detached from a dying patient?
7. Describe the cultural aspects of dying.

BIBLIOGRAPHY

Question Case I and II; AETCOM IMG Competency; NMC 2019.

Self-directed Learning: 2 hours

The students should read the research papers and write the conclusive summary of the paper.

1. **Farhud DD, Zokaei S. Conflict of Interest in Medicine and Health. Iran J Public Health. 2022 Jul;51(7):i–ii.**

2. Muth CC. (2017). Conflict of Interest in Medicine. JAMA, 317:1812.

3. **Huffman JC, Stern TA. Compassionate Care of the Terminally Ill. Prim Care Companion J Clin Psychiatry. 2003 Jun;5(3):131–136.**

4. **Mok E, Chan F, Chan V, Yeung E. Family experience caring for terminally ill patients with cancer in Hong Kong. Cancer Nurs. 2003 Aug;26(4):267–75.**

Introductory Lecture:1 Hour

After reading AETCOM Module from Year I to IV; Discuss points you would like to elaborate while handling death as doctor; Add to points below:

1. Empathy towards patients: Discuss your role.

2. **How will you address the emotion of family members after patient's death?**

3. **Comprehend the patient's experience at the time of death.**

4. **Is it rightful to patient deciding to die because of his health issue?**

5. **How would you respond if patient ask you to assist him in his death?**

6. **Describe the emotions which a doctor is likely to face on confronting death of patients.**

7. **Will you consider death of your patient as a defeat? Is it right for a doctor be emotionally detached from a dying patient?**

8. **Discuss the cultural aspects of death.**

CASE DISCUSSION

Points for discussion: After the self-study two-hour session—you can write appropriate answers for the cases below:

Case I

1. **As a doctor how should you deal with the emotions of patients and family facing death?**

2. **Can you comprehend the patient experience when he/she is dying?**

3. **As a doctor can you make the process of death comfortable?**

4. **Describe the emotions which a doctor is likely to face on confronting death of patients.**

5. **Will you consider death of your patient as a defeat? Is it right for a doctor be emotionally detached from a dying patient?**

6. **Describe the cultural aspects of dying.**

Case II

Points for Discussion

1. **Can patients have a choice for deciding to die? Do you think you as a doctor have a role in the death of patients? Will as a doctor you assist death?**

2. **Describe your role as a doctor while dealing with the emotions of patients and family facing death.**

3. **Describe the patient experience at time of death. Can you as a doctor make the process of death comfortable?**

4. **Describe your emotions as doctors when confronting death of patients.**

5. **Whether death is a defeat for the doctor?**

6. **Will it be appropriate to emotionally detached from a dying patient?**

7. **Describe the cultural aspects of dying.**

ASSESSMENT

1. Formative

Participation in sessions may be used as part of formative assessment.

Submitted narrative on socio-cultural aspects of death may be used as assessment.

Name of Student: ....

Participation in session 2:
The narrative is Excellent/Very Good/Good/Satisfactory/Poor

Signature: Faculty Incharge AETCOM ....

2. Summative

Write a note on assisted dying.

____

____

____

____

____

____

____

____

____

____

____

____

____

____

____

____

____

Disclaimer: All information in **Module 4.8**: Dealing with death, includes but not limited to, and is for information purpose only. The editor declares that the sincere attempt has been made to give standard accurate information in Module 4.8, but it is not a substitute for any legal or professional advice. The reader should seek advice from legal professional if they seek consultation and advice for any issue associated with fiduciary duty.

Module

4.9

Medical Negligence

Background: The present module has been designed to make student acquainted to the legal aspects of healthcare especially pertaining to medical negligence and consequences thereof and protective measures to protect oneself from such happening.

Learning Objectives: The students after reading the module should be able to:

1. Identifying, discussing and defending medicolegal, socio-cultural, professional and ethical issues in relevance to medical negligence.

MEDICAL NEGLIGENCE

Key Points

1. As a medical professional every doctor has to abide by the code of medical ethics and provide a standard medical care expected from an individual with similar expertise in profession with due diligence, care and devotion.
2. The doctor is expected never to be negligent towards his duties and responsibilities.
3. Any act of negligence by a medical professional is considered as breach as doctor–patient relation is considered to be a type of contract in which patient implies consent for treatment by a doctor on routine checkup while doctor is supposed to perform his professional duties diligently.
4. The doctor must get a written informed consent from his/her patient prior to starting any diagnostic procedure and/or therapeutic management.

The doctors, especially surgeons, should explain about any expected complication which may arise during course of operation and doctor must also obtain consent regarding any further treatment intervention the patient may require.

5. Usually no doctor would be negligent in his duty but the act may occur unintentially due to omission when doctor would have never intended to do so.
6. Usually doctors medical negligence has been observed in case of administering wrong injection by oversight especially the assisting nurse might have loaded the syringe for some other patient, or leaving a sponge/instrument in abdomen, or operating on wrong limbs/areas without reconfirmation before starting an operation, or not explaining the precautionary measures and the side effects of a sensitive drug while treatment and patient may land up in critical condition, etc.
7. As the services of the doctors come under the ambit of the Consumer Protection Act, 1986 and there are provision for seeking redressal from consumer court for any medical negligence committed by the doctor for any medical treatment.
8. A medical practitioner is expected to provide therapy pertaining to his expertise, for example, Allopath/Ayurveda/Homeopathy, etc. Supreme Court in its verdict in case of Poonam Verma vs. Ashwin Patel and others (Year 1996) 4 SCC 322, condemned a homeopathy practitioner for practicing allopath as quackery as concerned doctor does not have knowledge of that system of medicine and such a doctor is liable guilty of negligence *per se* and in such cases no further proofs are needed.
9. Doctor must strictly adhere to treatment for which patients have consented for. Any treatment beyond that may be breach in duty; it may lead to act of negligence as for the doctors responsibility in obtaining in informed consent but also a legal issue may arise if any complication occurs because of such treatment and patient may claim for compensation. In a case of Samira Kohli vs. Dr. Prabha Manchanda and others (2008) number CPJ 56 (Supreme Court.), where the doctor had obtained consent for diagnostic and operative laparoscopy only but later in course on operation table a total hysterectomy with bilateral salpingo opherectomy was performed. The appellant in this case was adult and not was mentally challenged or in incapacitated condition, hence it was responsibility of doctor to wait till the patient gained consciousness as patient was under anesthesia; obtained consent and then conduct further procedure as patients condition was not under preview of urgency. Supreme Court directed the doctor to pay Rs 25000/ as compensation to patient and was denied treatment charges.
10. Supreme Court in its landmark judgment in the case of the Indian Medical Association vs. V.P. Shanta and others (1995), had opined to have medical profession covered under the ambit of the Consumer Protection Act, 1986 for making all matters concerning ethics in medical practice and arising ambiguity be resolved.

11. But doctors need to be careful as at times there may be wrongly framed for negligence and penalized. This can be prevented if doctors obtained written inform consent for all diagnostic and therapeutic management, maintain confidentiality, maintain all records and discharge slip properly and strictly adhere to ethics in medical practice norms as framed by National Medical Commission.

BIBLIOGRAPHY

Pandit MS, Pandit S. Medical negligence: Coverage of the profession, duties, ethics, case law, and enlightened defense - A legal perspective. Indian J Urol. 2009 Jul;25(3):372–8.

Introduction of Case: 1 hour

Learning Method: The faculty in-charge should arrange an interactive panel discussion for medical students with lawyers for legal guidance and senior members of the medical profession for further insight into the topic.

The student should read the complete case from the link below and describe the content in space below as summary. Any one or all cases may be studied.

Case 1: Supreme Court of India

1. **V. Kishan Rao vs Nikhil Super Speciality Hospital ... on 8 March, 2010. https://indiankanoon.org/doc/1920027/.**
2. **Note:** In this case no negligence was found on part of the doctor.

Case 2: State Consumer Disputes Redressal Commission

1. **C. Parthiban, S/O ... vs Dr. Latha Chatruvedula, ... on 3 May, 2023, https://indiankanoon.org/doc/78608306/.**

Case 3: National Consumer Disputes Redressal

1. **Dr. (Mrs.) Indu Sharma vs Indraprastha Apollo Hospital on 22 April, 2015 https://indiankanoon.org/doc/64183895/.**

Case 4: State Consumer Disputes Redressal Commission

1. **Dr. Sunita Verma vs Smt. Sangita Dubey & Ors. on 8 April, 2015 https://indiankanoon.org/doc/171360953/.**

Self-directed Learning: 2 hours

The teacher should make the students read the following articles and write a conclusive summary of their learning:

1. **Dahlawi S, Menezes RG, Khan MA, Waris A, Saifullah, Naseer MM. Medical negligence in healthcare organizations and its impact on patient safety and public health: a bibliometric study. F1000Res. 2021 Mar 3;10:174. doi: 10.12688/f1000research.37448.1. PMID: 34113436; PMCID: PMC8156516.**

   The students can discuss the medical negligence in healthcare organizations and its impact on patient safety and public health.

2. **Luther GW. The Key Elements of Medical Negligence-Duty. Neurosurgery. 2021 May 13;88(6):1051–1055**

   The students to discuss the key element of medical negligence.

Discussion and Closure of Case: 1 hour

The students are required to write discussion summary in box below:

Case 1: Supreme Court of India

1. **V. Kishan Rao vs Nikhil Super Speciality Hospital ... on 8 March, 2010. https://indiankanoon.org/doc/1920027/.**

Case 2: State Consumer Disputes Redressal Commission

1. **C. Parthiban, S/O ... vs Dr. Latha Chatruvedula, ... on 3 May, 2023, https://indiankanoon.org/doc/78608306/.**

Case 3: National Consumer Disputes Redressal

1. **Dr. (Mrs.) Indu Sharma vs Indraprastha Apollo Hospital on 22 April, 2015 https://indiankanoon.org/doc/64183895/.**

Modern Trends in

Library and Information Science

-DR. D.C. OJHA FESTSCHRIFT-

Editors

Dr. Pawan K. Gupta
Hony. Director
Rajasthan University Library,
Jaipur

and

Tirth Das
Library Incharge
Dr. Raheja Library
Central Arid Zone Reserch Institute,
Jodhpur

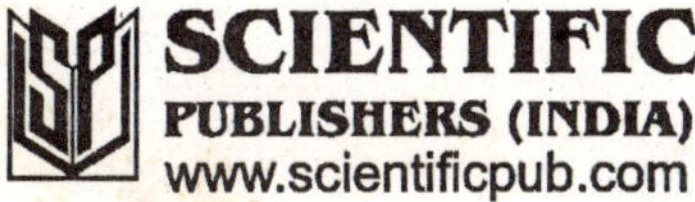

Published by:
Scientific Publishers (India)
5-A, New Pali Road, P.O. Box 91,
Jodhpur – 342 001 (India)

E-mail: info@scientificpub.com
www.scientificpub.com

ISBN: 978-81-7233-658-5

Lasertype set : Rajesh Ojha
Printed in India

This festschrift
is
fondly and respectfully
dedicated to

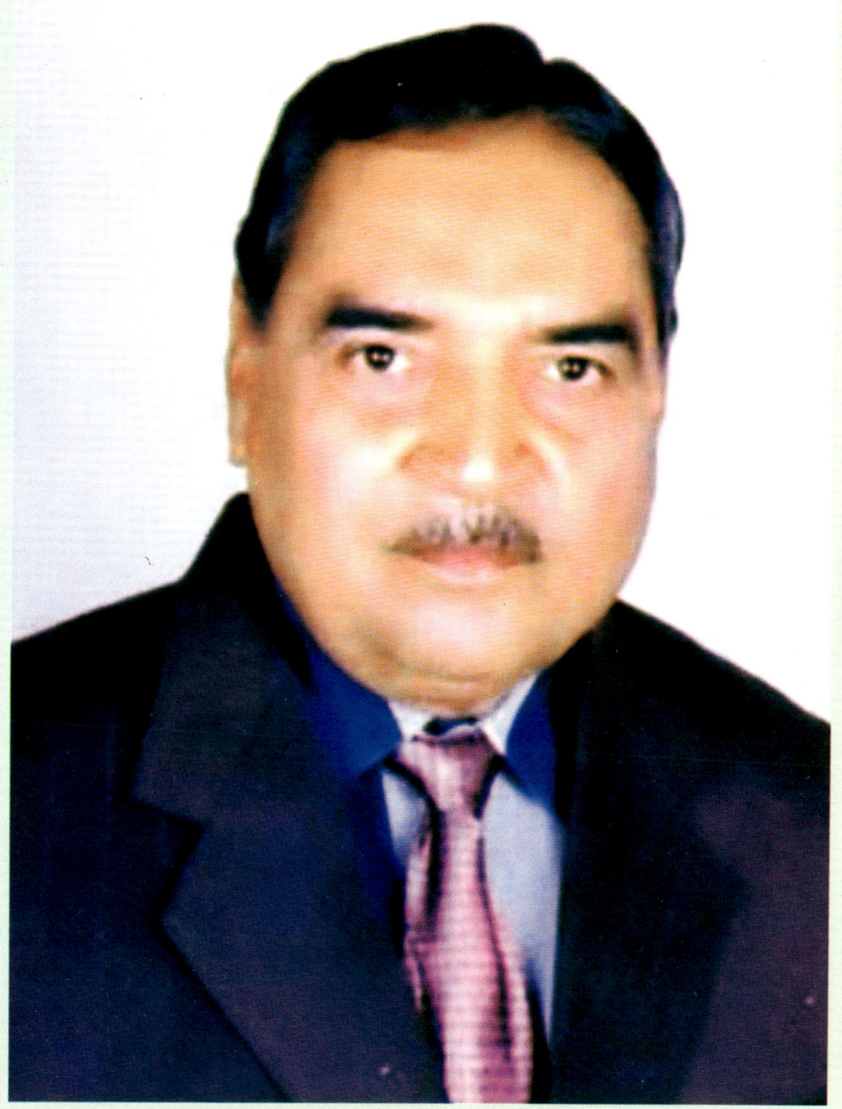

Dr. Dinesh Chandra Ojha

Prface

The word `Festschrift' is now no longer a new term. It is being used world wide. Since no English term for such a book had been in use, the German word Festschrift has been incorporated into the English language.... However, Festschriften are often titled something like Essays in Honour of .... or Essays Presented to ..... (Wikipedia). A Festschrift can be anything from a slim volume to a work in several volumes. *Aufstieg und Niedergang der romischen Welt* began in 1972 as a Festschrift to commemorate the 75th birthday of Joseph Vogt, a German classical historian; it was planned for four volumes but has reached to 89 volumes (several planned ..., but paused since 1998). The essays usually relate in some way to, or reflect upon, the *honoree's* contributions to their scholarly field, but can include important original research by the authors. Many Festschriften also feature a *tabula gratulatoria,* an extended list of academic colleagues and friends who send their best wishes to the *honoree* (Rounds & Dow). The Festschriften as a type of publication is growing now. Michael Taggart observes that Less than a dozen legal Festschriften had been published in the United Kingdom up to 1968, but since then more than a hundred legal Festschriften have appeared.

The present volume, a Festschrift is a humble presentation to Dr. Dinesh Chandra Ojha by his professional colleagues and friends to mark the occasion of his superannuation. Beginning his professional career in 1973 as a professional person in the Government Divisional Sumer Public Library, he never looked back. He, with his increasing appetite for learning, continued his professional education and completed his research degree from University of Rajasthan in 1989. He joined the Dr. Raheja Library, Central Arid Zone Research Institute (CAZRI-ICAR), Jodhpur, in 1978, where he worked for three decades in different capacities and relinquished the position of Head (Library & Information Services) in 2008. This has been a period of capacity building, differentiation, learning and application of ICT, in which Dr. Raheja Library and Dr. Ojha both continued on a fast track of unrestricted growth, resulting into a satisfying journey for Dr. Ojha and a source of inspiration and motivation for his colleagues. This was the period in which he drew the attention and was appreciated by the top brass of not only the community of scientists of CAZRI, but also the key persons in the Indian Council of Agricultural Research, and the top LIS professionals in the country.

As Rounds and Dow, more than three decades ago, have stated, "Rewards within the scholarly profession are limited, are often capriciously bestowed, and are frequently conditioned upon the expenditure of large amounts of time for trivial administrative purpose... More than it should be, scholarship is a life of devotion in which the only great reward is likely to be its own content... For such a life, Festschrift is the most honorable and the most appropriate of all possible rewards, because it serves or rather is intended to serve, the grand object of all scholarly devotion, namely the increase of scholarly interest and knowledge. At the same time a Festschrift is personal; a public and tangible tribute to one scholar by other scholars. This is what his friends have endeavoured to achieve - a bouquet for our associate and friend.

It is alleged that, more often than not, a collection of essays `represent conspiracies between academics with a duty to publish', however, the essays in the volume reflect interests and concerns of its authors. The unifying theme is the Modern Trends in Library and Information Science (L & IS), especially in Indian library scene, with its various facets and ramifications. The profession, as it can be culled out from the contributions, is in a constant transformation. It may be termed a phase of mutation rather than as of variation. L & IS professionals in India are seen as exploring the boundaries of application of modern information and communication technologies in all facets of library management and services. This is what is reflected in the contributions in this Festschrift. To name a few, contributors have talked about library software, open source software, library 2.0, RFID techniques, digital collection building, digital repository, e-resources, etc. It would be a fallacy to claim that these essays identify and evaluate exhaustively all the aspects or trends in L & IS in India, but they have potentially indicated the concerns of the members of L & IS profession in India and their reaction to the prevailing conditions. The authors have been able to analyse various issues, and give their expert comments and directions for future improvement. In all, this volume has 33 contributions, including the one giving `an intimate view' of Dr. Ojha.

Since a programme like this entails the services of a large team of specialists, we have been fortunate enough in attracting the quality in the contributions. A look into list of contributors is an indication of the level of confidence and attachment enjoyed by Dr. Ojha in the profession. We extend our particular thanks to the learned contributors and gratefully acknowledge their contributions. We must admit and state that we received an overwhelming response from professionals, which itself is a testimony of high esteem enjoyed by Dr. Ojha. On account of limitation of time and limitations on the volume of this publication, some contributions could not find a place in the Festschrift, and we offer special thanks to these friends. We were also constrained, obviously, to extensively edit some of the contributions, of course not at the cost of their content value.

For the general plan and supervision of the book, we are of course responsible and here again we are deeply aware of the value of part played by others. Our debt is immeasurable, to the expert friends and the members of the Felicitation Committee, for their constant guidance and encouragement during this project.

We, in particular, thank M/s Scientific Publishers (India), Jodhpur, without whose cooperation, the facile and neat publication of this volume would not have been possible.

We, on behalf of the numerous professionals, and friends of Dr. Dinesh Chandra Ojha, dedicate this volume to him on the occasion of reaching a milestone of superannuation after sixty eventful years of his life, and wish him a happy and healthy life, during which, we are sure, he will continue to contribute his might to the growth of L&IS discipline as well as this profession in India.

Jodhpur
Ram Navmi, 24.3.2010

Dr. Pawan K. Gupta
Tirth Das

Contents

Dr. D.C. Ojha: A Professional Journey

Anju Vyas

Librarian, Centre for Women Development Studies, New Delhi

FAMILY AND EDUCATION

Dr. Dinesh Chandra Ojha is one of the most well known and respected professionals in the field of Library and Information Science. Born on 16th June, 1948, he is the eldest child of his parents and has two brothers and three sisters. His initial education was done in the local schools where he was known for his brilliance in academics. In 1970 he did his graduation from Jodhpur University, now J.N. Vyas University, and also did his post-graduation from the same university in Political Science and Rajasthani in 1974 and 1984 respectively. His professional education started with B.Lib.Sc. in 1972 from Jiwaji University followed by M.Lib.Sc. from Banaras Hindu University in 1976. He was awarded the Ph.D degree in Library by Rajasthan University in 1989 on his research thesis entitled "Role of Libraries and Information Centres in Technology Transfer for Arid and semi Arid Regions of Rajasthan: A Critical Study" under the expert supervision of late Dr. C.D. Sharma, Director, Rajasthan University Library, Jaipur.

Dr. Ojha is married to Kalawati who is working as the Principal of a Railway School in Jodhpur. They are the proud parents of four beautiful and professionally qualified daughters. At the family front he is the most devoted son, brother, husband and a caring and loving father.

SPORTSMANSHIP

Dr. Ojha has been a very keen sportsman throughout his school, college, university and professional years. He is the first one to participate at an all India level in the "Wrestling and Body Building" competition on behalf of the Jodhpur University and Jiwaji University. He is the first and last to represent not only Jodhpur University but the whole Rajasthan in India's biggest Wrestling competition viz., "Bharat Kesri" and National Open". Football is still one of his favourite games. He participated in 7th "Arjun Shri of India" Best Physique Contest 1974 and was declared as `Mr. Muscleman of Rajasthan'. Dr. Ojha acted as Manager in Many All India Body Building Competitions and under his expert managership team won the champion trophy. In All India ICAR, sports tournaments he represented the CAZRI in `Kabaddi' team and also acted as Chief-de-Mission for CAZRI team. He used to perform many STRONG MAN FEATS like Breaking of Coconut with one blow, Bursting of Hot-Water Bottle, Tearing of playing Cards, Stopping of Two Motor-Bikes at a time etc. In one of the sports event at CAZRI, Dr. Ojha was declared as `He-Man'.

PROFESSIONAL CAREER DEVELOPMENT

Dr. Ojha started his career as the Assistant Librarian at the Govt. Divisional Sumer Public Library at Jodhpur and worked there from January 1973 to January 1978. While working in Divisional Public Library he prepared a printed catalogue of rare and reference books including manuscripts. He single handedly classified and catalogued 5000 old books and also moved the proposal for writing off 20 years old news papers, torn out books and magazines. He joined the Central Arid Zone Research Institute (CAZRI) at its Dr. Raheja Library in 1978 as the Sr. Library Technical

Assistant and retired as the Head, Library Services in 2008 after completing 30 successful and most satisfactory years. During his tenure at CAZRI-ICAR, Dr. Ojha has been instrumental in bringing the New Information Technology for the Library processes and services. He played the major role in the planning and construction of the new Library building and in shifting and making it operational. During the above period to give the modern look to the library, Dr. Ojha procured CD/Mirror Server with the capacity of holding 80 CDs at a time and provided connectivity to the 60 scientists of the Institute. He procured UNESCO Software CDS/ISIS for all Library Operations and also established LAN within the Library. Under his expert vision two international Databases namely AGRIS (1975) and CABI (1984) were procured and also introduced J-Gate Services.

Dr. Ojha has also been actively involved in teaching and research apart from being a practicing librarian. He has been teaching Diploma and B.LIS classes for over 20 years in Jodhpur. He has supervised one Ph.D and three M.Phil theses.

PROFESSIONAL WRITINGS

Dr. Ojha has always taken keen interest in expanding the horizons of his chosen field through his professional writings. He has a long list of articles/ papers which he wrote for the conferences, journals and books. Along with the professional writings he has been deeply interested in promoting Rajasthani culture through his writings and has written widely on various aspects of its rich heritage. He has written both in English and Hindi.

Dr. Ojha has also compiled a number of cumulative indexes to various scholarly journals and compiled many subject specific annotated bibliographies. He conceived the idea of bringing out a series viz., "Advances in Library and Information Science" under which 5 volumes devoted to different aspects of New Information Technology were brought out (Annexure 1).

PROJECTS

During his long inning at CAZRI, Dr. Ojha undertook various information projects and the ENVIS project from Ministry of Environment and Forest, Govt. of India is the most prestigious one among these. Started in 1991, the project is still going on till date. Under this project, the ENVIS (Environmental Information System) Centre on Desertification came up at CAZRI, Jodhpur. A number of statistical databases were created under this project and many publications and a regular Newsletter `DEN NEWS' and Abstracting Service are being brought out.

An active website - www.cazri.res.in/library has been developed under the subheads of - (a) ENVIS centre at CAZRI, (b) Activities, (c) Sub-committee, (d) Desert, (e) Publications (f) Statistical databases, (g) DEN Newsletter (h) DEN abstracts, (i) other ENVIS centres. The project is receiving the grant of Rs. 8 to 10 lakhs every year from the Ministry. It is worth while to mention here that Dr. Ojha worked as P.I. (Principal Investigator) since 1991 to the date of his superannuation i.e. 30.06.08.

SDNP Project

The SDNP (Sustainable Development Net-Working Programme) Project was sponsored for a period of two years by the Ministry of Environment and Forest, Govt. of India under ENVIS in collaboration with Indo-Canadian Environmental Facility (ICEF) on the thematic area Desertification. Under SDNP Project a database on Flora of Indian Desert of 694 species was prepared and a soft copy was distributed among all the ENVIS centres. The project which was started in Aug. 2005 was completed in May 2007.

NARZIC Project

The NARZIC (National Arid Zone Information Centre) Project was proposed in 1996 to the council (ICAR) for creating a database on Arid Zone Research and to develop a

Networking System among ICAR Institutes and agricultural universities working in the region. The project was approved by the council with a special grant of Rs. 3 lakhs. The centre was inaugurated by then D.G. and Secretary DARE Dr. R.S. Paroda.

AWARDS

Dr. Ojha has been conferred with various honours and awards for his multi-dimensional activities:

1. Best Librarian Award, 1992
2. Veer Durgadas Rathore Award, 1994
3. Roonkh Bhayala Awards for Environmental Information, 1998
4. Dr. C.D. Sharma Memorial Award, 1999

Name in International Biographies

It is really a matter of proud that considering Dr. Ojha's professional contributions of high repute, his name appears in the following internationally known biographical dictionaries:

1. Reference Asia
2. American Bibliography
3. Asia-American Who's Who
4. 20th Century Distinguished Who's Who
5. Best Citizens of India

Conferences/ Workshops and Training Participation

During his professional career Dr. Ojha has very actively participated in various Conferences/Workshops/ Seminars and Training Programmes from time to time. He has contributed a number of papers through these forums on various aspects of Library and Information Science. He has chaired sessions in some of these conferences. He also organized the 12th Rajasthan Library Conference during 10-

11 August, 2002 at CAZRI, Jodhpur. The National Symposium on Impact of Human Activities on Thar Desert Environment during 15-17th February, 2007 at CAZRI, Jodhpur was organized by him under the ENVIS programme.

Dr. Ojha has participated in 3 International, 15 National, and 10 state Conferences/ Seminars apart from many other forums.

Membership of Professional Associations/ Societies

Dr. Ojha associated himself with various professional bodies right from the beginning of his career and has been a life member of Indian Library Association (ILA) and Indian Association of Special Libraries and Information Centres (IASLIC) for over 35 years. He has also played a vital role in the regional professional bodies viz., Rajasthan Library Association by being the President for the period 1999-2000. He was elected as the Chairman of Indian Public Library Association (IPLA) for the year 1994-98. For over 10 years he remained secretary of the Association of Agriculture Librarians and Documentalists of India (AALDI) Bagalore from 1989-1999. Dr. Ojha was nominated as Chairman, Central Sectional Committee (Agricultural Libraries) by ILA, Delhi.

Dr. Ojha is held in high esteem in the professional circle and has been invited to be the member of various selection committees. He has been the Chairman for Assessment Committee of Technical Personnel (Library) in ICAR Institutes for the period 2004-2006.

Radio Talks

Dr. Ojha has been a popular speaker with the All India Radio, Jodhpur and have delivered over 30 talks in Hindi and Rajasthani. His love for Rajasthani culture and heritage is evident from the fact that most of these talks are related with its various aspects. Recently also, he has been with a classic work - `Marwar Ki Sanskritic Dharohar : Rajasthani Kahawaton'.

Summing UP

This brief overview is totally inadequate in doing full justice to present the multi-faceted and multi-dimensional personality of Dr. Dinesh Ojha. He comes across not only as an esteemed professional but more also as a very fine human being. He is a committed member of the community, ever ready to step forward to help and extent support to one and all both at the personal and professional levels. He has been an inspiration and role model to a larger number of youngsters in his community and has been a constant source of support to them.

It has been my good fortune to know him for over 30 years. I join the Library Community in felicitating him and wishing him a long, healthy and active life.

Annexure 1

Publications

1. Papers/ Articles in Journals/ Conferences

i. Ojha, D.C. (1976) Library Legislation in Rajasthan. Souvenior. Sumer Public Library, Jodhpur P. 7-11

ii. Ojha, D.C. (1978) College Libraries in Rajasthan. Proceedings. Master Moti Lal lecture series. Nagore. P. 5-8

iii. Ojha, D.C. (1979) Library Legislation and Adult Education. Seminar. Govt. Sr. Sec. School, Nagore, P.14-19

iv. Ojha, D.C. (1983) Role of libraries in 20 point programme. Proceedings of 7th RLA conference, Beware (Hindi) P. 11-14

v. Ojha, D.C. (1986) Ideal Staffing Pattern for ICAR Libraries: A case study of CAZRI library, Jodhpur, ILA Proceedings at Baroda. P.174-186

vi. Ojha, D.C. & Aminullah (1987). Use of computers in Libraries. Proceedings. 8th RLA Seminar, 26-28 April, 1987, Jaipur. P. 6-10.

vii. Ghosh, P.K., Ojha, D.C. and Bohra, H.C. (1988). Role of Livestock in the Socio-Cultural Mileu of the Rajasthan Desert. Proceedings. National Seminar on Integrated Socio-Ecological Development of Desert, CAZRI, Jodhpur. P. 19-21.

viii. Ojha, D.C. (1990) School Library Services in Rajasthan. Library Today. P. 4-7.

ix. Ojha, D.C. (1994). A Giant Remembered: Dr. S.R. Ranganathan. Indian Journal of Library & Information Science. V. 20 P. 20-23

x. Ojha, D.C. (1994). Prof. P.N. Kaula: My experience as student. The Lotus Petals. International Kaula Felicitation Committee, Delhi. P. 30-31.

xi. Ojha, D.C. (1996). CAZRI at a glance (Hindi). Jodhpur Info-Magazine. Aug.-Sept. 1996 P. 5-6.

xii. Ojha, D.C. (1997) Information Technology and Libraries. Proceedings. Pustakalaya Parisad, Jodhpur. P.16-19.

xiii. Ojha, D.C. (1999). CD Server: A Promising new library device for information storage and dissemination. Library Vision 2010. Proceedings. 45th All India Library Seminar (ILA), HAU, Hissar 23-26 Dec. 1999 P. 434-446.

xiv. Ojha, D.C., Sunita Arya and Tirth Das (1999). AGRIS Data Base : An Experience with CAZRI Scientist. Annals of Library Science And Documentation. Vol. 46(2) P.65-76.

xv. Ojha, D.C., Dave, R.K. and Sharma, K.K. (2000) "Impact of Information Technology on Libraries : A Futuristic Approach." In: Indian Library Association Bulletin. Vol. 36 (3) 87-92.

xvi. Ojha, D.C. and Arya, Sunita (2001). ENVIS Centre on Desertification. Souvenir. Symposium on Impact of Human Activities on Thar Desert Environment. CAZRI, Jodhpur. 15-17 Feb., 2001 P. 10-12.

xvii. Ojha, D.C. and Tirth Das (2001) Cost V/S Use Analysis : A Case Study of Journals at CAZRI Library. IASLLIC Bulletin. 46 (3) P. 133-145.

xviii. Ojha, D.C. (2002) Internet Service for Libraries. RLA Bulletin. 6 (1-3): 1-8.

xix. Ojha, D.C. (2004) Digital Libraries: A Need of Tomorrow. In CALIBAR (convention on Automation in Education and Research Institutions) proceedings. Jointly organised by Jamia Millia Islamia & INFLIBNET 11-13 Feb. 2004: 605-609.

xx. Tirth Das and Ojha, D.C. (2004). Progress of Public Libraries In India With Special reference to Rajasthan. RLA Bulletin Vol. 6-8 (4): 21-31.

xxi. Dave, R.K., Tirth Das, and Ojha, D.C. (2005). Development of Libraries In India : With Special Reference to Academic Libraries. RLA Bulletin Vol. 9 (1-4) P. 77-82.

xxii. Ojha, D.C. (2005) Digital Library: An Over view. Seminar on Development of Library-Palm leaf to Palmtop. Pustakalaya Parisad, Jodhpur. P. 1-8.

2. Papers/ Articles in Hindi

i. Ojha, D.C. (1985) Vissith Pustakalaya Aur Unki Samasyan. Ranganathan's 10th Death Anniversary Voume. ed. C.D. Sharma & Kailash Vyas. Print -Well P. 76-80.

ii. Ojha, D.C. (1987) Visseth Granthalaya Samaseyon our Samadhan. Granthalaya Vigyana ka Naya khitiz. ed. by C.D. Sharma and K.N. Vyas. Rachna Prakashan, Jaipur. P. 159-164.

iii. Ojha, D.C. (1993). Rajasthan Ma Pustakalaya Andolan ka Janak Dr. C.D. Sharma. Adhyatmik Punarjagran. 9.8.1993.

iv. Tirth Das and Ojha, D.C. (2002) CDS/ISIS Software ki Granthalayan Hattu Upyogita. Granthalaya Vegyana. 32 (1-2): 31-40.

v. Tirth Das and Ojha, D.C. (2002) Suchana Prodhyogiki Ke Vibhin Ayamo Ka Pustakalya Ma Mahatva. RLA Bulletin. 6 (1-3): 30-34.

3. Chapters in Books

i. Ojha, D.C. (1983) Current Awareness Services: Genesis and Utility. Developing Horizons in Library and Information Science, Vol. 1 ed. C.D. Sharma and K.N. Vyas, Printwell, Jaipur P.4-5.

ii. Ojha, D.C. & Aminullah (1986) A Draft Proposal for establishing Distributed Information Centre under Environmental Information System at CAZRI, Jodhpur. Advances in Library and Information Science. Vol. 2 ed. by C.D. Sharma and D.C. Ojha. Scientific Publishers (India), Jodhpur. P. 135-141

iii. Ojha, D.C. (1990). National & International Information System for Agricultural Science. Prof. K.S. Deshpande feliciation Volume on Current Problems and Trend in Library and Information Science. P. 251-260

iv. Ojha, D.C. (1990). Resource Sharing in Agricultural libraries of India. Advances in Library and Information Science, Vol. 2. ed by C.D. Sharma and D.C. Ojha. RBSA Publishers, Jaipur P. 85-96.

v. Ojha, D.C. (1992) NISSAT: An Over view: Advances in Library and Information Science. V.3 edited by C.D. Sharma and D.C. Ojha. Scientific Publishers (India), Jodhpur P. 168-178.

vi. Ojha, D.C. (1994). Importance of Information Communication Channels in Transfer of Farm Technology. Advances in Library and Information Science. V. 2 ed. by C.D. Sharma and D.C. Ojha. Scientific Publishers (India), Jodhpur. P. 129-139.

vii. Ojha, D.C. (1994). Libraries in Rajasthan. Resource Atlas of Rajasthan. DST, Govt. of Rajasthan. P. 176-177.

viii. Ojha, D.C. (1995). Computerisation of CAZRI Scientists publications using CDS/ISIS. Advances in Library and Information Science. Vol. 1 Rev. ed. Scientific Publishers (India), Jodhpur P. 233-250.

ix. Ojha, D.C., Arya, Sunita and Tirth Das (2000). Role and Impact of Information Technology in Libraries. Excellence in Information Technology. Dr. S.P. Sood Festschrift volume ed. by S.D. Vyas, Usha Pawan and Nirmal Swain P. 83-94.

x. Dave, R.K. and Ojha, D.C. (2005). "Digital Libraries and its Challenges. In Information Technology for e-libraries. Edited by K.N. Vyas. Raj. Publishing House, Jaipur. P. 59-70.

xi. Ojha, D.C. and Prajapati, M. (2004). Digitization of Dr. Raheja Library: A case study. Advances in Library and Information Science. Vol. 5 ed. by D.C. Ojha and D.V. Kothari. Scientific Publishers (India), Jodhpur. P. 135-145.

xii. Ojha, D.C. (2004) Digital Libraries: Myths and Challenges. Advances in Library and Information Science. Vol. 5 ed. by D.C. Ojha and D.V. Kothari. Scientific Publishers (India), Jodhpur P. 11-23.

xiii. Ojha, D.C. (2005). Internet Services for Libraries: An Over view. In Information Technology for e. Libraries edited by K.N. Vyas. Raj. Publishing House., Jaipur P. 1-10.

xiv. Tirth Das and. Ojha, D.C. (2005) Selection Of Library Software For Library Automation. In Information

Technology for e-Libraries. Edited by K.N. Vyas. Raj Publishing House, Jaipur. P. 146-157.

4. Articles relating to Culture

i. Ojha, D.C. (1982) Fairs and Festivals of Marwar. Souvenir. Durgawari, Jodhpur P. 4-5.

ii. Ojha, D.C. (1993) Ganesh Vahak Musak (Hindi). Rajasthan Patrika (Sunday) Dated 19.9.1993

iii. Ojha, D.C. (2001) Divya Vraksh Shami (Hindi). Kendra Bharti, June Vol. 9 P.10-11

iv. Ojha, D.C. (2002) Jodhpur ka Parmpragat Jalstrota (Hindi). Maru Krishi Chayanika, CAZRI, Jodhpur. 6 (1-3): 92-102.

v. Ojha, D.C. (2006). Bhartiya Vrat Sanskriti avam Paryavran Sanrakhsan (Hindi). Parijat. edited by Jaya Dave and S.N. Harsh, Jodhpur. 40-51.

5. Books Published

a. Reference Works: Indexes and Bibliographies

i. Ojha, D.C. and Kothari, D.V. (1979). Fifteen Years of Annals of Arid Zone. Scientific Publishers, Jodhpur P. 1-86.

ii. Ojha, D.C. and Kothari, D.V. (1981). Tropical Ecology: An Annotated Bibliography. Latesh Prakashan, Jodhpur. P. 1-130.

iii. Ojha, D.C. (1986). Indian Journal of Agricultural Science: A Comulative Index of Vol. 1-54 (1931-84). Deepal Publishers, Jodhpur P. 1-487.

iv. Ojha, D.C. and Vyas, A. (1983). Thirty Years of Phytomorphology: A cumulative Index Vol.1-30 Deepak Publishers, Jodhpur P. 1-264.

v. Rao, A.V., Ojha, D.C. and Saxena, A. (1998) 50 Years of Arid Zone Research in India: An Annotated Bibliography. Scientific Publishers, Jodhpur. P. 1-637

vi. Rao, A.V., Garg, B.K. and Ojha, D.C. (2000) Desertification: An Indian Scenario: An Annotated Bibliography. Scientific Publishers, Jodhpur. P. 1-284

b. Series

i. Sharma, C.D. and Ojha, D.C. (1987) Advances in Library and Information Science. Vol. 1 Computer Application. RBSA Publishers, Jaipur. P. 1-264.

ii. Sharma, C.D. and Ojha, D.C. (1989) Advances in Library and Information Science Vol. 2 Information Systems: Agriculture and Environment. RBSA Publishers, Jaipur P. 215

iii. Sharma, C.D. and Ojha, D.C. (1992) Advances in Library and Information Science. Vol. 3 Information Systems: Science & Technology. Scientific Publishers (India), Jodhpur P. 1-288.

iv. Ojha, D.C. (1993). Advance in Library and Information Science. V. 4 Information Communication. Scientific Publishers (India), Jodhpur P. 1-208.

v. Ojha, D.C. (1995). Advances in Library and Information Science. V. 1 Rev. ed. Computer Application. Scientific Publishers (India), Jodhpur P. 1-294.

vi. Ojha, D.C. and Kothari, D.V. (2004) Advances in Library and Information Science. V. 5 Digital Libraries. Scientific Publishers (India), Jodhpur P. 1-318.

c. Others

i. Ojha, D.C. (1980). University Libraries in India. Latesh Prakashan, Jodhpur. PP. 1-104.

ii. Ojha, D.C. and Others (1994).Library Organisation Administration and Reference Service. No. 2 Board of Secondary Education, Ajmer. P. 1-216.

iii. Ojha, D.C. (1995) Computer Application in Library and Information Science. Scientific Publishers, Jodhpur P. 1-337

iv. Ojha, D.C. and Kothari, D.V. (2002) Handbook of Libraries and Librarians in India. Scientific Publishers, Jodhpur. P. 1-381.

v. Ojha, D.C. (2010) Marwar Ki Sanskritik Dharohar : Rajasthani Kahavatein. Scientific Publishers (India), Jodhpur P. 1-460.

Information and Communication Technology (ICT) for Academic Libraries

Jagdish Arora

Director, INFLIBNET Centre, Ahmedabad, Gujarat

1. INTRODUCTION

Past three decades have witnessed unprecedented developments in computer and communication technology. Computers are being used increasingly to automate various activities in libraries with a suitable off-the-shelf general or specific-purpose software package that are now available in a wide range. Tremendous storage and processing potential of computers are being fully realized through existing communication and networking technologies. These two technologies are interdependent, inseparable and share a symbiotic relationship. The computer's ability to store and process vast amount of information and communication technology with its ability to transmit this information from one location to another converged to form "Information Technology" or "Informatics" or "Information and Communication Technology". The information technology refers to mosaic of technologies, products and techniques combined to provide new electronic dimensions to information and retrieval activities. The term information technology represents convergence of three strands of technologies, namely computer, microelectronics and communications. Information technology is used to describe products and services that came-up with rapid changes in computer and communication technologies and their fusion. Thus, technologies which improve the efficiency and effectiveness of an information system or service fall under the purview of information technology. Some of these technologies are available to the libraries for many years, while a few are now emerging as important tools for overcoming the barriers in the access and dissemination of information.

The emergence of Internet, particularly the World Wide Web (WWW) as a new media of information delivery, coupled with availability of powerful hardware, software and networking technology has further triggered large-scale commercial and non-commercial digitisation programmes the world over. Increasing number of publishers are using the internet as a global way to offer their publications to the international community of scientists and technologists resulting in large-scale appearance of STM electronic journals on the web. The internet and web technology provides an unparalleled media for delivery of information with greater speed and economy. Moreover, the web-based electronic information products not only eliminate paper, physical storage and transportation costs, it also offers a hosts of other possibilities for incorporating multimedia and hyper-link features to electronic documents hitherto very difficult through paper media. The web-based electronic information products are exerting ever-increasing pressure on the traditional libraries, which, in turn, are committing larger portions of their budgetary allocation for either procuring or accessing web-based online or full-text search services, CD ROM products, online databases, multimedia products, etc. The libraries and information centres, as consumers of electronic journals and online databases, are benefiting greatly from this technology-driven revolution. The information products of technological revolution, in turn, triggered major shifts in the traditional practices and policies of buying, storing and accessing journals.

Rapid changes in information technologies during past three decades have drastically changed the functions and activities of information professionals in libraries. Most functions in modern libraries are being performed using software packages that are now available off-the-shelf. Several libraries have their catalogues available on the internet with a web-based search interface along with links to resources either acquired through external agencies or created in-house. Most libraries are connected to the Campus network and subscribe to electronic resources to serve the information requirement of their academic community. Several libraries have taken-up small-scale digitisation projects for part of their collection. The librarians and information professionals are required to develop skills that are required to use, develop and maintain IT-based services and products used by today's libraries. The chapter deals with new information technologies, their products, services and applications in libraries. It describes web-based library services.

2. NEED AND PURPOSE OF INFORMATION TECHNOLOGY (IT) IN LIBRARIES

The application of information technology in libraries results in increased operational efficiency. The IT increases productivity of library staff. It relieves professional staff from mundane jobs that involves a lot of duplication so that they can be fruitfully be used for other user-oriented library services. It improves quality of services rendered by the library. Use of information technology ensures ease of functioning, accuracy and economy in human labour with greater speed. The exponential growth of information has made manual system redundant giving way to computerized information storage and retrieval tools. Effective and efficient handling of huge quantum of information is only possible by using computers, which have the added advantage of being highly accurate and efficient that adds value to information.

Moreover, the technology also helps in rendering services that were hitherto not possible using traditional means. The new information technology facilitates improved management of physical and financial resources. The advances in technology and its availability at lower cost, has also raised expectations of users from librarians and libraries. The new information technology, on one hand, facilitate wider access to information for the library users, on other hand, it facilitates wider dissemination of information products and services generated by the library. The availability of networks facilitates resource sharing and high-speed communication with other libraries.

3. DEVELOPMENTS IN COMPUTER AND MICROPROCESSOR TECHNOLOGY

Dramatic reductions in the size and cost of computer components and equally impressive gains in the speed, storage capacity and reliability of hardware components have expanded their use rapidly in all activities and functions of a library and information centre. Notable reductions in the size of microprocessors combined with dramatically enhanced capacity have added new dimensions to the computer new hardware technology. Initially, small silicon chips contained only few components and circuits, but the average number of components have doubled each year since 1965. Early small-scale integration efforts first gave way to large-scale integration (LSI) chips that contained thousands of components, very large-scale integration (VLSI) chips that contained hundreds of thousands of components and circuits, and now ultra large-scale integration (ULSI) chips came with millions of components and circuits.

A microprocessor, also known as Central Processing Unit (CPU) of a computer, is a complete computation engine that is fabricated on a single chip. Microprocessors are manufactured by different companies like Intel, Advanced Micro Divices (AMD), Motorola, etc. However, most widely used microprocessors are manufactured by Intel. The first microprocessor used in a PC was Intel 8080. Introduced in 1974, it was a complete 8-bit microprocessor on a single chip. Intel 8088 used in the IBM PC in 1979, was the first microprocessor that made its presence felt in the market. The PC market moved from the 8088, 80286, 80386, 80486, Pentium, Pentium-II, III, IV and now to Intel Dual Core and Quad Core. The new Intel Dual Core can execute any piece of code that ran on the original 8088, but the Dual Core runs about 3,000 times faster.

The capacity of a microprocessor is measured in terms of the number of bits it can send or receive and the number of bits it can process internally. The 8088 was an 8/16 bit processor, indicating that it can send or receive 8 bits of data and internally process 16 bits of data at a time. The 80286 was a 16/16 bit processor and 80386 chip had a 32-bit processor with a 32-bit data path and, as a result, was much faster than either the 8088 or the 80286 chip. The 80486 chip, introduced by Intel in late 1989, had a 32-bit processor. It has architectural enhancements, hence it performed better than the 80386 chip. The Pentium is a 32-bit processor with a 32-bit data path. It is three times faster than the 80486. The Pentium II and III had a 32-bit processor with a 64-bit data path. It was three times faster than the Pentium. The Pentium IV is a 32-bit processor with a 64-bit data path, and was introduced in 2000. It is four times faster than the Pentium. Currently, PCs and laptops are equipped with Dual Core which is a 64-bit processor with 64-bit data path and processing speed of 3.0 Ghz.

Like microprocessor technology, digital storage devices have also witnessed notable reductions in its size and cost with dramatically enhancement in capacity of storage. There are two types of data storage devices, i.e. removable data storage devices and non-removable data storage devices. The data storage devices come in many sizes and shapes. The storage devices can also be categorized based on media used for storage, for example magnetic storage media, optical storage media, metal-oxide semiconductors or flash memory devices (popularly known as Pen drives or USB drives).

Magnetic storage media are commonly used for large volumes of data (e.g., video, image, or remote sensing data). Large amounts of data are stored through tape drives because the capacity on the drives is huge - three billion (or three gigabits) of data per square inch can fit on a single magnetic disk. Hard discs, floppies, tapes, cartridges, etc. are example of magnetic media.

CD-ROMs and DVD ROMs are example of optical storage media which can again be of two types, i.e. (i) Write-once, read-many: data once written cannot be erased; and (ii) Rewritable: the data that is once written can be erased completely and the same storage device can be used again for storing different data. A typical disc used in a computer-based CD drive stores 650 MB. Digital Versatile Disk or DVD initially stood for Digital Video Disc. Like a CD, DVD is an optical storage system for read-only, recordable and rewritable applications. The DVD format provides several configurations of data layers, moving from 2D storage to 3D storage. Each configuration is designed to provide additional storage capacity. The similarity between the DVD and the CD gets smaller with each upgraded configuration, however, DVDs in contrast to CDs has storage capacity of 4.7 GB.

Metal-oxide semiconductors-based storage devices, popularly known as pen drives or USB drives or flash memory devices, is non-volatile computer memory that can be electrically erased and reprogrammed. It is a technology that is primarily used in memory cards and USB flash drives for general storage and transfer of data between computers and other digital products. Flash memory stores information in an array of memory cells made from floating-gate transistors. In traditional single-level cell (SLC) devices, each cell stores only one bit of information. Some newer flash memory, known as multi-level cell (MLC) devices, can store more than one bit per cell by choosing between multiple levels of electrical charge to apply to the floating gates of its cells. Flash drives are now available with 8 GB storage capacity.

Digital collections that are too large to store entirely on a disk use hierarchical storage mechanisms (HSM). In an HSM, the most frequently used data is kept on fast disks while less frequently used data is kept in nearline such as an automated (robotic) tape library. An HSM can automatically migrate data from tape to disk and vice-versa as required. Intelligent storage networks and snap-servers are now available in which the physical storage devices are intelligently controlled and made available to a number of servers. A number of RAID (Redundant Array of Inexpensive Disks) models are also available for greater security and performance. The RAID technology distributes the data across a number of disks in a way that even if one or more disks fail, the system would still function while the failed component is replaced.

4. DEVELOPMENTS IN COMMUNICATION AND NETWORK TECHNOLOGY

Communication technology, with its ability to transmit data and information from one location to another, serve as a tool to exploit potentials and ability of computer to store and process vast amount of information. A computer communication network is an interconnection of a collection of several computers from which the user can select the service required and communicate with any computer as a local user. A computer communication networks can be viewed as a collection of nodes with computing resources and nodal-switching computers that facilitate communication through a set of transmission links. Developments in communication technology have made it possible to interconnect geographically dispersed computing resources of different kinds and makes. Users can access the network through PCs and terminals attached to a node and messages traverse these networks through the switching nodes. Since computer communicates using digitized signals instead of electric signals, it requires different transmission facilities than those used for transmitting analogue electrical signals. It is, however, a common practice to use conventional telecommunication links for data transmission by converting digital signals into analogue signals using a process called "Modulation" and the device that performs the conversion is called the MODEM (MOdulator - DEModulator). Currently, terrestrial, satellite-based data networks, Integrated Service Digital Network (ISDN) and wireless networks are available that can handle all kinds of communication requirements (i.e. voice, data, telemetry, facsimile and video) without discrimination.

The computer networks can be grouped into four categories based on geographical locations of its computer terminals, i.e.

i. **Local Area Network (LAN):** LAN is a interconnection of many computers within a given local area, more often premises of a single organization building. A very high speed of data transmission can be attained within a limited geographic area. LANs are typically configured in a star, bus or ring. Low speed LANs use telephone wires or copper cables and optical fibre cables are used to achieve high-speed transmission of data.

ii. **Wide Area Network (WAN):** WAN is used to interconnect a number of widely dispersed computers in various cities of a country or different countries. WANs use communication media maintained by telegraph or telephone companies. These networks usually have land telephone lines, underground coaxial cables, microwave communication and satellite communications.

iii. **Metropolitan Area Network (MAN):** MAN refers to inter- connection within geographical limits of a city or town.

iv. **Gateways:** Gateways consist of software and hardware that are required to interconnect networks amongst them. Gateways contend with any differences in packet sizes, protocols and addressing methods between the two networks it connect. Gateways are also used to connect LANs to WANs and WANs, in turn, can be linked through gateways to create national and international data communication networks.

The communications networks can be grouped into the following three categories based on the technology and communication media used by them:

i. **Public Switched Telephone Network:** PSTN are managed by common carriers usually telephone companies / departments the world over. The PSTN generally provide two basic services, the normal dial-up connections to the subscribers and permanent leased connection between two subscriber's points. The permanent leased connections provide single traceable line between two subscriber points. The leased lines are generally less prone to noise than dial-up lines.

ii. **Public Data Network**: Analogous to the public telephone network, many domestic common carriers provide data communications services via a specialized network called a Public Data Network (PDN). Most Internet Service Providers (ISPs) use combination of PDN and PSTN for providing internet connectivity.

iii. **Integrated Services Digital Networks (ISDN)**: An ISDN is a network that provides end-to-end digital connectivity to support a wide range of services, including voice and non-voice services.

Computer networks use physical channels through which information is transmitted between computers in a network. Media may be classified as bounded i.e., wires (twisted pair telephone wires or UTP CAT 5), cables (co-axial) and optical fibres; or unbounded i.e., radio waves or microwaves.

Data communication is an integral part of the modern information storage and retrieval systems in terms of their online access. Today, network technology works on client-server architecture with middleware used for connecting software components or applications on clients and servers. Technique of packet switching, evolved in 1960s, is used for transferring data between computer systems with an objective to facilitate networked computers to communicate seamlessly across multiple, geographically dispersed locations. The Transmission Control Protocol (TCP) and Internet Protocol (IP), called TCP / IP suite, is the backbone of internet and other TCP /IP based networks. With developments in communication technology, institutions have options to set-up fibre optic-based gigabit LAN or wireless LAN. Depending on the geographical location, institutions have options to buy terrestrial or satellite-based internet bandwidth its combinations from a number of Internet Service Providers (ISPs).

5. LIBRARY AUTOMATION

The library automation refers to computerization or mechanization of all library activities. It deals with the design and development of process and system that minimize the necessity of human intervention in their operations. The library automation is defined as "integrated systems" that computerize an array of traditional library functions such as acquisition, cataloguing, circulation and serials control, etc. using an integrated library software. A computerized library and information system is a set of functional system encompassing:

- In-house Operations of the Library; and
- Other applications of the information technologies in libraries including information storage and retrieval.

An automated library is one where a computer system is used to manage one or several of the key functions of a library such as Acquisitions, Serials control, Cataloguing, Circulation and the Public Access Catalogue. An integrated library system or an integrated online library system is used for computerization of in-house activities of a library. Such application packages use a single bibliographic database and a set of interrelated application programs to support multiple library operations. Most integrated library softwares are modular in design consisting of a number of optional and basic modules. Most library packages typically incorporate modules for: Acquisition, Cataloguing, Circulation Control, Serials Control and Online Public Access Catalogue. Online Public Access Catalogue is often a principal motive for the implementation of integrated library software. Several off-the-shelf packages are available in the market that can be used for computerization of in-house activities of the library. These software packages are available for single user in a workstation mode (Windows 95/98/2000) as well in simultaneous multi-user environment on Windows and its variant / Unix / Linux / Sun Solaris Operating Systems. LibSys, SOUL, Alice for Windows, Slim +, Virtua, Librarians Suit, etc. are some of the important software packages available in India.

Libraries, besides using integrated library software, also use office automation software like word processing (MS Word), spread-sheet (MS Excel), database management systems (MS Access), presentation packages (MS Powerpoint) and graphic applications (Photoshop or Paint). Librarians and information professionals, therefore, require basic training in use of such general-purpose packages.

6. AUTOMATIC IDENTIFICATION AND DATA COLLECTION TECHNOLOGY

There are three important identification and data collection technologies that are used in libraries, namely, bar code technology, RFID and Smart card. These technologies are described below briefly.

6.1. Bar Code Technology

Bar code technology is being used in library and businesses for the past 30 years to minimize data entry errors, speed processes and reduce costs. Most books, journals as well as other consumer products in the market carry black and white thin and thick strips called barcodes. Barcode technology offers a mechanism that can be used for identification, location and tracking of items that are bar coded.

Barcode is not a new technology; it was introduced in 1940 although it was first applied commercially in 1960's as a method for tracking rail road cars. Since then, it has been used extensively in consumer industry, material handling, industries and libraries. A bar code is a machine readable code consisting of a series of bars and spaces printed in defined ratios. Bar code symbologies are essentially alphabets in which a different width of bars and spaces are combined to form characters and ultimately, forms a message. Because there are many ways to arrange these bars and spaces, numerous symbologies are possible. Common linear symbologies include UPC/EAN, Interleaved 2 of 5 (I of 5), Codabar, Code 39 and Code 128. While each symbology is in some way unique, the composition of a complete message (bar code) is regardless of the symbology used.

Barcode by itself is not a system but is an identification tool that enables accurate reading of data for sophisticated management systems. Use of barcode increasing accuracy in data collection, saves time and brings about the efficiency in library activities.

Bar code technology is being used in libraries all over the world especially for circulation of books as well as for several other functions including location control or book tracking, stock verification, receipt of issues of journals, cross checking of documents issued from the library, etc.

6.2. Radio Frequency Identification (RFID)

RFID (Radio Frequency Identification) is a term used for a radio-enabled device that communicates with or interrogates a tag or smart label, which is embedded with a single microchip processor and an antenna. The origin of the term lies in the invention of "tags" that reflects back or re-transmits a radio frequency signal. The two components of RFID are tags and readers. The tags or label is equipped with a single microchip processor, an antenna and an ID code that can be embedded in almost any object. RFID readers are radio-enabled devices that communicate with or interrogate RFID tags or labels wirelessly and obtain the ID code on the tags from a distance of several inches. The RFID readers can be fixed or made portable just like barcode scanners. RFID can also be referred as a high-tech version of the barcode.

In the past few years, the cost of RFID tags has come down drastically. Low cost RFID tags, typically costs less than Rs. 30.00 each for up to 1 metre range making the technology affordable as an alternative to the barcode, magnetic strip or printed label. RFID has advantages that include tolerance of mis-orientation and obscuration, lower cost over life and ability to "read". Most importantly, RFID tags are cheap enough to be disposable and thin enough to go even inside the sheets of paper in some cases.

An RFID tag is a means of storing and retrieving data through a radio frequency transmission to the chip inside the tag. An RFID tag is simply an integrated circuit (chip), which includes memory for data storage and a substrate backing material with an antenna pattern. The chip can typically hold up to 1,024 bits (128 bytes) of information. In a typical library implementation, each book is equipped with smart labels and library patrons are given library cards imbedded with smart labels. Tags or smart labels can be programmed to store (i) unique accession number of documents; (ii) class number of a document; and (iii) a unique security code for Electronic Article Surveillance (EAS).

While accession number is used for carrying out functions of circulation, stock verification and other library applications, class number can be deployed for sorting documents according to class numbers and segregating then into bins for different shelving areas. As mentioned earlier, the RFID tags can also be used as antitheft devices in libraries. Such applications of RFID are called Electronic Article Surveillance (EAS). New forms of RFID perform EAS functions as well, obviating the need for a separate device.

An interrogator, or reader, is a radio frequency device used to write data to and read data from the chip. Smart tags used in a library are passive, having no internal power source such as a battery. The interrogator provides enough RF energy to power and activate the tag to reflect or to present information stored on them. RFID tags transmit data, antennas receive or transmit the RF signal through the air and readers decode the RF information received from the RFID tag through the antenna. The data is then transmitted to the host application for necessary processing.

6.3. Smart Cards

A smart card, chip card, or integrated circuit card (ICC), is a pocket-sized card with embedded integrated circuits which can process data. Effectively, a smart card can receive input, process it and deliver the processed data as an output. There are two broad categories of smart cards; memory cards contain only non-volatile memory storage components and specific security logic. Microprocessor cards contain volatile memory and microprocessor components. The card is made of plastic, generally PVC. The card may embed a hologram to avoid counterfeiting. Smartcards are generally used as security authentication mechanism for single sign-on within large companies and organizations. A quickly growing application of smart card is as digital identification cards. In this application, the cards are used for authentication of identity. When combined with biometrics, smart cards can provide two- or three-factor authentication. The libraries generally use smart cards to identify and authenticate its patrons.

7. INTERNET TECHNOLOGY AND ITS SERVICES

The internet has revolutionised our society, our economy and our technological systems. Over the past century, important technological developments have created a global environment that is drawing people of the world closer and closer together. About fifteen years ago, most of the world knew little or nothing about the internet. The internet was then a private network accessible only to computer scientists and researchers who used it to interact with colleagues in their respective disciplines. It is estimated that about 60 million host computers on the internet today serve about 200 million users in over 200 countries and territories. Also, the total numbers of host computers and users have been growing at about 33% every six months since 1988 – or roughly 80% per year.

The Internet has revolutionised the computer and communications world like nothing before. The invention of the telegraph, telephone, radio, and computer set the stage for this unprecedented integration of capabilities. The internet is at once a world-wide broadcasting capability, a mechanism for information dissemination, and a medium for collaboration and interaction between individuals and their computers without barriers of geographic location. The internet represents one of the most successful examples of the benefits of sustained investment and commitment to research and development of information infrastructure. Beginning with the early research in packet switching, the government, industry and academia have been partners in evolving and deploying this exciting new technology. Today, terms like "Yahoo" and "Google" are common part of our vocabulary. Internet-based communication services, content creation and delivery tools applicable in libraries are given below.

7. 1. Internet-based Communication Services

Libraries use Internet-based Communication System while attending their day-to-day routine works. An Internet-based Communication System allows communication between computer users hooked into a network. Internet-based Communication System is used for communication between person-to-person, person-to-group and group-to-group. A document or message sent through electronic system may contain text, graphics, image, speech as well as other types of information. Major internet-based communication services are described below.

7.1.1. Electronic Mail (E-mail)

Electronic Mail, or e-mail, is a fast, easy and inexpensive way to communicate with other internet users around the world. It is the most popular and widely used services of the internet. E-mail is the term given to an electronic message, usually a form of simple text message that a user types at a computer system and is transmitted over some form of computer network to another user, who can read it. Email offers speedy and economical transfer of messages anywhere in the world. Sending e-mail messages are virtually free even to long-distance destinations. Most integrated library systems support e-mail-based communication to library users (for circulation and acquisition-related activities) and to the vendors / publishers (for placing orders, reminders, cancellation, etc).

7.1.2. Listserv

Listservs are electronic groups that typically centre around broad topics such as Digital Libraries or Reference Service, etc. Listservs of IFLA with the name IFLA-l, Digilib-l, LIBJOBS-l are good example of this. Every e-mail message sent to the listserv is distributed to all members of that listserv, which is potentially hundreds or thousands of people. It does not cost anything to subscribe to a listserver, but simply requires that the user sends an e-mail message to the appropriate address with the message: subscribe (listserv) Firstname Lastname. Each Listserv has one address where a user sends requests to subscribe, unsubscribe, search the archives, etc., and another address to send actual questions or responses to the readers of the list. Apart from organising discussions, job announcements and conference announcements are popular usage of Listservs.

7.1.3. Chat or Instant Messengers

Chat refers to any live discussions conducted using the internet, usually between more than two persons using their keyboard to communicate. Chat programs allow users on the internet to communicate with each other by typing in real time. It is a feature offered by many online services or Web sites that allows users to "chat" by typing messages which are displayed almost instantly on the screens of other users who are using the chat room at a given time. After entering a chat room, any user can type a message that will appear on the monitors of all the other users. Chatting is one of the most popular uses of the Internet. Generally the users remain anonymous by using nicknames or pseudonyms to identify themselves online.

A variation of chat is the phenomenon of the instant messenger. Instant messaging can be used to communicate privately with friends, relatives or co-workers. To send and receive instant messages, a user needs a connection to the internet and instant messaging software such as Gmail Messenger, Yahoo Messenger and MSN Messenger. The instant messaging software enables a user to set up a list of contacts who also use the same program. Once this list is set up, one can see each contact as they come online. A chat session can be started with them quickly and easily. Most conversations are typed text messages that are sent back and forth, though more advanced users can exchange voice, video, files and more.

7.1.4. Conferencing

One of the most exciting features of internet is to communicate, talk, and see groups of people in different locations around the world, without the expense of travel. Conferencing can take many forms, such as web chat, audio conferencing, video conferencing, multimedia conferencing, screen-sharing, etc. The conferencing programs, such as the popular CU-SeeMe, allow workgroups to use the internet to see each others' faces in small windows on the computer screen and to hear their voices through computer speakers. One can use desktop video and audio simultaneously or audio can be used alone or just use the screen-sharing capability without either audio or video.

7.1.4.1. Audio Conferencing or Internet Telephony

Internet telephony also called IP telephony is a combination of hardware and software that allows the internet to be used as a telephone carrier. Internet telephony is the conversion of analogue speech signals used on current telephone systems into digital data, allowing calls to be sent over the internet, bypassing long distance charges. While the internet was first devised as a way of transmitting data, it is now being used to make voice calls. Internet telephony is projected to explode as the costs plummet. After the costs of initial set-up and access to an Internet Service Provider, long-distance voice calls can be made via the internet free of charge, but current quality of voice transmission over the internet is not always as good as direct telephone service. There are also PSTN/Internet gateways that allow regular telephone callers to make Phone-to-Internet-to-Phone connections. There are PC-to-Phone connections and Phone-to-PC connections.

7.1.4.2. Video Conferencing

Video conferencing is one of the most exciting areas of development in telecommunications, with applications ranging from business to government to education to home and family. Video conferencing involves sending video signals as well as audio and computer data signals. Conferencing can be done one-to-one, one-to-many (called multicast), and many-to-many (called multipoint). While video conferencing, one can talk as well as see the people sitting miles away as if all are discussing in one room facing each other. One of the most popular applications is transmission on news from various locations by the TV news channels. It also has enormous potential for enhancing communications for small and mid-sized companies, as well as distance learning. However, video conferencing requires sufficient bandwidth to transfer video files of acceptable quality. Desktop conferencing, therefore, is not yet widely implemented for business and educational use. As bandwidth increases, desktop video conferencing is expected to blossom. The PictureTel and Vtel are two of the largest companies that sell video conferencing equipment.

7.1.4.2. 1. NetMeeting

Microsoft NetMeeting facilitates a new way of talking, meeting, working and sharing over the internet. It uses internet phone voice communications and conferencing standards to provide multi-user applications and data sharing over intranets or the internet. Two or more users can work together and collaborate in reach time using application sharing, whiteboard, and chat functionality.

NetMeeting can be used for common collaborative activities such as virtual meetings. It can also be used for customer service applications, telecommuting, distance learning, and technical support. The product is based on ITU (International Telecommunication Union) standards, so it is compatible with other products based on the same standards.

NetMeeting supports text chat, video shared whiteboard, transferring of files, directory of connected users.

Files, such as documents or pictures, can be exchanged. One of the problems with net meeting is the break-up in audio that sometimes becomes inaudible when using it on the internet, though it works fine over a high-speed company network. Net meeting is normally installed with Internet Explorer, or it can be download from http:// www.microsoft. com/windows/netmeeting/. There is a web site dedicated to Netmeeting at http://www.netmeet.net/.

7.1.5. News Groups

Another Internet service similar to listservs is a newsgroup. News Groups are like an International bulletin board. Each group is a forum for a different subject, where a subscriber can post his / her questions or answers. There are thousands of groups covering just about every area of interest. The difference between listserv and news group is that when a user joins a group, the mail is no longer automatically deposited into his mailbox. Instead a user is expected to go to the newsgroup himself to read it. Some listservs can also be accessed as a newsgroup. A good analogy to a newsgroup is a bulletin board, i.e. one can go to it, as opposed to having mail delivered to his / her desk. The mails from newsgroup do not get cluttered and it can be easily regulated how often messages are read. A drawback of a newsgroup lies in the fact that a user must remember to go out to the newsgroup to look for the information. There are hundreds of newsgroup communities. They centre on topics such as computing, news, recreation, social, and "alternative" topics. There are newsgroups dealing with virtually every topic under the sun and new newsgroups appear every day.

7.2. Internet-based Content Publishing and Delivery Services

The World Wide Web- known as WWW, W3 or simply, the Web help people to publish, organize and provide access to information on the internet. The WWW can be defined as a hypertext, multimedia, distributed information system that provides links to hypertext documents, as well as to many other internet tools and databases. The Web serves as a platform for several specialised content publishing and delivery services. Some of the important tools for content publishing and delivery services applicable to libraries and information centres are described below.

7.2.1. Blogs

A blog (an abridged form of term web log) is a website, usually maintained by an individual, with regular entries of commentary, descriptions of events, or other material such as graphics or video. Entries are commonly displayed in reverse chronological order (Wikipedia, 2008). Blogs are considered as lightweight publishing tools. Blogs provide control to an individual or group of individuals for publishing contents or making commentary on it. Technologically, blogs are easier to use, platform-independent, and accessible online over the internet. Broadly, blogs can be said to be online dairies, however, thousands of blogs are maintained by experts in different subject areas who are willing to share their knowledge, understanding and opinions with other people. Michael Casey, who coined the term "Library 2.0", for example maintains a blog on Library 2.0 called LibraryCrunch.

The most obvious application of blogs for libraries is to use it as a tool for promotion, publicity and for outreach services. Libraries can disseminate information to their users, make announcements for its new resources and events through its blogs. Blogs can be used to initiate debates and interaction amongst users and staff. Moreover, library staff and user can be encouraged to use Library blogs to get to know each other and interact at personal level.

7.2.2. Wikis

A wiki is a collection of web pages designed to enable anyone who accesses it to contribute or modify content, using a simplified markup language. Wikis are often used to create collaborative websites and to power community websites (Wikipedia, 2008). For example, the collaborative encyclopaedia, Wikipedia is one of the best-known wikis that has broken down one the golden rules of librarianship, i.e. content validation and authenticity of information. Wikis are also used in businesses to provide affordable and effective Intranets and for knowledge management. Ward Cunningham, developer of the first wiki software, WikiWikiWeb, originally described it as "the simplest online database that could possibly work" (Wikipedia, 2008).

Wikis can essentially be equated to open web-pages, where anyone registered with it can publish on to it, add to it, amend it and change it. As in case of blogs, Wikis do not have reliability as traditional resources. Inspite of this, their value as information resource cannot be undermined. Wikis are not only popular but de-facto source of information for people inspite of the fact that it is not validated or authenticated. The lack of peer review and editorship in case of Wikis is a challenge to librarians. Wikis as items in a collection, and the associated instruction of users in their evaluation, is certainly an important task for libraries.

Libraries can use wiki as a communication tool to enable social interaction among librarians and patrons. Users can share information, ask and answer questions, and librarians can do the same within a wiki. Moreover, a record of these transactions can be archived for perpetuity. Transcripts of such question-answer sessions would serve as a resource for the library to provide as reference. Furthermore, wikis (as well as blogs) will ultimately evolve into a multimedia environment, where both synchronous and asynchronous audio and video collaborations will take place.

7.2.3. Podcasting

The word "Podcasting" is derived from two words, namely "Broadcasting" and "iPod" (popular MP3 player from Apple Computer). Podcasting is defined as "process of capturing audio digital-media files that can be distributed over the internet using RSS feeds for playing-back on portable media players as well as computers. Users can subscribe to such feeds and automatically download these files directly into an audio management program (such as iTunes, Windows Media Player or MusicMatch) on their PCs. When a user synchronizes their portable audio device with their personal computer the podcasts are automatically transferred to that device to be listened to at the time and location most convenient for the user (Wikipedia, 2008).

Podcasts can be used with a variety of digital audio formats and play on almost any MP3 player or portable digital audio device - as well as any brand of desktop computer or laptop. Though podcasters' web sites may also offer direct download or streaming of their content, a podcast is distinguished from other digital media formats by its ability to be syndicated, subscribed to, and downloaded automatically when new content is added, using an aggregator or feed reader capable of reading feed formats such as Real Simple Syndication (RSS) or Atom. Several libraries use podcasts to support library orientations programmes.

Taking advantage of podcasting and other consumer technologies (e.g., PDAs, iPods and other MP3 players) as a deliver media of Library's content and services is a great leap forward for library profession.

7.2.4. Vodcasting

The "VOD" in Vodcasting stands for "video-on-demand". It is identical to podcasting. While podcasting is used for delivering audio files, vodcasting is used for delivering video content. Like podcast content, vodcasts content can be played either on a laptop or on personal media assistant (PMA).

7.2.5. RSS Feeds

RSS stands for Real Simple Syndication or Rich Site Summary. The technology, on one hand allows a web site (or e-publisher) to list the newest published updates (like table of contents of journals, new articles) through a technology called XML, on the other hand, it facilitates a web user to keep track new updates on chosen website (s). Like a personal search assistant, RSS feed readers visit pre-defined web sites, look for updated information and fetch it automatically on to the user's desktop. It provides users a way to syndicate and republish content on the Web. Users republish content from other sites or blogs on their sites or blogs, aggregate content on other sites in a single place, and ostensibly distil the Web for their personal use.

Libraries are already creating RSS feeds for users to subscribe to, including updates on new items in a collection, new services, and new content in subscription databases. They can also republish contents from other scholarly web sites on their sites.

8. DIGITIZATION

Digitisation is the process of converting the content of physical media (e.g., periodical articles, books, manuscripts, cards, photographs, vinyl disks, etc.) into digital format. A digital image, in turn, is composed of a set of pixels (picture elements), arranged according to a pre-defined ratio of columns and rows. An images document file can be managed as a regular computer file and can be retrieved, printed and modified using appropriate software. In most library applications, digitisation normally results in documents that are accessible from the web site of a library and thus, on the internet. Optical scanners and digital cameras are used to digitise images by translating them into bit maps. It is also possible to digitise sound, video, graphics, animations, etc.

Further, textual images can be OCRed so as to make its contents searchable.

Digitisation is not an end in itself. It is the process that creates a digital image from an analogue image. Selection criteria, particularly those which reflect user needs are of paramount importance. Therefore, the principles that are applicable in traditional collections development are applicable when materials are being selected for digitisation. However, there are several other considerations related to technical, legal, policy, and resources that become important in a digitisation project.

Several digital library projects are concerned with providing digital access to materials that already exists with traditional libraries in printed media. Digitization of printed material is practically the only reasonable solution for institutions such as libraries for converting existing paper collection (legacy documents) without having access to the original data in computer processible formats. Digitization is the natural choice for large-scale conversions for major digital library initiatives. Printed text, pictures and figures are transformed into computer-accessible forms using a digital scanner or a digital camera in a process called document imaging or scanning. The digitally scanned images are stored in a file as a bit-mapped page image, irrespective of the fact that a scanned page contains a photograph, a line drawing or text. A bit-mapped page image is a type of computer graphic, literally an electronic picture of the page which can most easily be equated to a facsimile image of the page and as such they can be read by humans, but not by the computers, understably "text" in a page image is not searchable on a computer using the present-day technology. An image-based implementation require a large space for data storage and transmission. There are several large projects using page images as their primary storage format, including project JSTOR (www.jstor.org) at Princeton University funded by the Melon Foundation. The project Jstor has a complete set of more than 1000+ journals scanned and hosted on web servers that resides at the University of Michigan and is mirrored at Princeton University. Using technology developed at Michigan, high resolution (600 dpi) bit-mapped images of each page are linked to a text file generated with optical character recognition (OCR) software. Linking a searchable text file to the page images of the entire published record of a journal along with newly constructed table of contents, indexes, permits high level of access, search and retrieval of the journal material previously unimaginable (Guthrie, 1997).

Capturing page image format is comparatively easy and inexpensive. It is a faithful reproduction of its original maintaining page integrity and originality. The scanned textual images, however, are not searchable unless it is OCRed, which in itself, is highly error prone process specially when it involves scientific texts.

9. ELECTRONIC RESOURCES

Electronic resources can be defined as resources in electronic format or computer-processible format that provide information or an indicator to the information and are generally accessible over the internet or stored on media like CD-ROM/DVD-ROM or other storage devices. The emergence of internet and the World Wide Web (WWW) in early 1990s, as a new media of information storage and delivery, came as a real boon for evolution of electronic resources. While searching bibliographic databases became popular, it created demand for actual content in full-text that became difficult for libraries to obtain. Coincided with evolution of World Wide Web (WWW), display technology evolved, cost of storage came down drastically and networks became faster. It became possible for publishers to deliver content, either as a bitmap page images or other structured formats such as HTML, PDF or RTF. Increasingly larger number of publishers started using the Internet as a global way to offer their publications to the international community of scientists and technologists given the fact that technology is in a position to deliver more content to more users at a significantly lower cost per user.

Electronic resources on the internet manifest themselves in numerous flavours and categories, although most of them emulate the traditional publishing while others are revolutionary in their design and approach. While the present trend to imitate and emulate the traditional models of scholarly communication may continue for some time, eventually the capabilities added by the new media would be used in more innovative ways. Some of the important types of e-resources are described below.

9.1. Electronic Databases

An electronic database consists of electronic resources integrated in highly organized fashion so as to provide controlled access to it by their commercial providers. The first databases were bibliographic in nature and were online version of existing indexing and abstracting services such as Biological Abstracts, Index Medicus, Chemical Abstracts, etc. By the year 1988, only half of all databases were bibliographic in nature. With introduction of a number of online databases containing textual information, news, statistics, commodity prices, etc., a third type of databases holding text of full-length documents started appearing. Several full-text of encyclopaedia, directories and articles from journals are now available online. Most of the publishers now provide access to their full-text journals through their web site or through other electronic publishing platforms. While there are a number of public-domain databases, most online databases require annual subscription for accessing them. Thousands of databases are now available on compact discs (CD-ROM) as well as on the Web.

9.2. Electronic Journals

Electronic journals, or "e-journals", are used for those journals and newsletters that are prepared and distributed electronically. Electronic journals may be defined very broadly as any journal, magazine, e-zine, webzine, newsletter or type of electronic serial publication which is available over the internet and can be accessed using different technologies such as WWW, Gopher, ftp, telnet, e-mail or listserv. Several traditional journals are now being published both on the Web and in print. Content lists for most of the journals are available on the Web or distributed to subscribers as an e-mail text messages or through technologies like RSS and Atom.

Internet-based electronic journals started to appear in the beginning of 1990. These journals were mostly delivered as an attachment to e-mail while their back issues were mounted on anonymous ftp sites and users were required to download them from these ftp sites. The libraries and information centres made them accessible through their gopher site. 1995 witnessed peak of Gopher technology which then dropped suddenly and dramatically by 1997. With advent of WWW technology in 1993, electronic publishing became more than a novelty, the web as a means of delivery of electronic information has grown steadily since then. As publishers experiment with different publication modes and models, the very definition of a journal is undergoing change in the electronic environment. New journals have evolved based on the graphic capabilities of the Internet that are available only in electronic form.

Like print journals, current and archival issues of electronic journals can be browsed through their content pages. Moreover, e-journals can also be searched not only on their metadata but also in full-text through sophisticated search interface. Currently, there are more than 50,000 peer-reviewed, scholarly electronic journals that are available on the internet.

9.3. Electronic Books

An electronic book is digital reading material that a user can view on a desktop or Personal Digital Assistant (PDA), laptop or on a dedicated, portable device with a large storage capacity and the ability to download new titles via a network connection. More and more traditional book publishers, as well as those catering to the professional and business communities, are launching their e-book collections.

The electronic books market consists of two distinct components i.e. (i) electronic books consisting of digital material or contents; and (ii) electronic book hardware including e-book reading appliance, PCs, laptop or PDA. The digital material or content that make an electronic book are simply textual and graphical files consisting of bits that can be transported any digital storage media or delivered over a network connection. It is designed to be viewed on some combination of hardware and software ranging from dumb terminals to web browsers, on personal computers to the new reading appliances.

More and more books are now being released on the web through enhanced interfaces that offer features such as increased search capacity within a book or entire collection of books, ability to highlight and flag a page, ability to make notes on text without damaging the book, ability to e-mail quotes from the books to other colleagues, etc. Most publishers like Springer, Wiley InterScience, Taylor and Francis, Cambridge University Press, Oxford University Press, etc. offer their e-book collections on subscription / one-time purchase basis. Besides, there are a number of e-books aggregators that make thousands of books available online for libraries and individuals at relatively lower cost. Three major e-books aggregators are Questia (http://www.questia.com/), Ebrary (http://www.ebrary.com/) and NetLibrary (http://www.netlibrary.com/). However, just like other e-resources, e-books come with restrictions such as limit on downloads, in terms of number of pages, i.e. one page at a time or one chapter at a time or no download at all.

9.4. Electronic Theses and Dissertations

Theses submitted to the universities as requirement for the award of Ph.D. degree constitute a useful source of information for the new and ongoing research. Doctoral dissertations submitted to universities and academic institutions are originally created in digital format using one of the word processing software packages like MSWord, LaTex, Word Perfect, Word Pro, etc. or one of the desktop publishing packages like Page Maker, Ventura, etc. These documents are undisputedly highly valuable collection especially in digital format that qualify to be an important component of a digital library. The documents composed on word processing packages / desktop publishing packages can be easily converted into PDF, Post Script or XML using appropriate software tools so as to host them on the web. Several universities and institutions have already implemented electronic submission of doctoral dissertations under the overall umbrella of an international digital library initiative called "Networked Digital Library of Theses and Dissertations" (NDLTD).

9.5. Digitized Print Material

Several digital library projects are concerned with providing digital access to materials that already exists with traditional libraries in printed media. Scanned page images are practically the only reasonable solution for institutions such as libraries for converting existing paper collection (legacy documents) without having access to the original data in computer processible formats convertible into HTML/XML or in any other structured or unstructured text. Scanned page images are natural choice for large-scale conversions for major digital library initiatives. Printed text, pictures and figures are transformed into computer-accessible forms using a digital scanner or a digital camera in a process called document imaging or scanning. The digitally scanned images are stored in a file as a bit-mapped page image, irrespective of the fact that a scanned page contains a photograph, a line drawing or text. A bit-mapped page image can most easily be equated to a facsimile image of the page and as such they can be read by humans, but not by the computers, understably "text" in a page image is not searchable on a computer using the present-day technology. An image-based implementation require a large space for data storage and transmission. There are several large projects using page images as their primary storage format, including project JSTOR (*www.jstor.org*) at Princeton University funded by the Melon Foundation.

Capturing page image format is comparatively easy and inexpensive. It is a faithful reproduction of its original maintaining page integrity and originality. The scanned textual images, however, are not searchable unless it is OCRed, which in itself, is highly error prone process specially when it involves scientific texts. Options and technology for converting print to digital and the process of Optical Character Recognition (OCR) are elaborated in section on "digitisation".

There are several other types of electronic resources such as e-prints, post-prints, technical reports, library catalogues, online courseware, educational materials, career sources, information on organizations, associations and so forth. Examples of various types of e-resources can be viewed on the web.

9.6. Audio, Video and Streaming Media

Streaming multimedia is sequential delivery of multimedia content, including video, audio or some other learning objects, over a computer network that is displayed (or played back) to the end-user as it is being delivered by the provider. The advent of the MP3 players and the iPod resulted in a greater effort to deliver downloadable media. Moreover, web documents are now coming with greater integration of text with media. Encyclopaedias now have articles with audio files, video clips and animation to illustrate a given topic.

Media can broadly be categorized into three category, namely (i) commercial movies that have greater copyright restrictions, (ii) educational media typically are lesser controlled and many a time are made available free-of-cost; and (iii) media targeted for individual users, such as movies and songs, that comes with restrictions in terms of copying and distributions.

9.7. Subject Gateways or Library Portals

The web, being a hypermedia-based system, allows linking amongst electronic resources stored on servers dispersed geographically on distant locations. The portal sites or gateways redirect a user to the holders of the original digital material. The librarians, being the earliest users of the web, started to gather and organize link to important web-based resources on various subjects.

A subject gateway can be defined as facilities that allow easier access to web-based resources in a defined subject area. The simplest types of subject gateways are sets of web pages containing list of links to resources. Some gateways index their lists of links and provide a simple search facility. More advanced gateways offer a much-enhanced service via a system consisting of a resource database and various indexes, which can be searched and/or browse throughout a web-based interface (O'Leary, 2000).

Subject gateways are also known as Subject-based Information Gateways (SBIGs), Subject-based Gateways, Subject Index Gateways, Virtual libraries, Clearing houses, Subject trees, Pathfinders, etc. Subject gateway is an important component of a library web site designed for the library users so as to help them discover high-quality information on the internet in a quick and effective way.

In the traditional information environment human intermediaries, such as publishers and librarians, filter and process information so that users can search catalogues and indexes of organized knowledge as opposed to raw data and information. Subject gateways work on the same principle, i.e. they employ subject experts and information professionals to select, classify and catalogue internet resources to aid search and retrieval for the users. Users are offered access to a database of internet resources descriptions which they can search by keywords or browse by subject area. A description of each resource is provided to help users assess very quickly its origin, content and nature, enabling them to decide if it is worth investigating further. In the process users get benefited from the expertise of librarians and subject experts with subject gateways rather than having to locate, evaluate, filter and organize the resources themselves. Specialized software are available as freeware or as priced software to create and maintain professionally developed subject gateways. Some of the major portal sites or gateways that provide access to electronic resources on the Internet are as follows:

WWW Virtual Library	http://www.edoc.com/
Internet Public Library	http://www.ipl.org/
Michigan Electronic Library	http://mel.lib.mi.us/
Penn Electronic Library	http://www.library.upenn.edu/resources/
BUBL Information Service	http://bubl.ac.uk/
Argus Clearing House	http://www.clearinghouse.net/
Internet Index	http://sunsite.berkeley.edu/InternetIndex/

10. INFORMATION TECHNOLOGY-BASED LIBRARY SERVICES

New information technology can potentially support a range of traditional and non-traditional library services. Most of the library services generated using information technology resemble closely to those generated manually with improvements and modifications to suit the requirements of automated services. Examples of some of IT-based library services are given below:

10.1. OPAC and WebPAC

Remote access to the Library catalogues (OPAC) was possible only through a telnet connection before the Web was launched. The web-based interfaces are now available for most of the integrated library software packages including Libsys. Web sites are increasingly providing links to their webPAC instead of telnet links to their Library OPAC. Exploiting the provisions of hyperlinking that the web provides, various searchable elements of a bibliographic record in a webPAC are hyperlinks to other records in the database. For example, an author is a hyperlink to all records in the database for that author, a series is an hyperlink to all serial title under that series; a keyword for a record is a link to all records in database having that keyword, etc. In effect, a web PAC adds software-based functionality to a conventional OPAC. A user has additional incentives to visit the library web page hosting webPAC. With web-based resources and services in place, many libraries are phasing out their dumb terminals. The library web sites are increasingly becoming a more logical gateway to the catalogue and other web-based library resources. The acceptability of web-based interfaces to the Library OPAC is much greater because web interfaces are familiar to the users with its graphical and navigational interfaces. The users can click complex subjects instead of typing them or remembering complex commands.

10.2. Information Alerting Services (IAS)

As the name implies, Information Alerting Services or Current Awareness Services (CAS) are produced by the libraries for their users to alert them about new developments in a given field of study. Information alerting services are issued periodically by the libraries either for internal distribution amongst staff and employees or externally to other users. The alerting service may be issued as a newsletter reporting new developments, programmes, forthcoming seminars and conferences, events, training programmes, etc. It may also consist of recent additions of books and other documents in the library for a specified time period. Most library integrated system facilitate generation of such a service organized according to subject category for a given time period. Alerting service may also consist of an indexing service issued by a library or a commercial publisher or a society that regularly indexes the contents of periodicals and some other publications systematically in a specified subject field. Such indexing services are issued at a regular interval. Abstracting services are essentially index-ing services wherein an abstract of articles are included in addition to its bibliographic details. Index India and Reader's Guide to Periodical Literature are examples of indexing services. Biological Abstracts, Chemical Abstracts and Index Medicus are example of abstracting services. Most indexing and abstracting services are now available as web-based databases with sophisticated search interface.

Selective Dissemination of Information (SDI) is a personal form of Current Awareness Service (CAS). It refers to the mechanism of selectively directing new items of information from primary or secondary sources to individuals based on their current interests in a particular subject. SDI is delivered based on a user interest profile which is matched with updates on databases for finding the items of interest for a given user.

Push technology and personalisation are more recent terms that are used in place of SDI.

10.3. Digital Reference Service

Reference service and imparting instructional training to the library users are key areas of activities for any library. The technology now allows reference librarians to reach out to the users using the network instead of waiting at the reference desk for users to come by. Besides, imparting instructions on mechanisms of using a library, a reference librarian is also involved in delivering reference service that require deep intellectual understanding of subject. Although automated libraries are not yet sufficiently advanced to offer interactive reference services, electronically-mediated reference services are increasingly available through libraries and information centres.

Digital reference service, also called "Ask-An-Expert" or "Ask-A-Librarian" services are Internet-based question and answer service that connect users with individuals who possess specialized subject knowledge and skill in conducting precision searches (Davis, 2000). As opposed to static web pages, digital reference services use the internet to place people in contact with people who can answer specific question and instruct users on developing certain skills. The people who serve as digital reference experts (also called volunteers or mentors) are most of the time information specialists, affiliated to various libraries.

10.4. Real-time Digital Reference Service: Library Chat Rooms

Several libraries have started experimenting with offering Real time Digital Reference Service, using chat software, live interactive communication activities, call counter management software, web contact software, bulletin board services, interactive customer assistance system or related technologies.

Many libraries are experimenting with internet chat technology as an innovative method to extend and enhance traditional and remote reference service. While digital reference service is asynchronous method of information delivery, the internet chat providing the benefit of synchronous communication between a user and a reference librarian (or mentor). Interactive reference services facilitate a user to talk to a real, live reference librarian at any time of day or night from anywhere in the world. Unlike with email reference, the librarian can perform a reference interview of a sort by seeking clarifications from the user. The librarian can conduct Internet searches and push websites onto the patron's browser, and can receive immediate feedback from the patron as to whether his or her question has been answered to his satisfaction. Most libraries currently involved in real-time reference service are part of a collaborative network so that they can share staffing and work around the clock to truly provide reference service any time. Library of Congress Collaborative Digital Reference Service (http://www.loc.gov/rr/digref/cdrshome.html) is one of such services. Several institutions including Cornell University, Internet Public Library, Michigan State University and North Carolina University are offering internet chat-based services using software like LivePerson, AOL Instant Messenger, Conference Room and Netscape Chat. The librarians have observed that their relatively new chat-based service logged significantly more questions in a relatively short time than their well-established e-mail digital reference service.

LiveRef(sm) (http://www.public.iastate.edu/~CYBERSTACKS/ LiveRef.htm) maintains an online registry of real-time digital reference services.

10.5. Electronic Document Delivery Services

The term "electronic document delivery systems" implies delivery of electronic version of a document that might involve reproduction of an electronic copy of a document if it is not available in electronic format. The libraries had been using fax machines for immediate delivery of photocopies of articles via telephone lines. The first use of electronic document delivery was based on scanning technology. With maturity of scanning equipment and technology, document supply services started scanning the documents as bitmap page images. Applications are built in such a way so as to automatically produce a hard copy together with a header page containing the address of the applicant which can again be sent by snail mail or facsimile. A software package known as "Ariel" is used in several libraries in developed countries for delivery of scanned articles via internet. The Ariel software is loaded on an internet-enabled computer can receive and send electronic information to other libraries which have installed Ariel.

Availability of most of the peer reviewed research journals in electronic format, inexpensive technology to scan articles and improved electronic delivery mechanisms are some of the enabling factors that have contributed to well-established electronic document delivery system now available commercially. More recently most of the secondary services that were available on CD ROM or through online search services are now available on the internet where the bibliographic references are linked to their full-text on the publisher's site. The technology has now been perfected and there are several electronic document delivery services that allow a user to download an article in full-text from their site or deliver them electronically as attachment to e-mails. Most electronic publishers and aggregators like OCLC, OVID etc. are offering full-text of articles through their web sites. Different vendors have various payment options; some charge each time the journal is used, whereas others provide open access for a set annual fee. A user who wishes to have the item delivered can enter a credit card number and specify a delivery method (postal, UPS, fax, e mail, etc.) and indicate whether it is a rush item (with a rush order fee attached.)

The ADONIS (Article Delivery Over Network information Systems) can be considered as a landmark development in electronic document delivery system. The project was launched by a consortium of five major publishers - Academic Press, Blackwell's Scientific Publications (merged with Wiley InterScience), Elsevier Science Publications, and Springer Verlag. The project uses combination of laser scanning, printing and digital optical storage technology for storage and retrieval of complete pages of over 650 scientific, technical and medical journal articles. The issues of journals are available on CD ROM with weekly updates for distribution to each centre in various countries licensed to use the system for document delivery.

10.6. Library Web Sites

Libraries are using web technology to create home pages as starting points or as gateways for searching information about the library. A home page reflects characteristics of an academic institution. It provides an opportunity to the library to propagate its services and facilities to the academic community worldwide. The home pages of libraries are increasingly used as an integrated interface designed to deliver detailed information about a library as well as to provide access to all computer-based services offered by a library.

Several library web sites facilitate virtual guide to the physical facilities including collections, services and infrastructure available in the library through their web sites. Most library web sites provide library layouts and floor plans to guide users to physical location of facilities and services along with link to relevant information.

Besides offering information, the library web sites of academic institutions invariably hosts subject gateways or subject portals that contains links to web resources for subjects of interest to the institution. Most of the IT-based library services mentioned in chapter are offered through the web sites of libraries.

The library web sites can have features like have Frequently Asked Questions (FAQ) along with their answers, library calendar listing events or show information for forthcoming events, Web forms for inviting feedback. Moreover, libraries may also use bulletin boards, threaded discussion forum and listservs to help promote and evolve web-based library services.

10.7. Web-based User Education

The www provides a dynamic environment for distributing information over a large network and web-based instructions is a suitable tool to do so. Web-based guides and teaching tools can be easily updated, accessed, and printed on demand. They may include colour graphics and screen-shots. The web-based user education provides a high degree of interactivity and flexibility to the users offering them the benefit of self-pace, graduated to teach from basic to highly advanced levels and designed in a wide range of formats that accommodate diverse learning styles. The proliferation of digital resources will generate greater demands on reference and instructional services. With availability of digital resources that can be used anywhere at any time, requirement for instructional and reference services would also grow. Failure to develop both the technological aspects and required service components would lead to under utilization of digital resources. The library web sites can use web-based user education for imparting training to users in the following areas:

i. Basic library skills along with glossary of library terms;
ii. Using Library OPAC/webPAC, locating books, magazines and other library materials;
iii. Instructions for searching CD ROM and web-based databases and other electronic resources; and
iv. Instructions on subject searching training, using Boolean operators and searching internet resources through search engines.

The web technology provides for incorporating both synchronous and asynchronous interactivity in the web-based user education.

11. DIGITAL LIBRARIES

The increasing popularity of internet and developments in web technologies act as catalyst to the concept of digital library. While the internet serves as the carrier and provides the contents delivery mechanism, the web provides the tools and techniques for content publishing, hosting and accessing. Today's digital libraries are built around internet and web technologies with electronic journals as their building blocks.

The libraries will not become digital libraries, but will rather acquire access to ever growing digital collections on behalf of their users. Majority of these collections are being made available by external sources like commercial publishers, collections mounted by scholarly societies, resources at other libraries, electronic journal sites, etc. The electronic journals have become the largest and fastest growing segment of digital collections for most libraries. The internet has long been a favorite media for experimenting with electronic publishing and delivery. The technology allows creation of fully digitized multimedia products and make them accessible through the internet. Technological changes, especially the internet and web technology, continue to attract more and more traditional players to adopt it as a global way to offer their publications to the international community of scientists and technologists. Most of the important publishers now have their web-based interfaces to offer full-text of their journals. The current electronic publishing market consists of traditional players offering electronic versions of their print journals as well as several new enterprises offering new products and services that are "borne digital". The market also has several subsc-ription agents in their new role as electronic aggregators.

Besides electronic journals, there are several online databases that are now available through the web including Medline (several versions), AGRICOLA and ERIC. Most online search services like STN and DIALOG also have their web-based interfaces. Reference works like encyclopedia, dictionaries, handbooks, atlases, etc. are also making their electronic appearance on the web. However, amongst electronic resources created exclusively for the web, imbibing all features and facilities offered by the new technology, include web-based educational tutorials called "online courseware". The online courseware is proliferating the web as a strong contender for distant education. Telecampus, Canada (www.telecampus.edu/) lists more than 12,000 online courseware available on the web. Moreover, highly specialized web sites are now coming-up in various disciplines which offer information in totality including all kinds of resources in electronic format, EI Engineering Village (http://www.ei.org/), ISI Electronic Library (http://www.isinet.com), IEEE / IEE Electronic Library (http://www.ieee.org/), Engineering Sciences Data Unit (http://www.esdu.com) are some of the important examples.

12. SUMMARY

Past three decade has witnessed unprecedented developments in computer and communication technology. Computers are being used increasingly to automate various activities in libraries with a suitable off-the-shelf general or specific-purpose software package that are now available in a wide range. Tremendous storage and processing potential of computers are being fully realized through existing communication and networking technologies. The application of information technology in libraries results in increased operational efficiency of library staff. It relieves professional staff members from mundane jobs that involve a lot of duplication and repetitive activities enabling them to fruitfully utilize their time for user-oriented library services. As such, it improves quality of services rendered by the library. Use of information technology ensures ease of functioning, accuracy and economy in human labour with greater speed.

Dramatic reductions in the size and cost of computer components and equally impressive gains in the speed, storage capacity and reliability of hardware components have expanded their use rapidly in all activities and functions of a library and information centre. Notable reductions in the size of microprocessors combined with dramatically enhanced capacity have added new dimensions to their usage in libraries and information centres. Like microprocessor technology, digital storage devices have also witnessed notable reductions in its size and cost with dramatically enhancement in capacity of storage. There are two types of data storage devices, i.e. removable data storage devices and non-removable data storage devices. The data storage devices come in many sizes and shapes. The storage devices can also be categorized based on the architecture and the design like magnetic storage media, optical storage media, mechanical storage media, flash memory devices, Pen or USB drives.

A computer communication networks can be viewed as a collection of nodes with computing resources and nodal-switching computers that facilitate communication through a set of transmission links. Developments in communication technology have made it possible to interconnect geographically dispersed computing resources of different kinds and makes. Users can access the network through PCs and terminals attached to a node and messages traverse these networks through the switching nodes. Today, network technology works on client-server architecture with middleware used for connecting software components or applications on clients and servers. Technique of packet switching is used for transferring data between computer systems. The Transmission Control Protocol (TCP) and Internet Protocol (IP), called TCP/IP suite, is the backbone of internet and other TCP/IP based networks. With developments in communication technology, institutions have options to set-up fibre optic-based gigabit LAN or wireless LAN. Depending on the geographical location, institutions have options to buy terrestrial or satellite-based internet bandwidth from a number of Internet Service Providers (ISPs).

Library automation is one of the most important applications of ICT in libraries. It refers to computerization or mechanization of all library activities. It deals with the design and development of process and system that minimize the necessity of human intervention in their operations. Most integrated library software are modular in design consisting of a number of optional and basic modules. These packages typically incorporate modules for: acquisition, cataloguing, circulation control, serials control and online public access catalogue.

There are three important identification and data collection technologies that are used in libraries, namely, Bar Code Technology, Radio Frequency Identification (RFID) and Smart Card. Bar Code Technology is being used in library for the past 30 years to minimize data entry errors, speed processes and reduce costs. Most books, journals as well as other consumer products in the market carry black and white thin and thick strips called barcodes. Barcode technology offers a mechanism that can be used for identification, location and tracking of items that are bar coded. RFID (Radio Frequency Identification) is a term used for a radio-enabled device that communicates with or interrogates a tag or smart label, which is embedded with a single microchip processor and an antenna. The two components of RFID are tags and readers. The tags or label is equipped with a single microchip processor, an antenna and an ID code that can be embedded in almost any object. RFID readers are radio-enabled devices that communicate with or interrogate RFID tags or labels wirelessly and obtain the ID code on the tags from a distance of several inches. The RFID readers can be fixed or made portable just like barcode scanners. RFID can also be referred as a high-tech version of the barcode. A smart card, chip card, or Integrated Circuit Card (ICC), is a pocket-sized card with embedded integrated circuits which can process data. Effectively, a smart card can receive input, process it and deliver the processed data as an output. There are two broad categories of smart cards, i.e. memory cards contain only non-volatile memory storage components and specific security logic. Microprocessor cards contain volatile memory and microprocessor components. The card is made of plastic, generally PVC. The libraries generally use smart cards to identify and authenticate its patrons.

The internet has revolutionised our society, our economy and our technological systems. Over the past century, important technological developments have created a global environment that is drawing people of the world closer and closer together. The internet is at once a world-wide broadcasting capability, a mechanism for information dissemination, and a medium for collaboration and interaction between individuals and their computers without barriers of geographic location. Libraries use internet-based communication system while attending their day-to-day routine works. An internet-based communication system allows communication between computer users hooked into a network. It is used for communication between person-to-person, person-to-group and group-to-group. A document or message sent through electronic system may contain text, graphics, image, speech as well as other types of information. Major internet-based communication services include: email, listservs, chat or instant messengers, audio conferencing or Internet telephony and video conferencing and news groups. Besides communication services, the web also help people to publish, organize and provide access to information on the internet. The Web serves as a platform for several specialised content publishing and delivery services including: blogs, wikis, podcasting, vodcasting, RSS Feeds, etc.

Digitisation is the process of converting the content of physical media (e.g., periodical articles, books, manuscripts, cards, photographs, vinyl disks, etc.) into digital format. A digital image, in turn, is composed of a set of pixels (picture elements), arranged according to a pre-defined ratio of columns and rows. An images document file can be managed as a regular computer file and can be retrieved, printed and modified using appropriate software. In most library applications, digitisation normally results in documents that are accessible from the web site of a library and thus, on the Internet. Optical scanners and digital cameras are used to digitise images by translating them into bit maps. It is also possible to digitise sound, video, graphics, animations, etc. Further, textual images can be OCRed so as to make its contents searchable. Several digital library projects are concerned with providing digital access to materials that already exists with traditional libraries in printed media. Digitization of printed material is practically the only reasonable solution for institutions such as libraries for converting existing paper collection (legacy documents) without having access to the original data in computer-processible formats.

Electronic resources can be defined as resources in electronic format or computer-processible format that provide information or an indicator to the information and are generally accessible over the internet or stored on media like CD ROM/DVD ROM or other storage devices. The emergence of Internet and the World Wide Web (WWW) in early 1990s, as a new media of information storage and delivery, came as a real boon for evolution of electronic resources. Coincided with evolution of World Wide Web (WWW), display technology evolved, cost of storage came down drastically and networks became faster. It became possible for publishers to deliver content, either as a bitmap page images or other structured formats such as HTML, PDF or RTF. Increasingly, larger number of publishers started using the internet as a global way to offer their publications to the international community of scientists and technologists given the fact that technology is in a position to deliver more content to more users at a significantly lower cost per user. Electronic resources on the internet manifest themselves in numerous flavours and categories, although most of them emulate the traditional publishing while others are revolutionary in their design and approach. Some of the important types of e-resources are: electronic databases, electronic journals, electronic books, Electronic Theses and Dissertations (ETDs), audio, video and streaming media and subject gateways or library portals.

New information technology can potentially support a range of traditional and non-traditional library services. Most of the library services generated using information technology resemble closely to those generated manually with improvements and modifications to suit the requirements of automated services. Examples of some of IT-based library services are: OPAC / Webpac. Information alerting services including CAS and SDI, digital reference service, real-time reference service, electronic document delivery services, library web sites and web-based user education. The increasing popularity of internet and developments in web technologies act as catalyst to the concept of digital library. While the internet serves as the carrier and provides the contents delivery mechanism, the web provides the tools and techniques for content publishing, hosting and accessing. Today's digital libraries are built around internet and web technologies with electronic journals as their building blocks.

The libraries will not become digital libraries, but will rather acquire access to ever growing digital collections on behalf of their users. Majority of these collections are being made available by external sources like commercial publishers, collections mounted by scholarly societies, resources at other libraries, electronic journal sites, etc.

Developments in information technology provide an opportunity to libraries and information centres to organize and offer new IT-based library services and resources to the users. The librarians can no longer stay behind the desk to wait for the users to come, assuming that the users would approach at the right time and for the right things. In an environment of self-service databases and online courseware, a user is likely to approach the librarian after he has already begun his search, but was not satisfied with the results.

The future will require the librarians to reorient themselves, think creatively and adopt new technology to generate services and resources where their skills of structuring and organizing resources are put to its best use.

If the librarians are committed to sustain their roles as providers and facilitator of information in the emerging and competitive space of higher education, they would need to adopt new technology, interact with users to learn about their requirements and expectations. The librarians have to join the academic community as facilitators and collaborators, guide the students through the complex maze of print and digital resources, teaching them how to search effectively and helping them judge the quality and usefulness of the information that they encounter. The opportunities are limitless especially in the chaotic scenario of Internet.

BIBLIOGRAPHY

Arora, Jagdish and Sharan Pal Kaur. Recent information technologies and its impact on dissemination of information. Annals of Library Science and Documentation, 39(1), 12-18. 1992 (Also published in Immuno-Informatics,1(5), 2-5, 1991).

Arora, Jagdish, Sharan Pal Kaur and Harish Chandra. Computer communication networks and their use: Basic tutorial and current scenario of networks in India. Microcomputers for Information Management, 9(4), 241-261, 1992.

Arora, Jagdish. Applications of new information technology in libraries and information centres. Granthana: Indian Journal of Library Studies, 1 (1), 6-96 (also published in: National Library Services: ICONLIS 2004: Papers of the International Conference on National Library Services (ICONLIS 2004), Kolkata, March 15-16, 2004 (ed. H.K. Kaul). Kolkata: National Library, p. 302-336, 2004.

Arora, Jagdish and Trivedi, Parul. Radio Frequency Identification (RFID): An automatic identification and data collection technology for libraries. International Information Communication and Education, 24(1), 7-19, 2005.

Cox, John E.. Publishers, publishing and the Internet: how journal publishing will survive and prosper in the electronic age. Electronic Library, 15(2), 125-131, 1997.

Davis, Eric T. An overview of the access and preservation capabilities in digital technology. (*http://www.iwaynet.net/~lsci/diglib/digpapff.html*)

Davis, G. Digital reference services: An overview. (http://www.suite101.com/article.cfm/9460/52394/)

Fox, E. and Marchionini, Gary. Towards a worldwide digital library. Communication of the ACM, 41(4), 29-32, 1998.

Guthrie, Kevin M. Jstor. From project to Independent organization. Dlib, July/August, 1997. (http://www.dlib.org/dlib/july97/07guthrie.html)

Lesk, M.. Practical digital libraries: Books, bytes and bucks. San Francisco, Morgan Kaufman, 1997.

Lynch, Cliford. From automation to transformation. Educause Review, 60 - 68, 2000.

Miller, P. Web 2.0: Building the new library. Ariadne, No. 45, 2005.

Miller, P. and Chad, K. Do libraries matter?: The rise of Library 2.0, Talis, 2005.

Miller, P. Library 2.0: The challenge of disruptive innovation. Talis, 2006.

O'Leary, M. Grading the library portals. Online, November, 2000. (http://www.onlineinc.com/onlinemag/OL2000/oleary11.html)

Schwartz, C. Digital libraries: An overview. Journal of Academic Librarianship, 26(6), 385-396, 2000.

Sloan, Bernard G. Services perspectives for the digital library: Remote reference services. Library Trends, 47(2), 1998.

Web Sites (Last visited on 7th Nov., 2008)

Wikipedia. WikiWikiWeb (http://en.wikipedia.org/wiki/WikiWikiWeb)

Wikipedia. Social bookmarking (http://en.wikipedia.org/wiki/Social_ bookmarking)

Wikipedia. AJAX (http://en.wikipedia.org/wiki/AJAX).

Indian Response to International Developments in ICT

P.S.G. Kumar

UGC Emeritus Fellow, Deptt. of Library and Info Science, RTM Nagpur University, Nagpur - 440 010

EMERGENCE OF COMPUTERS

First Generation

Charles Babbage first conceived of the Difference Engine and Analytical Engine in the early nineteenth century, as automatic devices to perform a sequence of operations. He could not have visualized the phenomenal developments that were to take place in the following century and a half. In fact, Babbage did not even succeed in completing his machine. It was only in 1944 that the Mark-I designed by Howard Aiken was built at Harvard University. This Automatic Sequence Controlled Calculator is widely regarded as the first computer. This was a mechanical machine unlike the electronic machine of today. Earlier to this, in Germany Konard Zuse is known to have developed the Zuse Z3 computer in 1941. But, little is known about this machine.

Second Generation

The first truly electronic computer was the Electronic Numerical integrator and Computer (ENIAC) designed by Mauchly and Eckert and completed at the University of Pennsylvania in 1946-47. ENIAC employed electronic components unlike the electro-mechanical components used by Mark-I, UNIVAC-1 by the same designers, became in 1951, the first commercially available large computer. Unlike encoded paper tapes used in Mark-I, in ENIAC operations were specified by connecting a groups of wires. But connecting wires and cables for small non-repetitives tasks was too high to be practical.

EARLY APPLICATION IN LIBRARIES

Indexing

Dissatisfaction with the pre-coordinated indexes have led people to devise post-coordinate systems which eliminate pre-ordering of the concepts, etc. In a post-coordinate system, the concepts will be kept separately and these can be coordinated by the user at the time of search. It should be noted that the process of coordination is there in both the systems, only they are done at two different stages.[1]

Important post-coordinate systems are :

(i) Mortimer Taube's Uniterm system,

(ii) Calvin Mooers Zator System,

(iii) Cordonnier's Selecto System.

Title Based Keyword Indexes

The use of computers in the field of indexing has increased with the pioneering work of Luhn of IBM on the KWIC (KeyWord In Context) index. Since then a number of variations of KWIC index like KWOC (KeyWord Out of Context), KWAC (KeyWord Away from Context), etc. have emerged.

Unit Record Systems

A large number of book catalogues were produced in the US in the 1940s using unit record machines. In a unit record system, the cataloguing information is keypunched and the punched cards are then sorted into a desired filing sequence using the sorters. Sorted cards are then processed using the tabulators to obtain either book catalogues or card catalogues.

Computer Based Systems

MARC Project

The introduction of computers in the late 1950s accelerated the use of automated techniques in the Library of Congress (LC). The appointment of King Committee to survey the Mechanization in Information Retrieval (IR) in 1958 can be regarded as a corner-stone in the progress towards automation at the LC. The final report of this survey funded by the Council for Library Resources (CLR) was published in 1963. This report envisaged the possibility of automating the entire bibliographic system of the LC within ten years. Encouraged by this report the CLR awarded a contract to LC for converting its catalogue to a machine readable form for the purpose of printing bibliographical products by computers. For this LC acquired two big computers, an IBM 1401 with four tape units and an IBM 1403 in 1963. This study was reported at a conference held in LC in January 1965. In December 1965, LC received a further graant from CLR for the development of a pilot operation to test the feasibility and utility of the distribution of machine readable catalogue data to user libraries. This project was called `MARC'.

COMPUTERS IN INDIA

Contribution of ancient India to computer technology

Aryabhatta, the ancient Indian mathematician, had no computer but some of the techniques which he developed are precisely the ones used in solving problems with today's computers.

There is an amazing similarity in the codes of artificial intelligence machines and the way the ancient grammarians of India paraphrased the Sanskrit language.

According to Subash Kak, Professor Electrical and Computer Engineering in the Lousians State University in the United States, computer designers in the west are now studying the works of Indian mathematicians to get a tip or two about writing software.

Aryabhatta's `Algorithm' called Kuttaka, meant to solve linear intermediate equations, was found to be "extremely efficient computationally", Kak said.

Similarly, the method of Brahmagupta, Jayadeva and Bhaskara II- which was rediscovered in Europe 1000 years later - was ``optimum in minimising the number of steps' for solving a problem.

Kak mentioned that a comprehensive analysis of the contributions of Indian grammarians had recently been made by an American computer engineer, Dr Rick Briggs.

In a paper published in the 1985 issue of Artificial Intelligence, Dr. Briggs said that ancient Indians developed a method for paraphrasing Sanskrit ``in a manner that is identical not only in essence but also in form with current work of artificial intelligence."

According to Dr. Briggs, ``Sanskrit grammarians have already found a way of solving what is perhaps the most important problem in computer science natural language understanding and machine translation."

Growth

The first computer system to come to India was the HEC-II computer brought by the Indian Statistical Institute in 1956. Esso was the first firm in India to use a computer for commercial purposes. This was in the year 1961.

Computers started appearing in a big way on the Indian scence in the mid-1960s. The Indian Institute of Technology, Kanpur and the Tata Institute of Fundamental Research, Bombay established computer centres in 1963-64. By 1970 there were about 120 computers installed in about 106 organizations scattered in 24 towns all over India. The number had gone upto 300 by 1975; and to over 600 by 1980. In 1982 alone, it was estimated, about 750 computers were to be installed in India.

COMMUNICATION TECHNOLOGY IN INDIA

``In ancient times those who controlled the roads and caravan routes held the power. In the fifteenth through the nineteenth centuries, control of the seas was a basis for power. In the twenty-first century whoever control the international electronic networks will surely wield the power." says Williams. Such is the potentiality of communication technology.

The New Era of Satellite Communication

1965 heralded a new era in communication with the orbitting of Early Bird telecommunication satellite by the United States. India started taking advantage of INTELSAT on completion of the ground station in 1974 at Pune.

By 1980 India had 24,77,000 telephone and 7600 telephone exchanges. There were 3,20,000 km wire lines, and 18,000 under-ground co-axial cables. Rs 60 crore were allocated to telecommunications in the First Five-Year Plan. In the Sixth Five-Year Plan, it was increased to 3000 crores.

Satellite Communication in India

India has developed sufficient technological capabilities to plan, design, build and test satellites for scientific experiments. Table lists India's achievements in this field.

Table 1. Growth in Telecommunication Service

S.N.	Facility	Unit	Position on 1-4-1948	Position on 1-4-1980	No. of times growth since 1-4-1948 (b/a)
1.	Telephone Exchanges	Number	321	7430	23.15
2.	Local Exch. Capacity	Lakhs lines	1.00	23.26	23.36
3.	Working connection (DELS)	-do-	0.82	20.14	24.56
4.	Telephone sets	Lakhs	1.68	26.15	15.57
5.	L.D. PCO	Number	338	13830	40.92
6.	Manual Trunk Boards	-do-	250	7106	28.42
7.	Trunk Automatic Exch.	-do-	Nil	18	infinite
8.	TAX Capacity	-do-	Nil	40300	-do-
9.	STD routes (pt to pt)	-do-	Nil	137	-do-
10.	L.D. Speech channels	-d0-	1426	59741	140.21
11.	Co-axial Cable system	Route km.	Nil	16641	infinite
12.	M/Wave system	-do-	Nil	16545	-do-
13.	Public Telegraph offices	Number	3324	24457	7.36
14.	Telex Exchange	-do-	Nil	136	infinite
15.	Telex Capacity	-do-	Nil	22015	-do-
16.	Telex subscribers connections	-do-	Nil	17983	-do-
17.	Voice Frequency Telegraph channels	-do-	450	17777	39.50
18.	Teleprints	-do-	615	36982	60.13

Source : Vijay Naval Patil, `Telecommunication Services in India : A Review and Perspective', *Yojana,* vol. 25, no. 11, June 1981, p. 12.

Table 2. Indian Satellite Series

S.No.	Project	Launched in	Objectives
1.	Aryabhatta	1975	Scientific experiments
2.	Bhaskara I	1979	Earth observations
3.	Rohini I	1980	Studies in stellite technology
4.	Bhaskar II	1981(from Soviet Cosmodrome)	Earth observations
5.	Apple	1981	India's first experimental communication satellite
6.	INSAT-1A	1982 (from USA)	Multipurpose satellite (Telecommunications, TV, Meterology)
7.	INSAT-1B	1983	-do-

India has made substantial progress in launching technology also. The first experimental Satellite Launch Vehicle SLV-3 (E)-01 was launched in 1979. The SLV-3 (E)-02 was fired into space successfully in 1980. A more advanced version of SLV-3 called ASLV (Augmented Satellite Launch Vehicle) which can launch a satellite of 150 kg has been designed and review has been completed. India has achieved success in launching a 600 kg class satellite with PSLV (Polar Satellite Launch Vehicle).

The INSAT Scheme

The INSAT-1 (Indian National Satellite-1) system is a multipurpose operational geostationary satellite system combining mainly three major subsystems, namely telecommunications, nationwide TW broadcasting, and meterological capacity. Unfortunately, the INSAT-1A system launched in 1982 had a premature end. However, INSAT-1B launched in 1983 is a success and it is being fully exploited for all the three major functions that are envisaged. The P & T Department has established thirty one earth stations for providing nationwide network.

INFORMATION SYSTEMS AND NETWORKS

International Information Systems

There has been rapid development of information systems and programs. Most of these are international in many respects. Those which are international in scope and coverage of materials were called international systems earlier. An information system or a bibliographical project is now international in many more respects. In fact, the national or international or universal has changed. In any system, now, there is a considerable amount of decentralization of efforts and activities. The input data created at different national focal points are merged and processed at the international centre and the processed data are sent back to national focal points for providing services to their immediate users.

Redesigning of National Services

National input ensures for each participating country, the receipt of a complete data base generated by the international agency. The usefulness of such a data base depends on the national services that can be planned and provided from them. The two most important services that are usually thought of in this context are SDI and bibliographical services - both on demand and in anticipation.

PARTICIPATION IN INTERNATIONAL SYSTEMS

Bhabha Atomic Research Centre

International Nuclear Informtion System Data Base : The International Nuclear Information System (INIS) is a computer based information system providing bibliographic description and abstracts of documents published in the field of nuclear science and technology. It is sponsored by International Atomic Energy Agency (IAEA), Vienna and started functioning in April 1970. The INIS Atomindex was started in May 1970. This is a semi-monthly and it covers the world's output in nuclear science and technology literature. As a by-product of this indexing and abstracting service, the magnetic tapes containing the INIS Atomindex are made available to the participating member states. These tapes containing machine readable files constitute the INIS data base. The INIS system is an example of an international data base with decentralized input and centralized output.

The Library and Information Services (L & IS) of the BARC, Bombay is the national input centre for INIS and receives the INIS output on magnetic tapes. The tapes are received by airmail every month and each tape contains two Atomindex issues. The INIS output tapes are half an inch in width and available as seven tracks with a density of 556 cpi or nine track with densities 800, 1600, or 2400 cpi. The INIS data base can be used for

A. Literature search,

B. SDI, and

C. Compilation of bibliographies.

The INIS-IRMS (Information Retrieval Management System) software package can be used for providing various information services. The processing of INIS data base at the L & IS, BARC was planned in two stages :

A. Providing SDI service.

B. Providing retrospective literature search.

SDI Service : The user is requested to give his subject interest in narrative form, underlining the terms which he thinks are important. The concepts are then identified and indexed using the INIS theasures. Using the index term-descriptors, a query is prepared. The set of cards punched accordingly is the user profile. This is run against the inverted file of descriptors using a computer program to find the document numbers which answers the final query positively. The extracted documents are sorted in ascending order using the fixed record length file, the bibliographic details of the documents in suitable format are printed. The abstracts are also included. The query cards and the number of documents retrieved are also printed. The user is requested to give a feedback on the print-out supplied to him. The user profile is updated on the basis of the feedback.

The retrospective search service could not be taken up immediately because of the additional storage capacity required and different set of computer programs needed for file updating and maintenance.

Indian Council of Agricultural Research

AGRIS Programme : The Sixteenth Congress of FAO held in November 1971 adopted a resolution endorsing the

AGRIS Programme and asked the Director General of FAO to pursue the system with all the means he had at his disposal and sought dditionl contribution from interested governments and organizations for the implementation. Thus, in August 1973, the first issue of AGRINDEX was brought out on a cooperative baasis. AGRIS is a computer based decentralized system with FAO as coordinating centre responsible for receiving, integrating, and processing bibliographic data submitted by national and regional centres all over the world.

In July 1974, the Government of India formally decided to participate in AGRIS Programme on a national basis through a national input centre under the Indian Council of Agricultural Research (ICAR). After an initial experimental carried out in November 1974, the Agricultural Research Information Centre (ARIC) began sending bibliographic data on AGRIS input sheets on a regular basis from May 1975 to the AGRIS data base at Vienna.

INS DOC

SDI Service

CHEM/SDI information retrieval system was started in January 1976 with Chemical Abstracts Condensates (CAC) and the CAN/SDI software by INSDOC, New Delhi, at IIT, Madras, with the support of Unesco. The DST provided additional financial support under the NISSAT programme. Presently it is being run by the INSDOC's Regional Centre of Madras using the IBM 370/155 computer facility at IIT Madras. The INSPEC and COMPNEDEX data bases were also added later.

On-line Service

RECON On-line Demonstration : For the first time in Asia, an on-line interactive computer demonstration of the ESRIN/RECON data base system at Frascati, Italy was arranged at the Tata Institute of Fundamental Research (TIFR), Bombay from 20 to 25 September 1976. The satellite communiction segment between Bombay and Rome was used for on-line linkage. It was done with the financial support of Unesco. About 700 scientists, engineers and others participated in this demonstration. The users could communicate with the data base being searched by using an interactive terminal.

NIC

Information System for Planning : The National Informatics Centre (NIC) under the Electronics Commission is responsible for establishment and development of computerized information system for planning. To achieve this NIC has built an intra-city computer network (NICNET) in Delhi by connecting six minicomputer terminals to the host Cyber-170 computer system using leased telephone lines and radio (VHF) frequencies. It has also planned to establish four data bases initially in the fields of A. Agriculture; B. Financial information; C. Manpower information; and D. Industry and technology. It has been planned to provide 60 interactive terminals in the various central and states government departments and ministries for on-line access. These Management Information Systems will be helpful for planning and policy making.

Data Communication

APPLE Experiment : APPLE (Ariane Passenger Payload Experiment), India's first experimental communication satellite was orbitted in 1981. It has a three-axis stabilized platform, an apogee motor and a C-band communication system. The National Informatics Centre has successfully conducted the Delhi-Ahmedabad satellite data communication experiment using APPLE. Large earth stations erected at Delhi, Ahmedabad, and Madras were used for computer interconnect experiments through APPLE.

INDONET : The Computer Maintenance Corporation (CMC) has an ambitious project in the area of communication, INDONET, which envisages the establishment of a grid of computer centres with adequate intercommunication facilities and sophisticated hardware for advanced data processing. A design of message-switching system with store and forward facilities for teleprinters named AUTOMEX has been successfully completed. These systems are of great advantage for on-line information retrieval.

SITE Program : In 1975-76, the Indian Space Research Organization (ISRO) carried out a short-term Satellite Instructional Television Experiment (SITE) with the help of USA's ATS-6 satellite loaned to India for a period of one year to evaluate the feasibility of providing satellite television to selected rural areas in the country. This was one of the largest satellite based mass communication projects ever undertaken. Direct reception TV sets were provided to 2400 villages spread over six states. SITE was designed as a total communication systems experiment involving the hardware delivery system consisting of the satellite, earth stations, studios, ground receivers and various links as well as the concomitant software system consisting of formative research, program production, evaluation and feedback.

Satellite Telecommunictions Experiment Project: The Satellite Telecommunications Experiment Project (STEP) was large-scale demonstration experiment conducted in 1977-79 using the Franco-German Satellite SYMPHONIE. The aim of this experiment was to gain experience in the field of domestic satellite telecommunication. Under the project, experiments in digital satellite communications, radio networking and television transmission were carried out.

PROGRAMMES

UNISIST

The idea of establishing a world system of scientific information which later became UNISIST originated in

India. At the Eleventh General Conference of the International Council of Scientific Unions (ICSU) held in Bombay in January 1966, a proposal was adopted to create a committee to examine the feasibility of a world scientific information system based upon achieving compatibility among existing and prospective programmes related to the storage and retrieval of science information. By then Unesco was also considering proposals for convening an internati-onal conference on the transfer of scientific and technolog-ical information. Realizing the need for cooperation for achieving the best results, the two organizations came together and created a UNESCO/ICSU Central Committee in January 1967 to carry out a feasibility study for a world science information system. After a three-years study, the committee submitted its study report in October 1970. The result was the establishment of UNISIST.

India and UNISIST

India has been actively participating in some of the UNISIST programmes right from the beginning. She was a member of the Steering Committee of UNISIST. Neelameghan of DRTC, Bangalore was also Chairman of the UNISIST Advisory Committee. India had hosted the Second UNISIST Meeting of Experts on Regional Information Policy and Planning in South and Central Asia in New Delhi from 18th March to 20th March 1976. Following this, the Unesco Regional Seminar on Scientific, Technical and Industrial Information Services was organized by INSDOC, New Delhi from 22nd March to 23rd March 1976. The Seminar felt the need for a Regional Task Group for developing and monitoring of regional programmes in library and information science. A Seminar, ``Library and Information Science Manpower Development in the Asian Region' was organized by the DRTC in collaboration with Unesco from 9th to 12th November, 1976. Further a short course on Scientific Editing for editors from countries covered by UNESCO/

ROSTSCA was held in New Delhi from 8th to 16th November, 1976.

NISSAT

Realising the urgency for a strong national information system, India made an appeal to Unesco for a short-term mission of a consultant to advise the INSDOC in these matters. Accordingly, Unesco deputed Dr. Peter Lazar during March-April 1972, who, after a thorough study, recommended the establishment of a National Information System for Science and Technology (NISSAT) for India. The Panel Group on the Information Sector of the National Committee on Science and Technology (NCST) of the Government of India in its report, prepared in 1973, also recommended the estblishment of NISSAT under the Department of Science and Technology (DST) Plan for 1974-79. A sum of Rs. 150 million was proposed for this scheme during the plan period. As a result, the planning of NISSAT was started in 1975 and was completed and approved by the Planning Commission and the Ministry of Finance for implementation since July, 1977. Its activities have been suspended recently.

Table 3. NISSAT'S SECTORAL CENTRES

S.No.	Sectoral Centre	Institution	Info. System
1.	Leather Technology		National Information Centre for Leather and Allied Industries (NICLAI)
2.	Food Technology	Central Food Technological Research Institute (CFTRI), Mysore	National Information Centre for Food Science and Technology (FOSTIS)
3.	Machine Tool	Central Machine Tools Institute (CMTI), Bangalore	National Information Centre for Machine Tools and Allied Product (NICMAP)
4.	Drugs and Pharmaceuticals	Central Drugs Research Institute (CDRI), Lucknow	National Information Centre for Machine Tools and Allied Product (NICMAP)

5.	Textiles	Ahmedabad Textiles Industry Research Association (ATIRA), Ahmedabad	National Information Centre for Textiles and Allied Subject (NICTAS)
6.	Chemicals	National Chemical Laboratory (NCL), Pune	National Information Centre for Chemicals (NICHEM)
7.	Glass and Ceramics	Central Glass and Ceramics Res Instt (CGERI), Calcutta	National Information Centre for Advanced Ceramics (NICAS)
8.	Crystallography	Deptt of Crystallography and Biophysics, Univ. of Madras, Chennai	National Information Centre for Crystallography (NICRYS)
9.	Bibliometrics	INSDOC, Delhi	Nationl Centre for Bibliometrics (NCB)
10.	CD-ROM	National Aero- space Laboratory	National Information Centre for CD-ROM

DEVELOPMENTS IN 1980s

National Centre for Telematics

In the Doordarshan news telecasted on 16th April 1984, it was announced that the Government of India will shortly establish a National Centre for Telematics in New Delhi which was envisaged to initiate systems for data, facsimile, teletext, videotext, telemail transmission in the country.

INDITEXT

*`Inditext'* : The Delhi Doordarshan introduced the home information system in Delhi on an experimental basis from 14th November 1985. This service called `Inditext' (Indian teletext) is available from 6 a.m. till midnight. The equipment was installed successfully at Doordarshan by Electronics Corporation of India Ltd. (ECIL), a public sector undertaking. It has also designed, developed and installed 100 receiver sets in the capital. The software was provided by the National Informatics Centre (NIC).

Just at the press of a button on a small Keypad (the size of a hand calculator) called decades a viewer can command his TV set to project Inditext or the normal programme. And if he does not want to disturb the normal programme, the teletext could be superimposed.

Various categories of Information selected for transmission include index, news, financial news, sports news, TV Choice, TV tomorrow, whether information, airlines, railways, city engagements, cinemas, travel information, quiz, etc.

DOT (Department of Telecommunication)

Creation of MTNL and VSNL

In 1985, the administration of Rajiv Gandhi introduced the first significant institutional reform in the sector. Telecommunication services were separated from postal services, the DoT was created under the jurisdiction of the Ministry of Communications to provide telecom services, and the Telecom Board (now the Telecom Commission) was formed to develop policy for the sector. In 1986, further restructuring led to the creation of two new companies : Mahanagar Telephone Nigagm Ltd. (MTNL) and Videsh Sanchar Nigam Ltd. (VSNL). While VSNL took charge of DoT international operations, MTNL took over the Department local services in Bombay and New Delhi.

Currently services are provided by the DoT, MTNL and VSNL, but both MTNL and VSNL are under the institutional umbrella of the DoT. Policy is drafted through a complicated and some obscure process in which the Ministry of Communications, the Telecom Commission, and the DoT have say. Institutional boundaries and policy making responsibilities are not clearly carried among these institutions. Although the Telecom Commission has the upper hand on regulatory recommendations, the actual implementation of policies is usually the outcome of political margin that involves not only these three institutions but also the Prime Minister's office, the Ministry of Finance, and the Parliament. As in the most democracies, these institutions often disagree on policies, slowing down any reform initiatives but providing legitimacy to the legislation that is implemented.

To de-politicize the current regulatory process somewhat, the government has passed a law transferring all regulatory functions in the sector to an autonomous regulatory body, the Telecom Regulatory Authority of India. This new agency will be non-statutory body operting under the jurisdiction of the Ministry of Communications, but it will presumably have considerable power and independence to buffer political influences from the executive branch, Parliament and other interest groups. The Authority's main tasks will include regulating everyday service provision and carrier operations, mediating among carriers and between carriers and customers, and enforcing legislation. More specifically, it will address issues related to standards for technical compatibility of networks and applications, pricing mechanisms and regimes and interconnection-related matters such as revenue-sharing agreements, access charges and time frames for interconnection.

OPTICAL/LASER DISCS

Optical/Laser discs brought yet another revolution in information and communication technologies. The use of online retrieval of bibliographic databases has reduced drastically with the use of CDs.

CD-ROM

Laser discs are one of read-only, write-once, or erasable and also one of analogue or digital. Read-only optical or laser discs are expensive to produce and the data on the discs cannot be altered. These discs are suitable as a computer storage medium, specially when the information needs to be amended and updated. These are, however, suitable for electronic publication of documents and graphics. The read-only analogue version is useful for storing video images and can hold digital data by converting it to analogue data.

Write-Once-Discs

Write-Once-Discs or WORMs (Write-Once-Read-Many) otherwise known as DRAW (Direct-Read-After-Write) have drives with a higher power laser than read-only. These discs can store digital files from work processor, documents, engineering and computer aided design drawings.

Erasable Discs

These will enable to erase a record, add new information, modify an existing one or manipulate the information in a way one needs. These will offer a much larger storage capacity than magnetic discs.

INTERNET

History of the Internet

During 1969 the US Department of Defence, through their Advanced Research Project Agency (ARPA) created an experiment. This was a Packet Switched Network over telephone lines. Out of this initial network Advanced Research Project Agency Network (ARPANET) one of the early forerunners of Internet was born. During 1970s the ARPA developed a set of rules, called protocols, that helped in connecting different networking connected to ARPANET continued to grow over the years. In 1982 ARPANET joined with MILNET (The Military Network) and a few others and it is said that the internet was thus formed from this consolidation of networks. As per the information available, there are 2,20,00,00 users by 1995 on the internet, and every month 1,50,000 new users are joining it. It is estimated that by the end of the year 2009, there will be 20 crore users on the Internet.

Uses of Internet

The Internet today gives access to an overwhelming amount of information, data and electronic information services provided by its ordinary users. At one end of the spectrum, there are personal `home pages' published by people the world over (for name-searchable collection see *Ahoy : The Homepage Gateway).* At the other end is official government information, for example, that provided by the *open-gov.uk* website, which provides a first point of entry for all UK government and public sector information.

To give a few examples, the Internet can be used to :

- exchange personal messages with colleagues, friends or relatives at other networked sites,
- engage in group discussions, exchange information and ideas with people who share a common interest, and seek information from them,
- automatically receive information on world events, leisure interests, and technical, business and professional matters by subscribing to electronic journals, conferences, newsletters and alerting services,
- look up information in reference works, databases and libraries worldwide,
- retrieve journal articles, books, computer programs, and graphic images, and transfer them to a personal computer,
- make use of computer facilities that are not available locally,
- download new software or updtes for existing applications,
- browse catalogues of goods and services and make credit-card purchases,
- participate in distance learning and academic conferencing,

- engage in read-time `chat' and multiplayer interactive games,
- communicate with individuals or groups by means of voice only or voice and image, and
- publish information for access by other internet users.

WWW (=World Wide Web) : *Documents and Links*

The WWW began as an attempt link researchers at CERN, the European Laboratory for Particle Physics, in Geneva, Switzerland. Around the same time that the Gopher and WAIS software were being developed, a small group of dvelopers led by Tim. Bemers-Lee at CERN proposed a network-based hypertext system for use at the institute.

The web combines two ideas which alone are useful and together have proven to be extraordinarily powerful: networked information and hypertext. By the time of its development, a number of systems that provided users access to networked information were available, anonymous FTP servers being the earliest and most used. Gopher being extremely approachable and opening up the world of networked information to many new users, and WAIS introduced many users to a full-text search engine for a networked retrieval system.

However, none of these systems provided a method of linking one piece of information directly to another within the body of a document. Such links are called hyperlinks and are a distinguishing feature of hypertext. Indeed, hypertext can be defined simply as a system of links of nodes, where the nodes may be documents that contain such links.

The WWW is a set of protocols that (i) allow for the location of any document on the Net through a naming system based on Universal Resource Locators (URLs); (ii) describe a way of placing links using URLs within text documents, called Hypertext Markup Language (HTML);

and (iii) specify a way to request and send a document over the network, the Hypertext Transfer Protocol (HTTP). With these standard protocols in place, one can set up a server and construct the responsibility of making the users aware of their role in fair use of the electronic access to the journaals. Davis and Reilly (1998) believe that the licensing of electronic journals requires legal expertise and skills beyond the training and experience of most librarians.

ELECTRONIC JOURNALS - INDIAN SCENARIO

In India, many research libraries and some university libraries are already accessing the electronic counterpart of the printed journals, which they are subscribing to. Most of these journals have the online access free along with the print subscription. For the last two or three years, many publishers and vendors were experimenting with their different pricing strategies to the libraries in India. Some of them started the offer of online access to the electronic journals free on a trial basis, wherever the libraries were subscribing to their print versions. As a next step, a few publishers offered their electronic journals for a nominal fee in addition to the print journals. The publishers were trying to arrive at a price, suitable to the libraries, especially for those in the developing countries (Louis, *et al.,* 2001).

While the libraries in North America and Europe were accessing the online journals, the libraries in India were still struggling to set up the infrastructure required for online access to journals. As a result, there is a delay in acquiring the electronic journals and databases in Indian libraries. Additionally, our library budgets do not give the flexibility to buy the much-required high-tech format of the information. Librarians are in a fix, as to how to manage accessing information within their budget. In addition, they are also expected to bargain for accessing more information. This is precisely what libraries in other countries have managed by establishing some formal networks like consortia, which have the ability to bargain collectively with the commerical publishers. The same concept or the trend has spread to our country in recent times. More and more publishers have shown interest and willingness to have a dialog with librarians in India. They expect the librarians to have a formal commitment among themselves before they start bargaining with the publishers. In the absence of standardized formal consortia arrangements within the country, it is a difficult situation for Indian libraries to accept the existing procedure for consortia models in other countries.

CONSORTIA APPROACH

Consortia are nothing but cooperative effort, which manages all the library services collectively. It has the purpose of exploring the need for libraries to make the most effectiveness of their funds collectively. This partnership fosters pride, determination and a sense of ownership between its constituent libraries and staff. Consortia are regarded as an effective strategy to increase the buying power of individual libraries over the shor term and as an opportunity to maximize the efforts of cooperative collection building for resource sharing over the long term (Richer, 1999). It is essential to understand the definition of the term ``consortium" which is a powerful cooperative strategy.

The following definitions from the available sources are the derivation from the basic term of ``consortium".

A Consortium is said to be ``a cooperative arrangement among groups or institutions, or an association or society" (American Heritage Dictionary)

Consortia in India

Libraries are taking the consortia to which they belong a great deal more seriously, than was the case a few years back. They offer libraries the ability to give users the access they are coming to expect and demand to a much broader range of materials than any one library could possibly offer.

SOME OF THE INDIAN CONSORTIA

1. FORSA (forum for Resource Sharing in Astronomy).
2. INDEST (Indian Digital Library in Engineering Science and Technology).
3. IIM Consortium.
4. UGC's INFONET.
5. CSIR Consortium.

OPEN ACCESS JOURNALS

Due to rapid growth in ICT, there has been tremendous scope to publish articles in a new breed of media, i.e. Open Access Journals (OAJ). The basic criteria of OAJ is to be available freely on the Web to any one to read, download, to save and down load either on Institutional Archives or Central Archives with no barriers of any kind. There are journals with online access but majority of them are accessible only on subscription. It has been estimated that there are about 5% of scholarly publishing journals which follow open access model. It is to be noted that OA journals also follow all rigorous treatment of peer review as of non-OA journals.

Characteristics of open access journals

The characteristics of open access journals as identified by Suber, P (2005) are :

- OA journals conduct peer review;
- OA journals typically let authors retain copyright;
- OA journals levy fee from the authors or his employer;
- Some OA journal publishers are not-for-profit (e.g. PLoS) and some are for-profit (e.g. BioMed Central or BMC); and
- OA journals are economically viable and disseminate information at a faster rate;

Indian Digital Repositories

Following institutions hve developed institutional repositories in India :

1. Indian Institute of Astrophysics;
2. IIM, Kozhikode;
3. Indian Institute of Science (IISc), Bangalore;
4. Indian Statistical Institute (ISI), Bangalore;
5. INFLIBNET, Ahmedabad;
6. Information Centre for Aerospace Science and Technology (ICAST);
7. National Chemical Laboratory (NCL);
8. National Informatics Centre (NIC), Delhi;
9. National Institute of Oceanography (NIO);
10. National Institute of Technology, Rourkela;
11. One World South Asia (OWSA);
12. Raman Research Institute, Bangalore;
13. University of Delhi, etc.

NATIONAL KNOWLEDGE COMMISSION

NKC is composed of honorary member of eminence, scholarship, academic and professional achievements, scientists and technologists with expertise in management and persons of vast experience, under the chairmanship of Dr Sam Pitroda of International reputation. The names of the other members are : Dr. P M Bhargava (Vice-Chairman), Dr. Ashok Ganguly, Dr Jyaniti Ghosh, Dr. Deepak Nayyar, Dr. nandan Nilekani, Dr Andre Betille and Dr. Pratap Bhanu Mehta. Established on 13th June 2005, NKC had time frame of three years from 2nd October 2005 to 2nd October 2008 to achieve its objectives.

The organisation structure of NKC is given in Fig. 1.

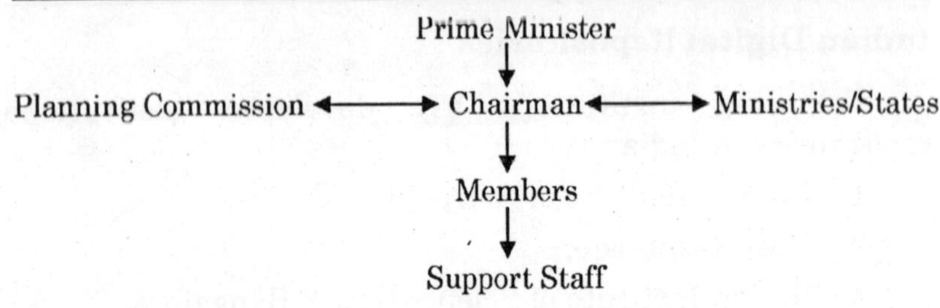

Fig. 1

NKC will be assisted by Technically Support Staff, Officers on Special Duty, a National Steering Group under the Chairmanship of PM. The group includes the Ministers of Human Resources Development, Agriculture, Commerce and Industry and Communication and Information Technology, State Minister of Science and Technology and the Deputy Chairman of the Planning Commission.

Three Advisers to assist NKC in their tasks are for Open and Distance Education, Public Information.

NKC Objectives

The overall task before NKC is to take steps that will give India the `Knowledge edge' in the coming decades, i.e. to ensure that our country becomes a leader in the creation, application and dissemination of knowledge.

- *Creation of new* knowledge principally depends on strengthening the education system, promoting domestic research and innovation in laboratories as well as at the grass roots level and tapping foreign sources of knowledge through more open trading regimes, foreign investment and technology, licensing;
- *Application of* knowledge will primarily target the sectors of health, agriculture, government and industry. This involves diverse priorities like using traditional knowledge in agriculture, encouraging innovation in industry and agriculture

and building a strong governance framework for public services;

- *Dissemination* of knowledge focuses on ensuring universal elementary education, especially for girls and other traditionally disadvantaged group, creating a culture of lifelong learning especially for skilled workers, taking steps to boost literacy levels, and using information and communication technology (ICT) to enhance standards in education and widely disseminate easily accessible knowledge that is useful to the public.

CONCLUSION

Libraries are one among the first to use computers for information handling. The first commercial computer UNIVAC -1 came into the market in 1951. Uniterm indexing system was developed in 1952 by using computers. The concept of post-coordinate system of indexing resulted with this invention. Appointment of King Committee by the Library of congress for mechanization in Information Retrieval in 1958 as a corner-stone in the progress towards automation in libraries in general and at the LC in particular. This committee envisaged the possibility of automating the entire bibliographic system of the LC. The concept of MARC was developed and improved by the LC which accelerated use of computers in library and information work.

The first computer system to come to India was the HEC-II computer bought by Indian Statistical Institute in 1956. Experiments in use of computers in information handling were started at TIFR, Bombay, INSDOC, Delhi, IIT, Kanpur etc.

1965 heralded a new era in communication with the orbiting of `Early Bird' telecommunication satellite by the US. India entered in the era of satellite communication in 1974 by using the services of INTELSAT. India Orbitted its first communication satellite in 1981 named `APPLE'.

With the use of satellite communication technology, scientific organisations started developing international information systems like INIS, AGRIS, etc, since 1974. These international databases were available online to users all around the globe. India is a participant in all these international information systems. By using these databases on tapes, Indian organisation started providing computerised SDI services since 1976.

RECON online demonstration made at TIFR, Bombay in 1976 encouraged may Indian scientific organisations to experiment and exploit online-retrievaal of information stored in for off places like USA, Italy, etc. But the prohibitive corps prevented them to fully exploit this technology.

Use of Optical/Laser discs for information started and retrieval revolutionised the concept of access to information. High costs of `online retrieval' took a back-seat.

Close to these developments internet and world wide Web brought information to the doors of almost each and every individual.

High costs of electronic journals still remains a problem. Efforts are being made to partially overcome these problems by `consortia approach'. UGC, CSIR, etc, are encouraging such efforts in India.

National knowledge Commission is going to provide a blue-print for making India a knowledge and leader among sister countries.

REFERENCES

1. Kumar, PSG. Computerization of Indian Libraries. New Delhi : BRPC, 1978.
2. Kumar, PSG. Fundamentals of information Science. Ed. 3. Delhi. Indraprastha, 2008.
3. Kumar, PSG. Information technology : Basics. New Delhi : BRPC, 2003.

Marketing of E-Resources in University Libraries(1)

M. Ishwara Bhat

Librarian, Birla Institute of Technology and Science,
Pilani 333 031 (Rajasthan)

ABSTRACT

In spite of advantages in terms of access and search capabilities, e-resources are underused in our libraries. Systematic marketing is to be done for their promotion of use. While a good ICT infrastructure is a prerequisite, it alone will not do. Proactive strategies are required and these need to be deployed imaginatively. Access to e-resources need to be made easier for both on campus and off campus users. Various methods have to be tried in order to grab the attention of the users towards the e-resources. User training will increase the confidence level of the users. Traditional awareness methods include : Personal visits, user training, brochures, posters and displays. Newer technologies from the Web 2.0 such as RSS alert services, Blogs, Wikis and Facebook make the interaction with the library not only interesting but also add more value.

1. USAGE OF E-RESOURCES IS NOT ENOUGH

Huge amount of money is spent on e-resources in our libraries and the trend continues. On the other hand, the number of titles coming in electronic format also has been increasing. As per a study commissioned by British Library, UK, it is estimated that by 2020, 40% of UK monographs will be available in exclusive electronic format while another 50% will be available in both print and digital[(2)]. British Library predicts a switch over from print to digital publishing by the year 2020, with 90 per cent of the British research monographs being published in electronic format by that date.

However, contrary to what many of us perceive, the use of e-resources in our libraries is much less than what we would like to see. The following two cases in my own institution illustrate the point.

In 2007-8, my university subscribed to an e-book resource having over 15000 high class text books at an annual subscription Rs 45 lakhs. The database was made available both to our on-campus and off campus students, totaling over 22000. In spite of having excellent infrastructure and internet connectivity all over the campus including staff residences and hostels, only 5385 users registered for this service. At the end of one year, we found that during the whole year, the total hours spent by all these users on this resource was only 8700 hours. Out of this, off campus students spent 7666 hours and on campus students spent 1034 hrs. Average time spent by each student reading the e-books in a year was just 1 hr 37 minutes.

Another example. In 2007, on specific requests by the faculty, we subscribed to seven high impact factor e-journals at the subscription cost US $ 11151. But at the end of the year, we were surprised to notice a total downloads of 1507 articles in the entire one year. One of these journals did not got even a single download!

According to a recent survey, 96% of Americans said that they had visited a library in person, but less than one third had visited their online library. Yet, increasing libraries are spending on online resources (Fagan, 2009).

As per the survey on `Perceptions of Libraries and Information Resources' undertaken by OCLC (www.oclc.org/reports/2005perceptions.htm. Acessed on 14.1.2009), which surveyed the information seeking behaviour of over 3300 respondents, only 16% of respondents had ever used free search engines like Google. The report concludes, `Majority of information seekers are not making much use of the array of information resources (online magazines, databases and reference assistaance, for example) which libraries make available to the communities'. The survey also showed that 39% of new information seekers learn about new electronic information sources through promotion or advertising as opposed to only 15% by message in the library sites. The librarian was ranked the lowest, at 8% as a source of information about e-resources.

According to another study called Pew Internet and American Life Project (www.pewinternet.org/pdfs/PIP College Report.pdf. Accessed on 14.1.2009), free search engines such as Google are the first choice of research for 80% of the respondents; the online library only for 6%. The study also showed that the information that costs money to obtain was cited by only one per cent of the respondents as a sign of reliability. 93% said that they do not trust information more if they pay for it. 90% of the respondents are satisfied with the most recent search for information using a search engine.

2. NEED TO INCREASE THE AWARENESS OF RESOURCES

One of the reasons for the slow uptake of e-resources is that its awareness among our users does not seem to be adequate as several studies indicate.

In a study of 143 faculty members in J D Institute of Engineering & Technology, Lohara, Maharashtra in 2007, 38% of faculty said that they were not using the e-journals because of lack of awareness (Labhasetwar, 2007)

In a study of 300 faculty members from IIT Delhi and IIT Kanpur in 2007, 35.66% of faculty expressed the lack of awareness of e-journals in the Institute (Nisha and Naushad Ali, 2007).

In an another study conducted in six universities of Karnataka state in which 845 research scholars participated, 37.86% of research scholars expressed the lack of awareness of e-journals (Gowda and Shivalingiah, 2007).

In one more study of 378 post graduates and research students in B A Marathwada University, Aurangabad, 29% of research scholars said that they were not familiar with the concept of e-journals (Golwal, Sonwane and Vaishnav, 2007).

Therefore, increasing the awareness of e-resources is one of the initial steps to enhance their use.

3. CHALLENGE OF INFORMATION DELUGE

What we witness now is the huge deluge of information on one hand and various communication media trying to grab the attention of the library users on the other. In this process, the user finds too little time to select information material which is reliable and is of good quality. In such a situation, the user tends to follow the ``Law of Least Effort'' nd takes recourse to ``Googling'' though this is not ideal. ``Googling'' provides brief information on any topic quickly and easily though it may not be comprehensive and of good quality.

The following paragraphs discuss some of the tried methods to promote the use of e-resources. Though the examples relate to university campuses, they are equally relevant to other situaations as well.

Wilson mentions that there are three aspects to successfully getting users to use the licensed e-resources : promoting them, making them easy to find on the library website, and providing seamless access to them (Wilson, 2004). We need to note that as of now, e-resources and print resources compliment each other. Also studies do indicate that users need both types of materials[3]. Therefore, the promotion of e-resources should not be done as an isolated activity. It has to be done in conjunction with the print resources under the overall promotion plan for library usage.

4. GOOD IT INFRASTRUCTURE IS A MUST

Good IT infrastructure in the campus is a basic prerequisite in our campuses and it transforms the information habit. Study by Moghaddham and Talawar (Moghaddham and Talawar, 2008) indicates that the free full text access from one's computer round the clock is considered a the most appealing feature by the scientists. On the other hand, various studies which probed into the reasons for not using the e-journals found out that lack of infrastructure, slow speed, lack of adequate computers, lack of printers, restrictions on the computer hours, etc constitute the major hindrance in the exploitation of e-resource in univeritie (Labhasetwar, 2007; Nisha and Naushad Ali, 2007; Gowda and Shivalingaiah, 2007; Golwal etc, 2007; Nigam and Sarmast, 2007).

5. ACCESS CONTROL

Access to e-resources within a campus has to be preferably through IP authentication since password hinders the usage. However, for those who wish to use the database outside the campus, password may be used. In this connection, ***Athens*** is a good innovation which provides a single user name and password to many online resources subscribed by the library. There are over 250 resources which are compatible with ***Athens*** (LEAHY). ***Athens*** is popular in UK universities though its user population is spreading to other countries as well. ***Athens*** provides the users access to the resources anywhere in the world. While the campus users access through IP authentication system without any identification, for those who wish to use the resources outside the campus, ***Athens*** goes a long way towards removing the barrier to use of the various logons and passwords.

6. GOOD LIBRARY WEBSITE

Library website is a shop window to the e-resources and it has enormous potential to attract people to the e-resources, yet it is very poorly used globally.

According to a survey conducted by OCLC in which over 3300 online information seekers participated, only one percent of them used library websites as a source to begin the information search(4). There are many guidelines for the development of library websites (Bhat, 2008). The following are some specific points which help in increasing the use of e-resources.

- Provide link to the library homepage from the university homepage
- Provide links to e-resources from the library homepage, prominently
- Provide both alphabetical and subject wise journal lists as well as vendor wise lists
- Provide telephone numbers and email addresses of library staff for any help
- Provide subject guides to online resources
- Provide facility to register online for training sessions

Since the library website showcases the library, it is important that it is promoted well so that we can ensure good traffic to it. Therefore, it is ideal if the link to the library website is given right from the homepage of the parent organization.

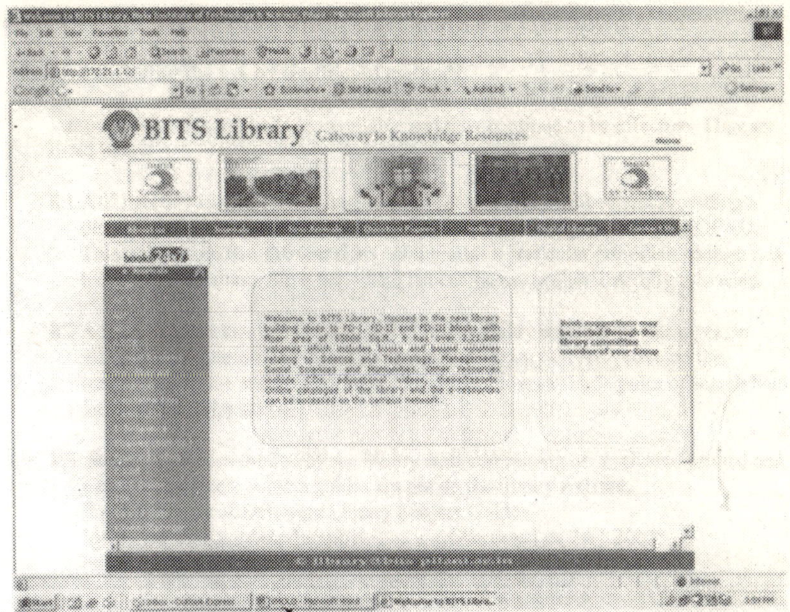

Fig. 1 : Library website wherein e-resources are prominently visible

Note : All e-resources are linked directly from library homepage in order to enhance their visibility.

7. INTERNAL MARKETING TO STAFF

Philip Kotler said, ``All employees in an organization are involved in the process of marketing and can either carry out or destroy the marketing"

It is essential that the library staff especially those who are in frontline are kept well aware of the various e-resources available and they need to know the strengths and limitations of every e-resources. Often when the user has an information problem, he/she may approach any library staff and not necessarily the librarian. Therefore, all profressional staff of the library be able to suggest alternative sources of information. Some ways of internal marketing to the library staff are :

(i) Run regular training sessions : Prepare a training package in order to cover all e-resources. These programs be run on regular intervals.

(ii) Encourage staff to experiment with online resources. Tell them that it is perfectly right to search online resources during their leisure time.

(iii) Involve staff in the selection and evaluation of online resources.

(iv) Encourage the staff to use the database for their own study and development.

(v) Involve maximum staff in vendor training sessions.

(vi) Create on online forum for staff to share ideas relating to e-resources.

8. PROMOTING THE USE BY TRADITIONAL METHODS

Various traditional methods are available and they continue to be effective. They are listed below :

8.1 A-Z lists of journals : Providing a list of e-journals subscribed and providing a direct link to the journals either from the library homepage or from the OPAC. This will ensure that the user does not miss out a particular periodical though it is hidden in a database. Such periodical list can be made alphabetically title wise.

8.2 Access e-books through library OPAC. Some library automation packages do allow the integration of e-books metadata with library OPAC provided the metadata is in the standard format. Integration allows a single point of search both for print and e-books.

8.3 Subject guides compiled by the library staff comprising of evaluated printed and e-resources. These subject guides are put on the library website.

E.g. University of Delaware Library Subject Guides

http://www2.lib.udel.edu/subj/(Accessed on 24.1.2009)

http://www.lib.polyu.edu.hk/ (Accessed on 25.1.2009)

Some libraries bring out course specific subject guides as given in the following website :

http://library.csusm.edu/guides.asp (Accessed 25.1.2009)

8.4 Banners, posters, brochures, bookmarks, emails etc : Use of printed brochures, flyers, posters, bookmarks etc should not be underestimated. Such flyers, brochures, bookmarks etc be made freely available in various service points in the library. Posters be pinned in library, hostels, faculties meeting places etc. Various e-journal publishers have brought out templates of banners, posters, brochures, bookmarks, e-mails and press releases which can be used for publicizing their e-books. These communication toolkits can be customized by putting your library logo, address etc.

Examples :

http://www.proquestk12.com/productinfo/marketingkits/ELKIT.shtml (Accessed on 25.1.2009)

http://www.oclc.org/netlibrary/marketingkit/ads.htm (Accessed on 25.1.2009)

http:// library.netlibrary.com/MarketingKits.aspx (Accessed on 25.1.2009)

Inflibnet Centre, Ahmedabad has designed good posters which are provided free to all participating institutions. Besides, they can be downloaded from :

http://www.inflibnet.ac.in/downloads/

(Accessed 26.1.2009)

These communication tools are excellent for awareness creation. Many vendors and publishers might come up with similar posters and brochures in order to promote the use of their own products.

8.5 Publicize in the physical library. For instance, put posters about online journals in the journals stack area. Similarly, display information about e-books in physical stack area. Amidst bookstacks of Science, one can display major online databases in the area of Science. Similarly, in case the library subscribes to online archives of newspapers, proper signs may be put up in the newspapers reading hall of the library.

8.6 Book dummies in the physical library. In case both printed and e-reference book are available, put a dummy book adjacent to the physical book. This will catch user's eyes. The publishers of the online ***Kompass*** provide a `big black box' to all subscribing libraries (Shepherd, 2006). The box mimics the well known printed ***Kompass Directory*** and it invites users to use the online ***Kompass***.

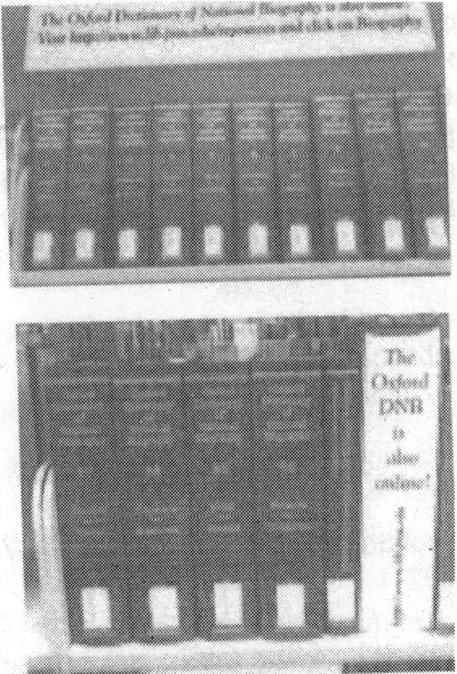

Fig. 2. Signages and book dummies in the physical reference section

8.7 Library newsletters (printed or electronic) can be used for providing general messages about library services, such as new databases added, training progrms, new facilities etc. Also information about databases may be provided on the library newsletters. However, it has to be noted that the newsletters are only passive means of promotion, similar to printed brochures which are waiting to be picked up.

8.8 Various in-house magazines are brought out by student bodies, academic associations etc. Write ups on subject specific online resources will attract the students and researchers.

8.9 Research reports culled out from the online databases may be distributed to key academic staff. This provides good publicity for the online resources. Similarly key reports may be mailed to senior academic discreetly.

8.10 Encourage users to review databases. Such particip-ation will encourage users who in due course, will become `Library Ambassadors'.

9. PERSONAL INTERACTION WITH USERS

Face to face interactions in the form of training programs, personal visits, launch events, user meets, library stalls etc make a good impact.

Study by Elsevier (Dewhurst, 2008) has found that the impact is always noticed more if there is a physical interaction between the user and the information marketing people (compared to communication through brochures, email or web etc). Realizing this, Elsevier has packaged the markting strategy with On Site Awareness Programs, Student Ambassador Program and User Training with local language trainers. Elsevier runs a very interesting program named Student Ambassador Program under which they train a few students in using their e-resources. These students in turn, train other students (Elsevier, 2005).

Importance of training programs has been emphasized by a study by Punjab University (Dhingra and Mahajan, 2007) wherein 48% of respondents mentioned that lack of training was an impediment for the effective use of e-resources.

Certain face to face interaction methods are given below:

9.1 Visits to departments. Visits to departments and laboratories are still needed in order to get noticed.

9.2 Subject specific training programs : These will be welcomed by the departments. Similarly, presentations might be offered to various Subject Associations such as Physics Association, Pharmacy Association etc.

9.3 Through events in the institution: Events in specific subjects may be used to promote e-resources in the related area. For instance, Engineers' Day may be used to promote the resource ***Engineering Village*** database. Therefore we need to have a good overview of what is happening around in the campus.

9.4 User Meets: Regular user meets or Open Houses may be used to publicize online resources.

9.5 Competitions : Interesting competitions may be organized involving intensive use of online resources. Vendors might be too happy to sponsor these competitions.

9.6 Launches: Launch events for specific e-resource may be organized and it will attract good publicity.

9.7 Library stall in Institute events: Library stalls in Institute events will create awareness for various e-resources available in the library.

9.8 Training sessions, Workshops relating to specific resource be run. Eg ***Use of Capitative Plus***. Similarly workshops relating to resources of particular subject. eg ***Use of Physics Databases*** will be welcomed by the concerned department.

9.9 Marketing of the databases by vendors: Many of the vendors offer training in order to promote their databases. Some databases such as ***Chemical Abstracts*** need intensive instruction by the trainers and vendor's help has to be availed in order to exploit all the features of the database.

10. PROMOTION THROUGH THE WEB/INTERANET

10.1 E-mails - global: Emails to all library users indicating new subscriptions, launch events, training programs will promote awareness. Emails are very proactive. Emails have to be short, specific news items, which could be read quickly. The periodicity could be preferably weekly or bi-weekly. More frequent ones are likely to be ignored by the user. Emails be sent only to the subscribers and there has to be facility for cancelling the subscription.

10.2 Targeted emails: This is preferable. The message has to be tailor made. Examples include contents of new e-books added with a link to the book's website by which the user would hopefully `hook' into investigating more deeply through the hyperlinks provided. This service is very effective, though time consuming.

10.3 Screen messages on computer terminals: Screen savers on computer terminals may be used to give powerful messages, announcements etc.

10.4 Online Information Tutorials: Online information tutorials on how to search information, evaluating and organizing information, citation, ethical and legal issues relating to electronic information tools etc will be useful. Some database producers such as Proquest, Lexis/Nexis, OvidSP, PubMed etc bring out Video tutorials which can be linked from the library site.

Example : New York Institute of Technology Library

http://iris.nyit.edu/library/video.htm
(Accessed 26.1.2009)

10.5 Table of contents : British Library in UK provides an electronic table of contents service named Zetoc covering 20000 e-journals and 16000 conference proceedings. This service is made available free for members of JISC sponsored Higher Education institutions of UK. Other institutions are encouraged to subscribe to this service[(5)].

10.6 RSS Feeds : Using RSS Feeds, one can get e-alerts from the favorite e-journals. Applications may include : Current awareness services to keep oneself up to date, RSS Feeds of new article references, news alerts from different subject databases. Other library related uses may include RSS Feeds of new book titles based on selected keywords, and subject related library events. Many e-resources provide RSS Feeds. Examples include IEEExplore, Lexis/Nexis, Proquest, Nature, Proceedings of New York Academy of Sciences, American Chemical Society Journals etc.

10.7 Wikis : Wikis can be useful to share documents. University of Huddersfield Library, UK has prepared a Wiki document providing information on the various electronic resources available in the library with ample hyperlinks.

http://library.hud.ac.uk/wiki/Main Page
(Accessed 25.1.2009)

10.8 Blogs: Blogs encourage interactivity between writer and audience by allowing readers to post comments and questions about the entries. These blogs can be on general topics or they can be subject specific. Libraries can use blogs in order to announce new e-resources, provide subject guides, announce library events, e-book reviews, etc. Blogs serve handy for students to chat with librarians and for librarians to notify about library products and services.

Example : Georgia State University Library

http://homer.gsu.edu/blogs/library/
(Accessed on 25.1.2009)

Indira Gandhi National Open University

http://libraryservicesignou.blogspot.com/
(Accessed on 25.1.2009)

10.9 Facebook : ***Facebook*** is a free access social networking site. Users can join the network to interact with other people. North Warwickshire and Hinckley College uses the ***Facebook*** for promoting the library services.

http://www.facebook.com/pages/North-Warwickshire-Hinckley-College-Library/46001030909 (Accessed 25.1.2009)

11. CONCLUSION

Marketing is a continuous activity in the library and every library staff needs to be trained in this activity. While good ICT infrastructure is a prerequisite for the effective use of e-resources, there has to be a well organized plan for the promotion of use. Various methods need to be explored in order to make the e-resources visible. Traditional methods such as launch events, personal visits and training work-shops need to be continued. Printed brochures, posters, newsletters do create awareness and provide the much needed publicity. E-mails and alert RSS alerts bring the information for the personal attention of the user. Newer methods by using Web 2.0 which include Blogs, Facebook, Wiki are interactive and they make the visits to library site interesting.

12. NOTES

1. This article is based on a paper presented at the International Caliber 2009 Convention on Automation of Libraries in Education and Research Institutes held at Pondicherry on 25-27 February 2009 organized by Inflibnet, Ahmedabad.
2. Source : Scholarly Communication available at : (Accessed on 21.1.2009)
3. In a recent survey of 719 faculty and 648 research scholars in six universities of Karnataka, 55% of the respondents stated that they wanted to see both print and electronic resources in the libraries. While 24% preferred the print version, 8% preferred the e-resources. (Ref.: Vishala, B.K. and Bhandi, M.K. E-

resources : new models for content delivery - preference to forms of journals by academicians of universities of Karnataka : a survey report. *E-content management : Challenges and strategies,* ed by Jagdish Arora *et al.* Ahmedabad, Inflibnet Centre, 2009, pp. 407)

4. Quoted from WILLIAMS, Lessley. Making `E' visible. Library Journal June 15 2006 Available at : http://www.libraryjournal.com/article/CA6341888.html (Accessed on 14.1.2009)

5. Source: http://zetoc.mimas.ac.uk/ (Accessed on 19.1.2009)

13. REFERENCES

Bhat, Ishwara. Designing efficient home pages for special libraries. In Shaping the future of special libraries, ed by S M Dhawan *et al.* New Delhi, Ane Books, 2008, p 420-435.

Dewhurst, Charlotte. How marketing can help increase the value of e-resource investments : five key findings. Library Connect Newsletter. 2008, 6 (1), pp. 1.

Dhingra, Navjyoti and Mahajan, Preeti. Use of electronic journals: A case study of Panjab University Library. In Proceedings of International Caliber 2007, Ahmedabad, Inflibnet, p. 744-755.

Elsevier. How libraries are training users on e-resources : Best practices. Library Connect. 2005, 6(1), p. 8.

Fagan. Jody Condit. Marketing the virtual library. Computers in libraries. 2009, 29 (1), pp. 49.

Golwal, Madan D, Sonwane, Shashank and Vaishnav, A.A. Use analysis of electronic journals. In. *Digital Media and Library Information Services,* Kolkata, IASLIC, 2007, p. 663-669.

Gowda, Vasappa and Shivalingaiah, D. Training needs of researchers in the changing information environment : a case study of university libraries in Karnataka. In. *Digital Media and Library Information Services,* Kolkata, IASLIC, 2007, p. 398-403.

Labhasetwar, Milind K. Use of electronic journals by the faculty members of JDIET Yavatmal. In. *Digital Media and Library Information Services,* Kolkata, IASLIC, 2007, p. 375-377.

Leahy, Phil. Athens access management system (Availabler at : http://72.14.235.132/search?q=cache:azi96BbBYKUJ: www. athensams.net/~/media/at hens/ppt/britishcouncil_ march03% 2520 ppt.ashx+Athens+access+management+ system&hl = en&ct = clnk&cd = 5) (Accessed on 22.1.2009)

Moghaddam, Golnessa Galyani and Talawar, V.G. Use of scholarly electronic journals at the Indian Institute of Science : a case study in India. Interlending and Document Supply. 2008, 36 (1), p. 15-29.

Nisha, Faizal and Naushad Ali, P.M. A comparative account of the use of paeriodicals in Indian Institute of Technology, Delhi and Indian Institute of Technology, Kanpur with special references to electronic journals. In. *Digital Media and Library Information Services,* Kolkata, IASLIC, 2007, p. 391-397.

Shepherd, Nancy. Putting it on the shelf. Gazette. 28 July - 10 August 2006, Available at : *www.media.xrefer.com* / x/about/ whitepapers/xrefer-rtlo.pdf (Accessed on 26.1.2009)

Wilson, Paula A. Take it to street. Netconnect, July 2004, p. 12-15 12.

Evaluation of Indian Software Packages for Librarians

C. Lal and K. Kumar***

* Agra College, Agra (Retd.)
** Librarian, Govt. College, Chharra, Aligarh (U.P.)

INTRODUCTION

This age is said to be a computer age, as computers are being used in each and every area of human life. Libraries are not exception of it. Use of computer in libraries is called computerization of libraries. Thus for computerization of any library, computer is an essential tool, which consists of various types of other components. To make these components workable, the computer machine needs instructions. These instructions to the computer are provided by the softwares, where software is a set of instructions to the computer. Through these set of instructions (i.e, softwares) the computer does various activities and operations of the liberaries. Softwares are written or developed to enable the computers to do desired activities and operations of the libraries. In this way, we may say that, besides computers, softwares are also very essential means for computerizing any library.

1. WHAT IS A SOFTWARE ?

As we know that hardware is the collection of physical components of a computer whereas software means the general purpose of hardware of a computer system is made to perform specific tasks. Software contains the complete and unambiguous description of each task, in terms of the available operations of a computer. In other words, software may be defined as a set of programmes for a computer. Each programme is a complete specification of the processing to be performed on supplied data, expressed in terms of the available operation of a computer.

2. TYPES OF SOFTWARE FOR LIBRARIES

The software can be broadly categorized into two types : (i) System Software (ii) Application Software. The System Softwares are otherwise known as operating systems which are set of programmes inbuilt in computers to run the computer whereas Application Softwares are used in the computer to perform specific applications. In the case of libraries application softwares are used to automate house keeping operations such as Acquisition, Technical processing, Circulation, Serial control etc. Today, quite a good number of library software packages are available for libraries for their house keeping operations and information storage and retrieval functions.

The softwares for libraries can also be categorized according to their functions which are as follows:

(a) Basic Software: Basic software packages are available for performing operations such as data entry and validation, sorting and mergining of files and editing data. A data entry and validation package allows the user to define a format to be displayed on VDU of the computer. Sort package are designed to sort a specified file of records into order according to a particular field value or key. Editing packages are likely to contain commands to insert, delete, print and replace specific lines of text. Sophisticated packages offer full screen editing facilities and automatic input and output.

(b) Word Processing Software : In libraries word processing softwares are used in the preparation and updating of manuals, library guides and in the generation of some forms, compilation of lists, production of catalogue cards and so on. These are able to permit the uses to manipulate the text, as it is necessary in alignment of margins, in addition and deletion of paragraphs. They also provide search capabilities.

(c) Database Management Systems (DBMS) - These are essentially programming frameworks and can offer good storage and retrieval. They are mainly intended for programmers to interact with and thus may need a programmers in order to make them usable to libraries. This is specially applicable in case of network and hierarchical models of DBMS. In market, three types of DBMS are available to a micro-computer uses :

(i) File Management systems,

(ii) Relational DBMS,

(iii) Network and hierarchical DBMS.

(d) Text-retrieval Packages - Text-retrieval is defined as the storage and subsequent retrieval of records from a computer system. The records being essentially textual rather than numerical, tabular or graphical. An unique feature of this type of software packages is user interfaces, which allows a non-programmer to understand and use them directly without any difficulty. These are also very much useful in search and indexing functions.

(e) On-line Searching Retrieval System - Each major online system has its own software which supports its activities on a host computer, which now has began to offer private file facilities. Private file facilities are expensive since a telecommunication charge is imposed every time a host computer is used. The second category of these software systems enables more interaction with an external database and permit the development and editing of search profiles and search outputs locally.

(f) Library House Keeping Softwares - There is a variety of packages, which are specially designed to support library house keeping routines. Some of them are integrated packages covering many functions while others concentrate on specific functions of the libraries.

3. SOFTWARES FOR LIBRARIES

A single software will not serve all the purpose of a library, because in library different types of activities and operations are performed. Therefore, need to have bunch of softwares for performing different activities and operations of the library. For the purpose a large number of various types of foreign and Indian softwares are easily available these days in the market. For performing different activities and operations of the libraries, a list of following types of softwares is given :

- Operating Systems : Windows 95/98, NT, UNIX, DOS.
- Automation Systems : Libsys, Sanjay, Soul, Maitrayee, CDS/ISIS, etc.
- Word Processing : MS-Word, Word Perfect, Word Star etc.
- DBMS : Foxpro, D-Base
- Scanning software : Odyssey, Power look, Vistascan etc.

4. AVAILABLE LIBRARY SOFTWARES (INDIAN)

As our study is limited to Indian softwares, so we present here a list of such softwares, which are important and being used in Indian libraries. These softwares have been developed by professionals or computer experts for in-house use of library automation for specific functions and activities. Some agencies have also developed them on a commercial basis for general application in libraries. The list of Indian softwares is given below :

IMPORTANT INDIAN SOFTWARES FOR LIBRARIES

SN	Software's Name	Name of the Company
1.	LIBSYS	Libsys Corporation, New Delhi.
2.	LIBRA	Ivy Systems Limited, New Delhi.
3.	LIBRIS	Frontier Information Technology, Secundrabad.
4.	LIBMAN	Datapro Consultancy Service, Pune.
5.	LIBRARIAN	Soft & Computer Pvt. Limited, Pune.
6.	WILISYS	Wipro Computer Limited, Bangalore.
7.	MAITRAYEE	C.M.C. Limited, Calcutta.
8.	NIRMALS	Nirmal Institute, Trichirapalli.
9.	GRANTHALAYA	INSDOC, New Delhi.
10.	Golden LIBRA	I.V.I., Delhi
11.	TRISHNA	NISDUS, New Delhi.
12.	ILMS	DESIDOC, New Delhi.
13.	DELMS	DESIDOC, New Delhi.
14.	SANJAY	DESIDOC, New Delhi.
15.	SOUL	INFLIBNET, Ahmedabad.
16.	PALMS	Dr. R.C. Prasad :
17.	ODYSSEY	S.R.A. System Limited, Madras.
18.	BASIS PLUS	Information Dimensions Inc.
19.	LIBRATOR	C.M.C. Limited Calcutta.
20.	NILIS	Amita Consultancy Limited, Mumbai.
21.	TULIB	Tata Omisis Limited, Mumbai.
22.	DELSIS	Delhi Library Network, New Delhi.
23	DELDOS	Delhi Library Network, New Delhi.

5. EVALUATION OF SOME IMPORTANT LIBRARY SOFTWARES (INDIAN)

Different types of softwares are available which allow us to automate the activities of the library. Here we give brief account of some of the Indian library softwares, which are in use:

5.1 LIBSYS

Libsys is an integrated library management software, which was introduced by Libsys Corporations, New Delhi. It is a fully integrated multiuser library software designed to run on a wide spectrum of hardware/software platforms in client-server environment. This software runs on DOS, Windows, UNIX etc. platforms. It is very easy to operate and the library staff can begin to use it quickly without knowing much computer skills. It ensures high productivity because of minimal data entry requirements, maximum possible integration of functions and powerful search & query facilities.

Libsys software package covers almost all functions of a library. It has six modulus. They are Acquisition, Cataloguing, Serial and Circulation control, OPAC etc. The **acquision** module is meant for ordering of materials, receipt monitoring, invoice processing, etc. The **cataloguing** module provides facilities for various catalogues, indexes, bibliographies, CAS, SDI, import and export of bibliographic data etc. **Serial** modules controls the periodical subscription and keeps track of the scheduled arrival of serials. The **Circulation** module performs functions related to circulation, bindery record management, display of recent additions etc. Searching the bibliographic database is facilitated of **OPAC** module. This module allows to collect the information on recent additions to the collection; allows users to find the materials issued out to them and materials on reserve.

5.2 Sanjay

Sanjay is the library automation software, which is designed by DESIDOC with the support of NISSAT. It is augmented version of CDS/ISIS for catering to the needs of the libraries. It is an integrated package that enhances the capabilities of CDS/ISIS by interfacing Pascal programmes. This package performs the library management functions such as acquisition control, online catalogue management, circulation control etc. It has been organized into two modules namely User Module and Maintenance Module. The **user module** helps library staff to carryout the routine operations like circulation control, acquisition control, serial control and assist the users to have online access to the catalogue. The **maintenance module** restricts the access right to a limited set of users as authorized by the database administrator. It is also used to enter new data. Access to this module is restricted with PASSWORD. It has the provision to safeguard data against accidental loss. Some of the features of this package are as under :

- The package is capable of handling numerical operations like calculations of budgetary allocations and expenditure.
- It provides linking of two or more databases for a single application, like linking an acquisition system with the online catalogue and circulation system.
- The inserted files are updated automatically whenever a change is made in the database.
- It has a set of 70 pascal programmes and 25 special menus.
- Faster response time.
- New menus can be inserted in between the existing menus without affecting their functions.

5.3 SOUL

The SOUL (Software for University Libraries) is a windows based library management software designed and developed by INFLIBNET Centre, using client - server architecture, which adds extra advantages for example high storage capacity, multiple access to single database, various levels of security etc. to the software. This software was designed after a comprehensive study of different library related functions practised in university libraries. It is an user friendly software and is quite easy to work. The inbuilt network feature of the software allows multiple libraries of the universities to function together and access to distributed databases installed at various university libraries. Access to authority files on servers as well as selection box in various fields of records is one of the unique features of the software.

The SOUL software comprises of six modules namely Acquisition, Catalogue, Circulation, OPAC, Serial Control and Administration. The **Acquisition module** enables library staff to handle major functions concerned with acquisition of library materials, such as suggestion management, ordering, cancellation and reminders, receiving, payment including fund control, duplicate checking etc. **Catalogue module** is used for retrospective conversion of books, technical processing of books received from Acquisition section, printing a range of records for verification, searching by title and accession numbers, the authority files for publishers etc. The **circulation module** takes care of all possible functions dealt in a university library setup. Starting from membership management to maintenance of status of library items can be handled using this software. The circulation transaction viz. issue, return, renewal, reserve, recall and hold can be done successfully. Reminders for overdue, inter library loan have also been covered. The OPAC module is a window to the library collection. By using the user friendly menu, user can search for an item available in the library by author, title, corporate author, conference name, subject descriptor, class number etc. It also serves as a gateway for accessing internet, Union databases or any other external sources. The **serial control module** handles effectively the complex job of keeping control on serials. It handles functions such as suggestions, subscriptions, payment including fund control, check of user, issue arrivals, reminders generation, binding management, search status of every item, master database management report generation etc. The **Administration module** is used for creating new users and giving them right for accessing different modules of this software. In this way, we see that the SOUL as a software package is a total solution for library automation and management. It is available free of cost to university libraries in our country.

5.4 Palms

Palms i.e, Prasad Automated Library Management systems is a menu-driven, user friendly single and multi-user networking package, which runs under DOS environment. It was developed by a Scientist of Library and Documentation of G.B. Pant University, Nainital, and is distributed by M/s Nutan Software & Publishing Company, Almora (UP). The Package is very useful to automate both small and large libraries. It is useful to scientists as well as researchers in maintaining the references concerned with their field of research. The main features of this package include report generation, utilities and tools, automatic book number system, data production, data management, fast speed, querry facilities, information services, such as SDI, CAS and bibliographic services and the compatibility with other software packages etc.

5.5 Maitrayee

This software package has been developed by CMC (Computer Maintenance Corporation) Ltd. for Calcutta Library Network. It is designed to work in UNIX environment and uses TCP/IP for networking and supports MARC Communication format. It enables library computerization, resource sharing, standardization, connectivity and modularity. It provides facilities for all jobs relating to house keeping and information storage and retrieval functions. This software has following modules :

- Acquisition and accounting
- Cataloguing
- Circulation control
- Serial control
- SDI Service
- OPAC
- Budgetary control
- Periodic jobs
- Network service
- Central host service
- Keyword etc.

5.6 Nirmals

It is an integrated library management software which was developed by Nirmal Institute of Computer expertise Tiruchirapalli. It has the mechanism for data validation, integrity check and access security at every strategic point. This package has following functional modulus :

- Acquisition module
- Bibliographic control module
- Circulation control module
- Serial control module
- OPAC module
- Desktop information system module
- Union public access catalogue module.

5.7 Librator

This software is a comprehensive library management package developed by CMC Limited, Calcutta. It is designed according to the International Standards for data security and data management with the help of eminent library professionals and computers experts. It includes all operations of the libraries. It is fully automated and suited to both small as well as large libraries. It performs functions like acquisition, cataloguing, circulation, serial control, union catalogue, querries and reports, inter library loan, e-mail etc. It helps the librarians in entering networks for resource sharing. It supports UNIMARC.

5.8 Golden Libra

It is a library management software package which is developed by I.V.I., New Delhi. It runs on IBM PC/XT compatibles. It has been tested at the British Council and American libraries. It is provided with a stock module to give the status of the books at a given periodicity including the valuation of books. The functions of the software package are as under :

(i) Keeping track of subscription, storage and retrieval of book and periodicals.

(ii) Generating reports on various matters such as over due periodicals, list of books and magazines and reports to publishers and members for non-receipts of books and periodicals.

5.9 Odyssey

Odyssey is a comprehensive Document Image Management System and is based on client-server architecture. It was developed by SRA System Limited (Imagine Division), Madras, which provides easy methods for storage, sharing and retrieval of documents. It takes information from various sources such as scanner, faxes, computer created documents and other ASCII files. It was on advanced database engine to store, retrieve and provides multiple searching mechanism like Boolean operators, keywords, Wild cards etc. As it is developed with modular and open-ended design, therefore it can easily be integrated with other application software systems.

5.10 TLMS

TLMS i.e, Total Library Management Services is a library automation package, which was developed by OPAC infosys Pvt. Ltd. Pune. This software has some unique features such as Z39.50 standard client server, Internet and Intranet facility, provision for virtual library, virtual audio/video facility, SQL database, graphical representation of statistics, WEB OPAC, multimedia help, digital camera support, presence of Chat room, bulletin board etc. It has got the feature of auto cataloguing where one can enter the ISBN number in TLMS Web site and Web server returns the catalogue information. The Web OPAC allows the user to search the library catalogue through Internet. The article scan facility allows to scan the article and catalogue it and make available image through the OPAC. In short, TLMS provides many facilities, which are not available in other Indian library automation softwares.

5.11 Librarian

Librarian is a library management software package developed by Soft-Aid Co. Pune, with the help of computer professionals, in consultation with experienced library professionals. This software can be operated under LAN and can accommodate data of 10,000 members and 1,50,000 books. It has the capacity of handling 5,000 transactions per day. This package can be used in receipt and issue of books, in search by author and title as the books, list of overdue books and in tracing the borrower names etc.

5.12 Libris

Libris is a comprehensive, user friendly and menu-driven library software package. It was developed by Frontier Information Technologies Pvt. Ltd., Secunderabad. The software package covers all the functional activities such as acquisition, cataloguing, circulation, serial control, enquiries and library administration.

5.13 Libman

This software package was developed by Datapro Consultancy Services, Pune. It is designed specially for small and medium libraries. It is a menu-driven package and can be used under MS-DOS environment. It provides the facilities of creation of databases of books, members, issue and return, inter library loan, generation of overdue lists, computerization of figures etc. It has some features also such as facilities of automatic retrieval data files, double level access etc.

5.14 Libra

This is a multiserver, multi-lingual, user friendly package, which is developed by IVY Systems Limited, New Delhi. This package facilitates house keeping operations such as acquisition, circulation control, cataloguing and online retrieval.

5.15 Granthalaya

This software package is developed by INSDOC, New Delhi. It is based on MS-DOS environment but is now available in UNIX and LAN versions also. It is a flexible package to suit any type of library.

5.16 Trishna

It is one of the versions of CDS/ISIS software package which was developed by NISTADS, New Delhi. It supports data creation, storage and retrieval in Indian Languages.

6. SOFTWARE DEVELOPMENT

The discussion made above reveals that quite a number of Indian library software packages are available to librarians, but each of these softwares has its own merits and demerits. Hence it is the duty of the librarian to assess the positive and negative aspects of the software package and select an appropriate one which is suitable for his library. Now the question is arised whether a librarian himself should go for a library package or go for purchase of a commercially available package in the market. The software developed by himself (by librarian) and that available from market have their own merits and demerits.

(a) Self Developed Software Package - Self development of the software for library functions is a very difficult task. There are many problems which a librarian has to face before and after the development of a software and it is because of the complexity of the information procedures in the libraries. It is easier to develop the same for other functions like accounts and inventory control but very difficult for library operations. The software developed by the librarian, are not usually developed scientifically and tested by time in its use. But of course, the cost is less in the development of such packages. Whereas in the case of commercially available packages, they are developed as a result of team research and tested by time and most of these packages have general application and are suitable for all types of libraries. But the cost is high in the case of commercially available packages. So in the light of experts opinion and experience, it is better to go for purchase of a commercially available package.

(b) Commercially available package - A large number of software packages are commercially available in the market these days, which meets of the requirements of the library. Now let us try to understand as to why we should use a commercial package. There are so many advantages of commercially available packages, which are as under :

(i) The development of a software package is very expensive which requires atleast 4 to 5 years of programming efforts. The investment cost for initial creation of the package is spread over many users and any one user pays only part of this total cost.

(ii) Since a package is to be sold it must be visible in the market place which requires that the package be well documented with, for example, user manuals, text data. Guidance on the setting up of system employing the software must be readily made available.

(iii) The supplier with a number of clients has sufficient maintenance income to justify the establishment of a sound service.

(iv) Packages which have widely been used, will be thoroughly tested, in several different environments, and thus any weakness or fault can be quickly identified and corrected.

(v) So many desirable features are incorporated into a commercial package, which has been refined after application in several organisations, but these features are not apparent to the new user. Such features include security PASSWORD, back up, restart and recovery programmes and integrity checkling and skills and voice level assistance.

(vi) Another important merit found by the use of a software package commercially available is the existence of a user group allowing the organisation to compare its experiences of using the package with others. This certainly provides valuable information, which can be utilized for developing improved strategies for using the package more efficiently and also for extending the use of the package to new areas.

All the above mentioned points certainly point out to the advantages involved in the use of a commercial software package. Thus we see that the advantages associated with use of a commercial software is packages. But while selecting commercially available software package, following general guidelines should be in mind.

(i) Locate and evaluate a knowledgeable dealer or sales person.

(ii) Thoroughly examine the documentation for the software you are considering.

(iii) Arrange for a demonstration of the software.

(iv) Prepare yourself before the demonstration.

(v) Put the programme through its spaces.

(vi) Evaluate the quality of the supports you can expect from the dealer or vender.

7. SELECTION OF SUITABLE SOFTWARE FOR LIBRARIES

A large number of various types of software packages are available these days in the market. Now the question before librarian is, which library software package should be purchased out of the large number of packages that are commercially available in the market. What are the criteria or check list to be considered in the selection of software package? Computerisation of a library requires a lot of money, manpower and materials. The computerised library system may affect positively or negatively the efficiency of a library because of the particular software package used by library. Hence an objective assessment or evaluation of the packages is required in the choice of a particular software for automation. Obviously, a number of factors have to be considered prior to the selection of the software package.

(a) Hardware - A library must select to purchase softwares symmetrical to already exist hardwares or that software should be selected for which the cost of the hardware is less. Hence, to give attention about the hardware of the computer is necessary.

(b) Cost - To give attention on the cost of the software is also very important, as each library has limited funds for buying software. It is also to be kept in mind that the cost, that is being paid for software would equally be useful or not. Because the full success of the library automation is mostly depends on the qualities of the used software, hence a good software decreases the cost of the working of the library.

(c) Operating system - The operating system is also a considerable point to be considered for suitable selection of the software package. Each operating system has its own qualities. Some of them are more convenient and some are not so. Therefore, keeping in mind the qualities of all operating systems, the software should be selected.

(d) Programming Language - While selecting a software, its programming language should also be kept in mind. A software has how many facilities, this depend on the language in which the software is written. All programming languages have their own qualities.

(e) Data Storage Technique and Search Response Time - When a user wants to get information about a document in a computerized library, how much time the computer will take in searching the document, depends on so many things such as size of the file arrangement, operating systems, hardware platforms etc. Data storing technique also pays role in determining the time taken in searching of the information. It has been felt that the speed of searching of the structure of inverted File is quicker than the structure for simple File.

(f) Library Services - Even the services provided by all the libraries are mostly similar but even then they differ at some instant. Some of the libraries provide specialized services. Hence, it is essential to observe the services, which are providing in he library to the users, whether they all are taken care in the software or not. It is necessary that all are combined in the software. It is not necessary that all of the services are available in all the softwares.

(g) Updateness - Updateness of the softwares is always necessary. For this the facility of changing the software according to requirement is also necessary. The experiences show that software developed by private agencies are more up-to-date.

(h) Easy in use - The library should opt such type of softwares, which are easy for use. The using guidelines should also be simple.

Thus we see that, in general, the selection of the suitable software in the libraries is a very difficult task, therefore, the libraries should be very careful in selecting a suitable software. In fact, the selection of a software should be considered with the following aspects :

- Objectivity of the library,
- Collection of the library,
- Services to be generated from the library,
- User friendly nature of the software,
- Cost, compatibility of the software,
- Authoritativeness of the firm; and
- After sales service support etc.

8. CONCLUSION

A software is a set of programmes, by which a computer performs various types of general as well as specific library operations. This article is intended to give a brief account of some of the important Indian Software packages only, which are largely being used in our libraries. The articles also provides certain guidelines and the criteria for the selection of suitable library software packages developed in our country only. Thus the matter contained in this article will help those who are going to use and select software packages for their libraries to computerize various library operations,.

REFERENCES

1. Lal, C. and Kumar, K. : Descriptive Questions in Library and Information Science. New Delhi; Ess Ess Publications, 2004.

2. Malwad, N.M. : Selection Criteria for Library Automation Software. DESIDOC Bulletin. 15 (2); 1995, p. 17-25.

3. Devarajan, G. : Information Technology in Libraries. New Delhi : Ess Ess Publications; 1994, p. 48-52.

4. Khan, M.T.M. : Information : Organisation and Communication. New Delhi : Ess Ess Publications; 1998, p. 248-254.

5. Basu, Karabi : Information Technology Management : Tools and Techniques (In IASLIC Proceedings : Special Publication No. 39). 1999, p. 125-127.

Information Management in DRDO Libraries

R.S. Rathore

Scientist, Defence Laboratory, Jodhpur

ABSTRACT

Information is emerging as a critical resource for users at all level : education, research and development, advancing the frontiers of knowledge and improving the quality of day to day life. Digital Libraries, employing a multitude of new technologies, are bringing about a revolutionary improvement in the way libraries and organisation deliver information. Digital medium has reduced space requirements of libraries and the direction of sharing of resources has surpassed all earlier effort in this direction. Digital Libraries networking is the best possible solution for cost effective utilisation of resources. The paper explains DRDO Rapid On Line Network Access (DRONA). This network provides easy access to data interchange and secure communication within the organisation. It also prevents the possibility of leakage of information. A firewell PC is used for protecting the network from illegal access. DRONA provides host of network services. DRDO Libraries/TICs (Technical Information Centres) are integral part of this dedicated network. Inspite of all technological developments, management is of paramount importance.

1. INTRODUCTION

Library is as old as man himself. Library is a place which collects, organises, provides and maintains documents for a particular type of users. Depending upon its function it may be called a Public Library, Academic Library or a Special Library. The function of a Public Library is mainly to meet the cultural and recreational needs of the society. Public is its users. The function of an Academic Library is mainly to meet the educational and research needs of teachers and students of an academic institution. In such libraries, service is based on demand and initiative of the user. In most of the cses the service is confined to the documents and not to the specific piece of information. The users are mostly self-helpers. There is hardly any information service or product offered by these libraries. Compared to a public or an academic library, a Special Library is unique in its functions, services and products. The collection of a special library includes all types of documents, depending upon the requirements of users. A special library is generally attached to research organisation, industrial institution or a government department. They are limited to subject coverage, and aroused only by specialised clientele, like chemists, doctors, engineers, scientists, managers etc. Besides performing such functions as collection, processing, storage, their main emphasis is on information retrieval and dissemination. They provide service to the user both in anticipation as well as on demand. They also conduct retrospective searches for the users. Bibliographies, current awareness, state-of-the-art reports and accession lists etc. are their main information products.

The digital revolution has altered our all walks of life and libraries are not exception to this. The last five decades have witnessed tremendous advances in information technology and its application. The latest technologies offer cheap computer processing power, cheap mass storage, inexpensive access to high speed networks and retrieval devices which give us the ability to create, manipulate, store and transfer large quantities of information in digital form at low costs. Electronic publishing and resource sharing activities have become very easy and convenient today. These changes have resulted into the evolution of libraries into digital libraries.

Library and information professionals have always responded to the opportunities and challenges of the developments in information technology with a high degree of enthusiasm and professionalism. The optical storage technology offered the CD-ROM and the library community was the first to find the best application which at once is economical and highly useful for its user community. The online database and the OPAC also are such examples that utilised the high-performance of computers.

2. INFORMATION MANAGEMENT

A library is a specific type of information system. Its activities can be classified into sub-systems like acquisition, processing, service and maintenance, and each activity can further be sub-divided in terms of tasks and procedures as various operation/functions. For example, acquisition can have specific procedures or operations like, initiation, authorization, activation, recording, reporting and cancellation as suggested by Thomas to complete a particular task. All the library sub-system components (i.e. acquisition, processing, service and maintenance) collectively perform the functions of obtaining, receiving, recording, arranging, disseminating and preserving of documents and information.

An Information Centre is a place which acquires, organises, analyses, synthesises, stores and disseminates information. Broadly speaking, there is not much difference between the functions and services of an information centre and a special library. However, according to Meltzer, a special library is an information centre, with the added function of analyzing and synthesising the information needed by users. In brief, an information centre is a special library with more concentration and emphasis on advanced information services through review and evaluation for the use of its clientele. On many occasions, it is also found that an information centre has a wider variety of non-standard information containing documents, such as in-house management information, company sales and production figures, engineering drawing, personnel data, etc. All DRDO libraries/Technical Information Centre (TIC) have such literature in their collection and coming under this category. Today, we have variety of information centres such as Discipline-Oriented Information Centres and Mission-Oriented Information Centres.

2.1 Management Approach to Library and Information systems

Every organisation has its some objectives or goals. It needs some system or tool which can utilise its resources (men, material and money) effectively to achieve these objectives. This system, which leads, guides and directs the organisation to achieve its pre-determined objectives is called Management.

It is not that earlier the ``Art of Management" was not there. In fact, it was there at all the times in different forms and in different organisations. The only difference is that this art, system, practice, experience or philosophy was not widely known to the public. This came to light very recently through various communication means when it crossed the barriers of people, organisation, languages and countries to which it was originally confined. Tody, these managerial functions and principles are universal and applied to all types of organisations depending upon situation or environment to provide effective results. Libraries and Information Centres are not exception to it. As shown in Figure given on next page, there is considerable parallelism of functions between a business enterprise system and an information system. Both have definite objective, both apply management functions in terms of planning and employment of man, material and money; both apply basic management principles and approaches to achieve the pre-determined objectives, and both interact with the consumers for evaluation, revision or setting of new objectives or goals for the organisation. The only basic difference is that in a business enterprise system the efficiency is measured in terms of ``profit or" monetary gains," whereas in library or an information system, the efficiency is measured in terms of ``service". So, in a business enterprise, the objectives or goals that are set, are ``profit oriented", wheres in library or information system the objectives or goals are ``service-oriented".

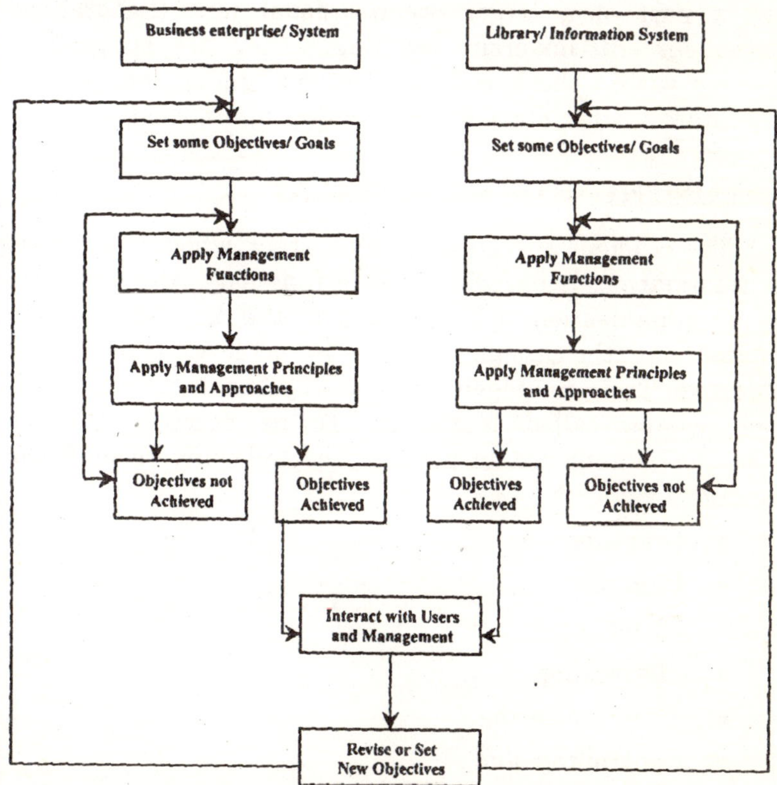

Fig. 1. Parallelism of functions between a Business Enterprise System and a Library/Information System.

There is lot of confusion over the terms Administration and Management. The functions of both are different, but interrelated. Administration concerns itself with such aspects as establishing primary objectives, formulation of strategies or long-range plans, laying down of specific major policies and procedures, and approval of necessary budgets and project; whereas, Management, basically carries out the plans and policies laid down by the Administration within the allocated budget to achieve the pre-determined objectives.

Normally, all librarians or informtion officers in their respective roles are managers rather than administrators. The reaason being that all libraries or information centres are a part of a larger organisational unit (Laboratory/ Establishment/University, etc.) and they are suppose to operate within the specified objectives, guidelines, policies procedures, rules, etc. laid down by the administration.

2.2 FUNCTIONS OF MANAGEMENT

The efficient operation of any system, whether business or information, is based on certain functions. At every level in an organisation, management is the key person who carries out the assigned tasks to achieve a particular objective. Thus, management of any system is done through key person, called Managers. To be successful, every manager is required to perform the following seven basic functions :

- Creating
- Planning
- Organising
- Motivating
- Communicating
- Controlling, and
- Decision-Making.

All above mentioned seven functions are equally important but decision-making is function of paramount importance in management. A good manager has to make effective decisions continuously at all stages of creating, planning, organising, motivating, communicating and controlling. Manager executes an action by decision-making. Delay in decision-making delays the achievement of planned objectives. Decision-making keeps the organisation dynamic and moving continuously forward towards the achievement of set golas.

The above mentioned functions of management play key role in modern library and information management. The information sources, budget and the information requirements of users cannot be managed effectively if they are not tackled with proper management functions. To be a successful librarian or an information manager, one should understand and practise the various management functions for efficient and effective working. It may be mentioned that these managerial functions are inter-related and during the course of action, they interact individually as well as simultaneously, as shwon in Figure -2.

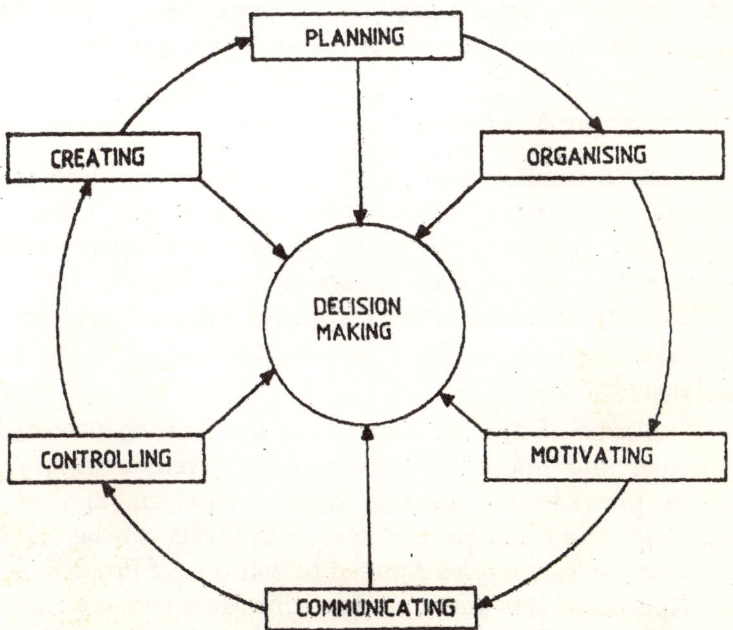

Fig. 2. Interaction of managerial functions

2.3 APPROACHES AND TRAITS OF MANAGEMENT

Like management functions and principles, the various approaches and traits of management also play important role in the efficient functioning of an organisation. The emergence of various approaches is linked with the size of the organisation itself. The size of an ambitious organisation is never static; it grows with time. With the growth of the size of the organisation, the managerial problems and their complexity also grow. Various management approaches have been developed by different people at different times to meet different situations, such as human relations approach, participative aapproach, operations research approach, systems apprloach, network analysis approach, management by objective (MBO) approach, organisation development approch and many others. Almost all the approaches are primarily based on scientific principles and human behaviour. Even now these management approach are practised in organisations in one form or the other. All above mentioned approaches can be grouped into two main approaches; the Systems Approach and the Behavioral Approach.

2.3.1 Systems Approach

Modern management is based on scientific methodologies and principles to provide efficient solutions to complex managerial problmes. It works on such principles as-first defining the problem, then analyzing it, and finally finding a solution to it in terms of work analysis, job analysis, service analysis, efficiency analysis, development analysis and cost analysis etc.

The area of System Analysis is the mother of systems approach and many other techniques. Systems Approach can be viewed as a part of System Analysis applied to problems. The other part of system analysis can be viewed as a Body of Techniques Applied to Solution of Problems. As an ``Approach" it is based on Scientific Management Theory; however, as a Body of Techniques", it is based on Mathematics, Operations Research and the use of Computer. Systems Approach is simple to follow for a library or any other library-like information system. A typical" Information System' model, is shown in Fig. 3. The system has four major components-Communication, Storage processing and Feedback. Each component can further be divided into small sub-systems.

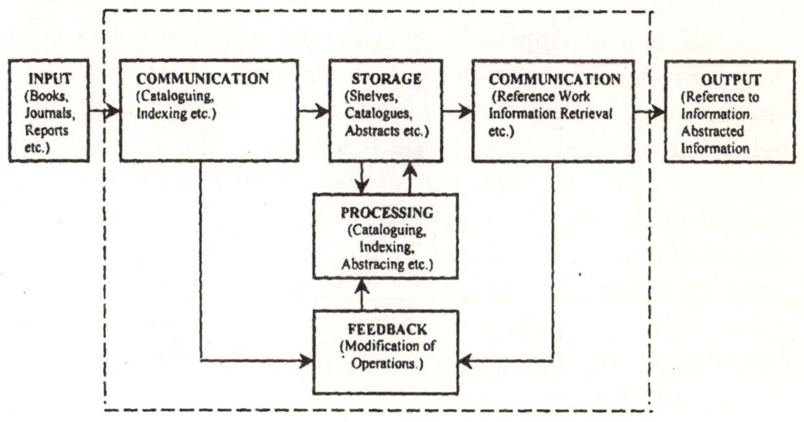

Fig. 3. Typical Information System Model

TYPICAL INFORMATION SYSTEM MODEL

The documentary information is communicated as an ``input" through catalogue or indexing to the storage unit, and the desired information is then again communication to the user as an ``output" after proper processing. According to Morton F. Meltzer, the Systems Approach to an ``Information system; involves five basic steps :

- Setting the goals, objective or plans of system to be achieved.
- Determining the problems that must be solved to achieve these golas.
- Listing the alternatives by which these problems may be solved and the goals may thus be achieved.

- Deciding which of the alternatives offers the optimum results.
- Implementing the plan with a ``feedback system' to make necessary adjustments, as goals and values change over a period of time.

2.3.2 BEHAVIORAL APPROACH

Behavioral Approach of the manager also plays a dominant role in achieving the planned objectives of an organisation. Behavioral approach is mainly based on behaviour of the manager and leadership. The term Leader and Manager are not the same, rather `Leadership' is having many important qualities of manager. Thus, a good manager may be a good leader but a good leader may not be good manager. More generally, leadership is defined as ``an inter-personal process of information, the thinking and activities of an individual or a group towards the achievement of desired goals."

The concept of leadership is described differently by different people in different terms based on the following main aspects :

- Leadership of Traits.
- Leadership of Activities.
- Leadership of Skills.
- Leadership of Styles of Behaviour.
- Leadership of Situation.

Depending on the above aspects, a manager can have a variety of Leadership.

2.33 Combined Approach : Systems-Behavioral Approach

Both, the System Approach and the Behavioral Approach, can be conveniently applied in combination to any Information System Management with little modification. In any Library-type infomation system, there are four major inter-related activities or functions which are normally carried out. These are :

- Planning and Development.
- Processing and Organisation.
- Service and Dissemination.
- Maintenance and Evaluation.

There are normally, five major Independent Components (5 Ms) in the design of an information system which interact closely and functionally to perform the above mentioned activities. These are :

- Mottoes (i.e. Goals or Objectives).
- Materials (i.e. Building, Facilities, Furniture, Equipment, Documents and Information).
- Manpower (i.e. Staff and Users of the System).
- Money (i.e. Budget for Build-up, Operation and Maintenance of the System).
- Moment (i.e. Time, Situation, Environment, Future, etc.).

To be more specific, these five major system components can be broken into ten distinct requirements or elements which are essential for an ideal information system. These are :

(a) Goals for the system, which form the existence of the system itself.

(b) Budget, which converts plans into cautions and actions into achievements.

(c) Functional Building, various facilities, proper organisation and dissemination of information.

(d) Facilities, Furniture and Equipments through which staff produces information services and products to the users.

(e) Manpower, which actually operates the system.

(f) Information Material, which forms the basis of an information system.

(g) Users' Information Requirements, which provides continuous feedback and dynamism to the system.

(h) Environment in terms of men, material, money supply, purpose, commitments under which the system is required to be operated.

(i) Time in terms of achievements of results, progress or meeting information requirements of the users. All activities must be time-bound.

(j) Future in terms of gains of the system. Growth and development of an information system is based on the present goals that are set keeping future in view.

All the elements and activities interact together for the achievement of desired result, goals or objective of the system. In this interaction, both system elements and behavioral elements are corrdination, controlled and directed by the management towards the accomplishment of pre-planned goals or results, as shown in Figure given below. Management keeps the whole Information System Co-ordinated, Controlledand unidirected from Initial Planning to Final Achievement and Evaluation of Results.

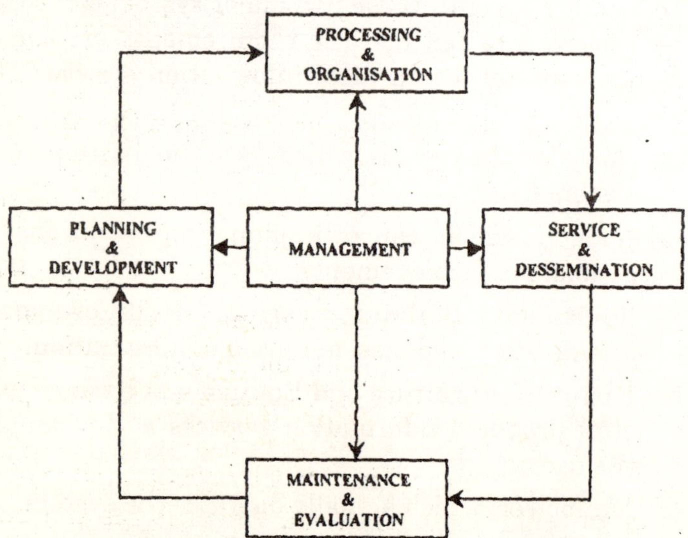

Fig. 4. Uni-Directional Information System

3. DRDO LIBRARIES AND THEIR ROLE IN R & D

Information is a vital resource for research and development. Scientists need information on the work being done or already done elsewhere to corroborate their work. Such information made available at the right time, in the right form would result in more efficient and fruitful R & D programmes. Realising this each of the DRDO Laboratories established a good Library/TIC. Some of the DRDO Laboratories Library are termed as Technical Information Centres (TIC) of the Laboratory.

Some Libraries have changed their name as Knowledge Centre. Today, Libraries/TICs of D R D O are the central information agency for collection, processing and dissemination of scientific and technical information of interest to the laboratory. The term library will be used for all these names as their prime function is library and information work. There are fifty one Laboratories and in each laboratory minimum one library exists. Each Library/TIC is in specific subject and all of these libraries are involved in information processing. These laboratories are spread around all the four corners of the country as given below

Information in the field of defence science is not available in abundance and accessibility to the sources of such information is also restricted. Yet, there is great demand for such information from the defence scientists. Of course, the information requirements of defence scientists vary with their roles. Research scientists or production engineers emphasize on specific information or data relevant to the projects allotted to them. The evaluating authority needs information on broader aspects of the project work. Top managers and policy makers require information covering a still wider spectrum of project work in the light of national and international developments. In order to ascertain these diversified requirements, it is necessary to build strong information system for defence scientists individually or group wise or labroatory wise. The information needs of different categories of defence scientists are discussed along with the role of library in catering to such needs.

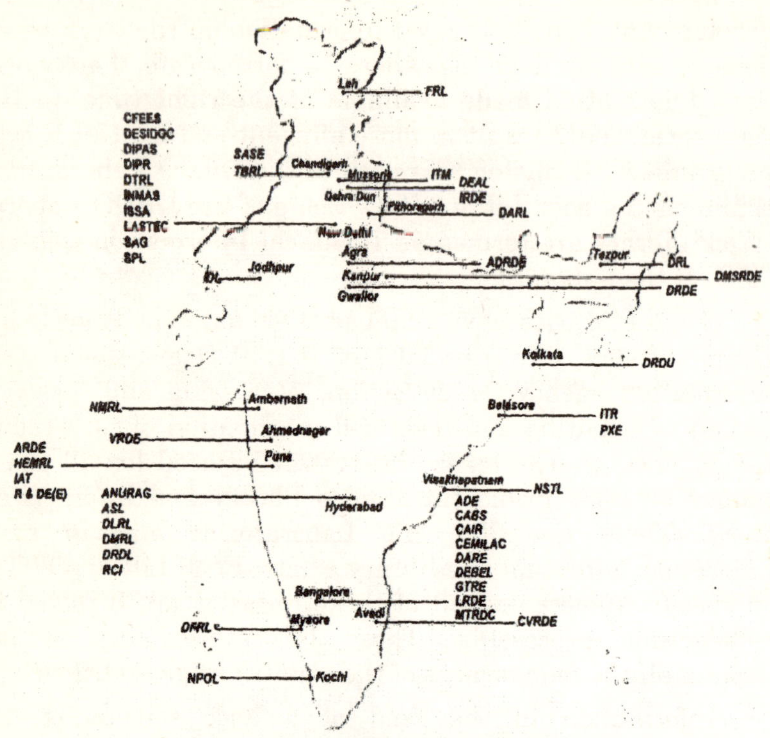

Fig. 5. DRDO Laboratories

3.1 Information Requirement of Defence Scientist

Science applied to defence is generally known as defence science. Defence science has grown to embrance an ever-widening area. It differs only in respect of its limited clientele and restricted accessibility. There is also difference in the working environment. Most of the research work in the defence is conducted under the veil of secrecy. In certain key areas, the information is not allowed to come out of the concerned department. The case of defence science is somewhat different from the other sciences even in the age of information explosion. In India, the defence science sector comprises the research laboratories/establishments under

DRDO, the public undertaking in the Ministry of Defence, the production units and some other subordinate institutions under the same Ministry. In some developed countries, it has been extended to the private sector.

The modern trend of dependence on science for fighting wars gave rise to class of scientists and technologists who can be termed as defence scientists. Their duty is to make defence system successful by solving the scientific and technological problems faced by the armed forces. Apart from solving the problems, defence scientists also keep watch over global developments in the field of defence science and bring them to the notice of the policy makers. All these operations require a powerful information system, capable of storing relevant information and disseminating it in proper form as per the requirements of the defence scientists. Defence scientists can be broadly grouped into three categories according to their functional roles :

(a) **Working Scientists** : Scientists of establishments belong to this category. They carry out the work required for the projects allotted to them. They are the ``workhouse" in the defence R & D. Numerically, they are superior to other categories.

(b) **Evaluating Authority**: The second category of scientists are working in technical directorates at the DRDO headquarters. They provide necessary guidance and review the progress of the sanctioned projects. They are responsible for transferring the successful project work to production units.

(c) **Top Manager** : Policy planners and decision makers constitute the third category. They coordinate the research work in the light of national and international developments.

The information requirements of defence scientists mainly depend on the role they play. Working scientists require information/data about the projects allotted to them. Scientists working at DRDO HQrs require information on broader spects of the project. They also require information about similar type of work conducted elsewhere in the country or abroad. Top managers also require project oriented information in brief along with information about the present and future needs of the armed forces in the light of national technological capability and international developments.

3.2 Phases of Projects

All defence scientists need information on project but in different forms. DRDO has a large number of laboratories engaged in scientific and technological researcdh for end products required for the armed forces. Defence scientists are engaged in these laboratories in various research projects. These projects are either user sponsored or suggested by the scientists from the laboratory group. Distinct steps of a complex project may be described as follows :

(A) Preliminary Project Formulation : In this phase, broad objectives are translated into preliminary practical alternatives. The end results of this exercise is a recommendation that feasibility studies be undertaken on one or more of the alternatives. For this pre-project study and formulation stage, the scientists require general infomation about the project. At this stage, they need review articles and state-of-the-art reports about the project. Any information of similar type of work conducted elsewhere will be helpful to the scientists.

(B) Feasibility Study and Report : At this stage, a bit detailed information is needed. If there are several methods of achieving the end, then all the alternatives have to be studied and the basis of selecting the proposed one should be given. Exhaustive information is necessary for better reporting.

(C) Detailed Project Report : The report contains in brief details about (i) the general description analyzing the environment to which the project belongs, (ii) project descriptions giving analysis of alternatives and detailed description of the accepted one, (iii) technological aspects covering technology/process to be used and availability of know-how, (iv) financial aspects stating the estimated cost including foreign exchange, (v) manpower requirement, and (vi) system plan. Detailed and extensive information covering all the aspects of the projects report is necessary at this stage.

(D) Progress of Project Work : After sanction of the project work is carried out as per PDC (Probable Date of Completion). The progress is reported periodically. At this stage, scientist requires specific information and data about the project.

(E) Final Stage : After completion of the project, the research product, equipment/store developed, undergoes user trials. After successful trials the design characteristics are finalised and this information is sent further for use in connection with production. Relatively less information is required at the final stage in comparison to the earlier stages.

The scientists rather generate certain amount of data at all these stages. These are to be verified with available similar data. The information supplied has to be very specific and correct. From the above, the following general observations can be made in respect of the information requirements of defence scientists :

(i) More information is required at the operational/ working level than at the planning stage.

(ii) The higher the hierarchical level, the greater is the requirement of information about national and international developments.

(iii) Some information may be required during several or all steps of the management cycle.

(iv) Information has time dimension. It becomes outdated rapidly and new information is required to take the place of the old.

(v) There is a precise need for better rather than more information.

Scientific and technological information holds the key to successful research work. The right type of information should be made available as and when required. But in practice there is always a gap between the available and the needed information. Prof. Finagle has aptly described the situation as :

"Information we have is not what we want
Information we want is not we need
Information we need is not available."

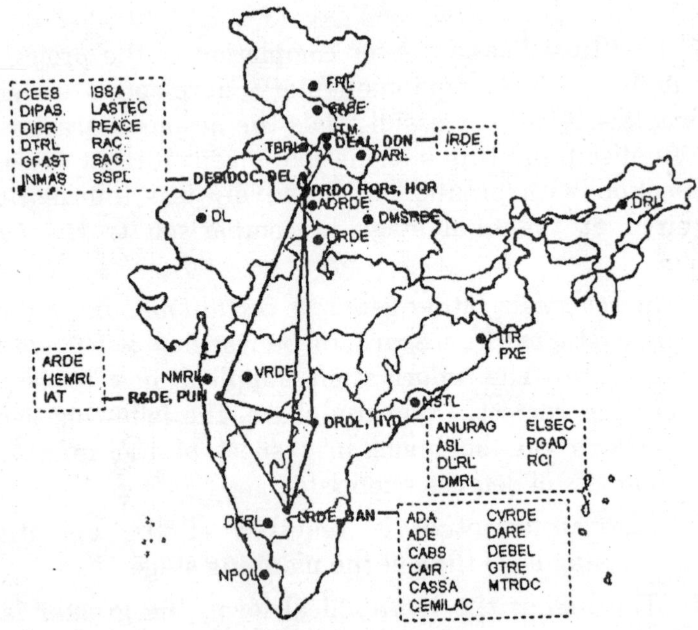

Fig. 6. Drona Network

4. DRDO NETWORKING

DRDO Laboratoriesare networking with dedicated network of DRDO which access is denied to outside world. This dedicated network of DRDO is DRONA. DRONA stands for DRDO's Rapid Online Network Access. It is intended to connect all laboratories of DRDO. These are about 54 laboratories connected to this network. These laboratories are geographically spread over 23 places in the country apart from the DRDO HQs at New Delhi. The data and resources available on this network will be accessible to geographically spread users. All the laboratories have set up their own LANs to enable their scientists to access the DRDO network. Figure given on pre page expresses the geographical topology of the DRONA Network.

4.1 Network Architecture

The Whole network is divided into Main Nodes and Sub Nodes. (A particular laboratory is designated as Main Node or Sub Node). There are about six Main Nodes to which other sub nodes are connected. The Sub Nodes which which are geographically nearer are connected to one Main Node. Each Main Node hosts CISCO 3640 Router and it is called Main Router centre (MRC). MRC forma the backbone of DRONA. Each sub router hosts a CISCO 1601 Router and it is called Sub Router Centre (SRC). The SRC caters to both intra-city and inter-city connections with the MRCs. Functionality of both these CISCO 3640 Routers and CISCO 1601 Routers are same. The difference lies in the number of ports they have. Routers are basically computers that sends your messages to their destinations along thousands of pathways.

Each Main Node has routers with more ports for connectivity, while the Sub Node cater to the requirement of a single laboratory. All MRCs are hosting WIN NT Server provided with Network Management System Software for monitoring the network. It is known as Network Management System (NMS). The NMS allows for monitoring and control of the traffic on the whole network. It logs all the transactions for later examination. It is possible to set or modify the access parameters of all the routers from NMS system itself. This facility is centralized enforcement of security on DRDO network.

4.2 Data Communication in DRONA

The communication is achieved through ISDN (Integrated Service Digital Network) Line provided by the DOT. Alternatively services like Dialups/INET/VSAT/ Microwaves are used where ISDN services are not available. ISDN uses digital signal for transmissions. It also has the advantage of setting call faster over Public Telephones. The ISDN connectivity will be provided up to a gateway to the Local Area Network (LAN) of the individual laboratories, through a firewall.

In DRONA, communication has been designed in such a way that a remote SRC cannot contact diectly to another remote SRC. Communication between SRC's is possible only through MRC's. So if an SRC wants to communicate with another remote SRC it has to contact (dial) the MRC to which it is connected the MRC on receiving the request, will dial the nearest MRC to which it is attached. If more than one MRC's are connected, then it will choose the shortest path of transmission Routers decides the path of transmission as discussed earlier. Once shortest route is determined, it will connect to that MRC. This MRC in turn contacts the requested SRC. All the MRC's have dedicated connection to DRDO HQ's. Each request for connection between MRC's and SRC's goes through the firewall PC. Firewall PC checks the IP address of the incoming packet (data). If the incoming packet is illegal, firewall will discard it.

4.3 Security Mechanisms

The security measures provided on DRONA can be classified into following categories.

- Network Security.
- Firewall.
- Data Encryption.
- Computer System Security.

4.4 Services Provided by Drona

Being R & D Network, DRONA provides all network services. At the same time it has restricted some services which can cause security hole in the network. DRONA software development team has designed a DRONA interface software for accessing various network services. The network services are divided into allowed services and non-services. The following are the allowed services currently provided by DRONA.

(a) Electronic Mail.

(b) File Transfer.

(c) Website for Laboratories.

(d) Home Page for Scientists.

(e) Bulletin Boards.

(f) Library Information Service.

(g) Corporate Databases Access.

(h) Project Monitoring.

5. CONCLUSION

Management is a complex task of getting workers to contribute effectively towards the attainment of their organisation's goal and objectives. Managing is, therefore, concerned with the relationships of managers with their sub-ordinates at various levels of the organisation. If an organisation is to function effectively and efficiently, it must attract people, hold people and motivate people and in this task the manager with supervisory responsibilities plays a unique role.

In the modern period, information has emerged as a key resource which has got an over riding influence on all other resources. Naturally, Information Technology which is concerned with the storage, processing, retrieval and transmission of information has come to stay with us. The primary impact of Information Technology is that it enables the managements to have better access to information wherever it is available. This helps them to take right decisions at the most appropriate time.

Modern libraries have already accepted that their major goal/objective is the provision of information. Libraries are facing multifold challenge to accomplish this goal. This is primarily because of the varied nature of information. Inter-disciplinary nature of information can be considered as another dimension of information. It means the same information is most often required by the people from different subject disciplines. It seems information is becoming more and more inter-disciplinary in nature.

The same phenomenon when explained from user's point of view, it can be said that the information required by a user lies scattered in a variety of documents in the same subject field and at times, even in different subjects fields. This nature of information is referred to as `scattering of information' in the literature. As a result, there is growing tendency among the people to search the literature of different (related) fields to get required information. This nature of information also poses several problems to the librarians in the provision of information service. While searching for information, the librarians cannot confine to only one discipline. Most often sources from other related fields must also be searched to get the relevant information.

As a cardinal principle management of information must place customer needs at the higher level of priority. It is not the convenience of the staff or the manager but it is the need of the user that is important. Credibility amongst users should perhaps be the most important criterion to judge good management of libraries and information centres. Library automation eventually leads to networking of libraries. The information technology has brought together libraries and has resulted in the concept of library without walls, meaning thereby that the resources of all libraries in a network are available to the whole user community. DRDO Libraries/Technical Information Centres

(TICs) are providing services to their clients i.e. defence scientists by utilizing their laboratory resources, LAN, DRONA and INTERNET with best of their capabilities.

REFERENCES

HODGE (Bartow). Management Information Systems. 1984. Roston; Virginia.

BOMMER (Michael R W) and CHORBA (Ronald W). Decision Making for Library Management. 1982. Knowledge Industry Publications, Inc., New York.

JONES (Noragh) and JORDAN (Peter). Case Studies in Library Management. 1988. Clive bingley; London.

UMAPATHY, (K S). Problems in Library Management. 1984. Vikas; N. Delhi.

SINGH (Mohinder). Library & Information Management; Theory & Practice. 1988. International Book Traders; Delhi.

WHITE (Herbert S). Library Personnel Management. 1985. Knowledge Industry Publications, Inc.; New York.

ROBERTS (Stephen A). Cost Management for Library & Information Services. 1985. Butter worths; London.

HARRISON (Colin) and BEENHAM (Rosemary). The Basics of Librarianship. 1987. Clive Bingley; London.

SRIDHAR KEN (M C). Patterns of user visit, movement and length of stay in a special library : a case study. *Annals of library science and documentation.* 36, 3; 1989; 134-133.

GHOSH (S B). S & T. Information system and service in Hungary. *Annals of library science and documentation.* 35, 2; 1988; 45-57.

LAHARI (Ramansu). The human side of the library : A profile of manipur. *Annals of library science and documentation.* 35, 2; 1988; 84-92.

GOPINATH (M A). Librarianship in Library Management. IASLIC Bulletin. 35, 4; 1990; 135-142.

D.R.D.O. Newsletter. 14, 1; 1994.

BANDHYOPADHYAY (A) et al. Information needs of Defence Scientists. *Proceedings of National Conference on Scientific*

Information for Defence. N. Delhi, 25-26 February'8G, DESIDOC, N. Delhi. 1988. p. 49-53.

BREMBER (V L) and LEGGATE (P). Linking a medical user survey to management for library effectiveness. *Journal of Documentation.* 41, 1; 1985; 1-14.

D.R.D.O. Defence Research and Development Products Processes Technologies Handbook. 1986. D.R.D.O.; N. Delhi.

VIJ (Rajeev). Infomation needs of Research Scientists. *AGLIS Journal*. 8, 1-4; 1990; 23-31.

LAZAR MATHEW, (T) *et al.* Modern technologies for biomedical information handling. 2000. INMAS; Delhi.

RATHORE (R S). Information management in DRDO Libraries/ Technical information centres. 1995; Ph.D. Thesis of University of Rajasthan, Jaipur.

DRONA Manual. D.R.D.O.; New Delhi.

DRDO Booklet. Vigyan Rail (Dec. 03-Aug. 04). D.R.D.O.; New Delhi.

Evaluating Information Technology (IT) Skills of the Users of Banasthali University Library : A Study

Praveen Babel* and S.D. Vyas**

*Librarian, WISDOM Library, Banasthali University, Banasthali - 304 022 (Raj.)
**University Librarian, NALSAR University of Law, Hyderabad - 500 078 (AP)

ABSTRACT

This study investigates the availability of IT skills among the users of Banasthali University Library. Library users (Students and Teachers) of the Banasthali University library were given questionnaires to provide information about Information Technology skills. Reveals that among the ICT-based services, e-mail is used by the large percentage of the users. Reports that library users were satisfied with the application of ICT, but they face problems due to slow speed of Internet and lack of IT skills. Study proposes a variety of measures of formal orientation and training in ICT to prepare effective users. Provides tables and diagrams to prove that there is an urgent need of developing IT skills among the users of academic institutions

1. INTRODUCTION

The Banasthali University was established in the year 1935. The Banasthali University Library supports teaching and research and provides bibliographic and reference services to the students, scholars and teachers. There is a Central Library and six Departmental Libraries in the university. Presently the collection of the Central Library is more than 1,65,000 documents, comprising books/ reference books, reports, bound issues of periodicals and 550 print current journals. Apaji Institute of Mathematics and Applied Computer Technology Library subscribes to AIEEE and ACM e-journals. Department of Management Library (WISDOM) and Faculty of Education also subscribe number of journals.

The Banasthali University library (BUL) introduced computers in 1999. The library acquired CDS/ISIS package of DOS version and later window version was acquired from NISSAT. In the beginning the library staff used the computer facilities available at Computer Science Department for practice as well as developed sample records of books and journals. The book records and a list of current serials compiled on CDS/ISIS were sent to INFLIBNET, Ahemdabad. However actual library automation work began in July 2000 when six computer systems, one server, two printers and UPS system were installed in the Central Library with a grant of Rs. 6.5 lakhs received from INFLIBNET/UGC. It also purchased UGC funded software SOUL in 2000. BU library later acquired commercial software LibSys in the year 2004. Later BU library has also acquired a file server with 23 nodes and three printers. At present seven computer systems are housed in Computer Room where in house database preparation work is going on. Two terminals have been put to use for students and teachers to access OPAC, two computers are at the circulation counter for issue and return work and three are installed in Technical Section for technical processing of books. The library also has 10 Bar-coding machines; one scanner and two photocopy machines. All the Assistant Librarians have their separate PCs in their office. The computers are used mainly for housekeeping, user services, management support activities, Internet and printing of catalogue cards. The computer application has helped the library to clear the backlog of cataloguing books. Circulation activities have been computerized with barcode to achieve speed and accuracy in maintaining the circulation records. To facilitate the payment of fines, debt collection has been integrated with the circulation system. The library has provided Online Public Access Catalogue (OPAC), which is a bibliographic database of books and periodicals available in the library. OPAC can be accessed through author, title or class number, etc from any library under local area network All Departmental libraries are inter connected with accessing catalogzed database of libraries with server located at the Apaji Institute of Mathematics.

In matters of IT, Banasthali University authorities were always ahead of other universities of the state. Today Banasthali University Library and its Branch Libraries are fully automated. The credit for it goes to the University authorities, Central Library and the Computer Science Department staff for their full co-operation.

2. PURPOSE OF THE STUDY

The following are the purpose of the study:

- To study the use of information technology by users in the University Library.
- To evaluate IT skills of the users of the University Library
- To find out the problems of the users while accessing OPAC databases as well as e-databases.
- To study the level of users satisfaction in the use of IT.
- To seek users suggestions for the improvement of the IT based services in the University Library.

3. METHODOLOGY AND ANALYSIS OF DATA

This study examines the Application of IT at the Banasthali University Library. To conduct the present study, the survey method was chosen for which a questionnaire was designed (Appendix-I). Questionnaire and interviews represent the most common methods of data collection in social sciences research. The study is an outcome of a sample of 500 library users of students and teachers of Banasthali University Library (300 students and 200 teachers). Out of the total number of respondents, 200 students and 120 teachers responded, which is suppose to be a most satisfactory response. The chi-square test is used to point out the association between the attributes and simple percentage method has been used for the analysis of this study.

4. ANALYSIS OF THE SURVEY STUDY

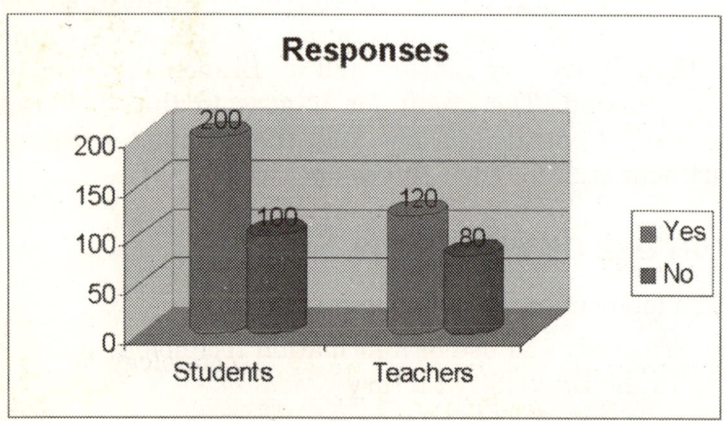

Table 1. Purpose of Using Information Technology

Reason	Total	S	%	T	%	
Study	167	97	48.5	70	58.33	T=Teacher
Updating Knowledge	264	154	77	110	91.66	
Doing Research Work	200	100	50	100	83.33	S=Student

Writing Papers and Presenting Paper	214	114	57	100	83.33
Entertainment	150	100	50	50	41.66
Total		565		430	
Pearson Chi-square value 11.170a			df = 4 P= .025		

The chi-square test proves that there is significant difference between students and teachers in the matter of purpose of using of IT. Users indicate that main purpose of using IT is updating knowledge as well as writing and presenting papers in the seminars/ conferences. 77 per cent students and 91.66 per cent of teachers responded saying that they use technology for updating knowledge while 57 percent student and 83.33 per cent teachers say that they use computers for writing and presenting papers, 50 per cent students and 83.33 per cent teachers use computers for research.

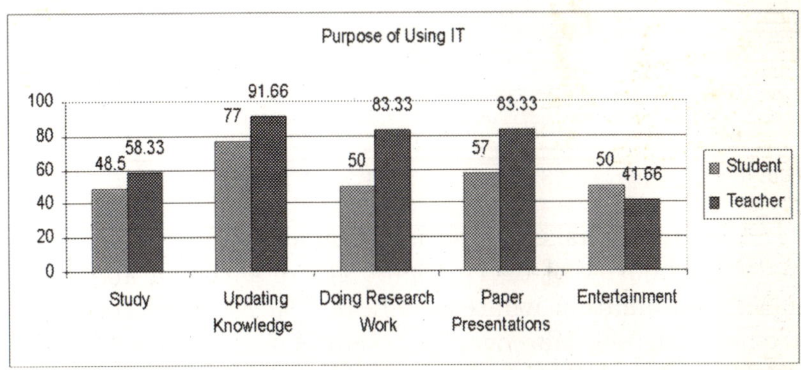

Table 2. Awareness of Library Automation

		Total	S	%	T	%	
1	Yes	244	154	77	90	75	S = Students
2	No.	48	18	15	30	25	T = Teachers
	Total		172		120		
Pearson Chi-square Test = 10.871a				df =1		P = .001	

Awareness of users regarding technology indicates that 154 (77%) users are aware of the automated services whereas only 18(15%) respondents reported that they are not aware. The above Table 2 shows that students are more aware of technology than teachers which shows young generation is technology proficient irrespective whether they are teachers or students.

Table 3. Library Automation and users satisfaction

		Total	S	%	T	%	
1	Satisfactory	250	160	80	90	75	S = Student
2	Not satisfactory	36	6	3	30	25	T = Teacher
	Total		166		120		

Pearson Chi-square = 28.950a df=1 P = .000

Users were asked for satisfaction about the library automation. Majority of users 160(80%) are satisfied about the library automation whereas only 6 (3%) reported that they are not satisfied. Moreover 117 (58.5%) users are highly satisfied with the OPAC facility provided by the library where as, 14 (7%) users are not satisfied but they have not assigned any reason for it.

Chi-square test reveals that the satisfaction between the teachers and students toward library automation is quite significant. Students are highly satisfied than teachers. The main reason of this difference is that students adaptation to new technology is quick. It is due to exposure as well as training.

Table 4. Availability of Internet Facility

	Place	Total	S	%	T	%	
1	Library	124	94	47	30	25	S = Students
2	Computer Center	192	122	61	70	58.33	T = Teachers
3	Home	77	37	18.5	40	33.33	
4	Internet café	38	28	14	10	8.33	
5	Hostel	34	34	17	0	00	
	Total		315		150		

Pearson Chi-square = 35.706a df=4 P = .000

The various groups of users access Internet facilities at the library, the computer laboratories and at the home. Although a few users 37(18.5%) have Internet facility at home and 34 (17%) users at the hostel. A major proportion 94 (47%) of users have used the facilities provided in their library. 122 (61%) users say that they have to use the Internet facility at computer laboratory because the university wants centralized access by the users. However, they feel that the right place would be libraries to offer IT services and they express it to the librarian and his staff rather then expressing it to the management.

Chi-square test reveals that there is a different place of Internet surfing by users is significant. A good number of teachers and students are using Internet facility at computer laboratory as shown in the Table 4.

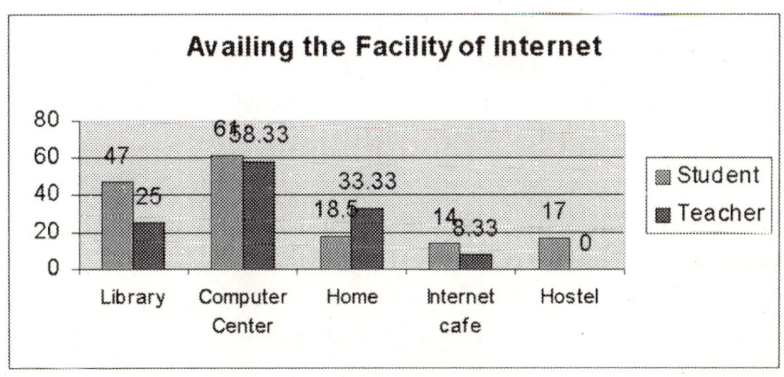

Table 5. Frequency of Using the Internet

	Frequency	Total	S	%	T	%	
1	Daily	227	137	68.5	90	75	S = Student
2	Once a week	71	51	25.5	20	16.66	T = Teacher
3	Once a fortnight	00	0	0	0	00	
4	Once a month	00	0	0	0	00	
5	Rarely	30	20	10	10	8.33	
	Total		208		120		

Pearson Chi square = 3.222a df=2 P = .200

Respondents were asked about the occurrence of frequency of accessing Internet. 137 (68.5%) respondents say that they use Internet facilities daily while 51 (25.5%) per cent say that they use them once in a week. Users are overlapping in to the other frequency option of use, some 20 (10%) users of the humanities and social sciences indicated that they use internet rarely.

Chi-square test shows that there is different frequency of internet access between the users is significant

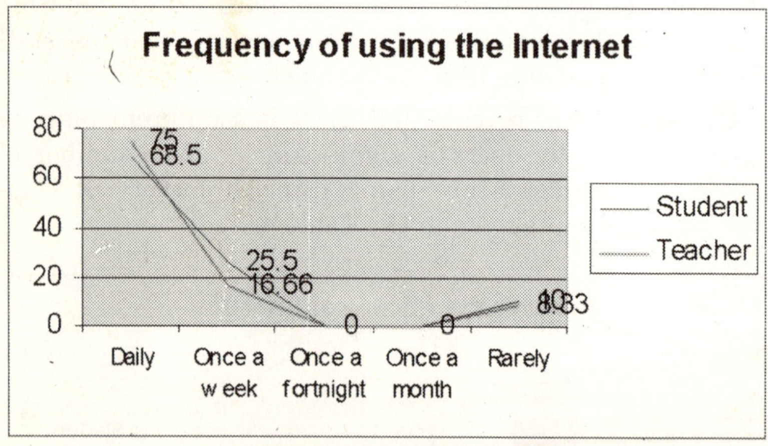

Usually browsing is done for different purposes. Education is most important purpose the variables as majority 163 (81.5%) of users answered that they use internet for education. 149 (74.5%) users use it for E-mail while 103 (51.5%) users use internet for updating their

knowledge. 29 (14.5%) users access internet for other work. The above analysis shows that there is no marked pattern of using the net by the respondents.

Table 6. Purpose of Utilization of Internet

	Purpose	Total	S	%	T	%	
1	Education	283	163	81.5	120	100	S = Student
2	E-mail	199	149	74.5	50	41.66	T = Teacher
3	Updating of Knowledge	123	103	51.5	20	16.66	
4	Any other	59	29	14.5	30	25	
	Total		444				

Pearson Chi-square = 40.898a df=3 P = .000

Chi-square test shows utilization of IT is significant. Category of the users is strong point of this significant difference.

Table 7. Use of Search Engines

	Search engine	Total	S	%	T	%	
1	Google.com	289	169	84.5	120	100	S = Student
2	Yahoo.com	170	120	60	50	41.66	T = Teacher
3	MSN.com	20	20	10	0	00	
4	Alta vista.com	43	23	11.5	20	16.66	
5	Any other	44	34	17	10	8.33	
	Total		366		200		

Pearson Chi-square = 23.793a df=4 P = .000

Important search engines are Google, Yahoo, MSN, and Alta-vista. It is observed that 169 (84.5%) users use Google as the most used search engine, followed by Yahoo 120(%), MSN 20 (10%), Alta-vista 23 (11.5%) and any others 34(17%).

Chi-square test shows that there is different frequency of the use of search engine between the students and teachers which is quite significant.

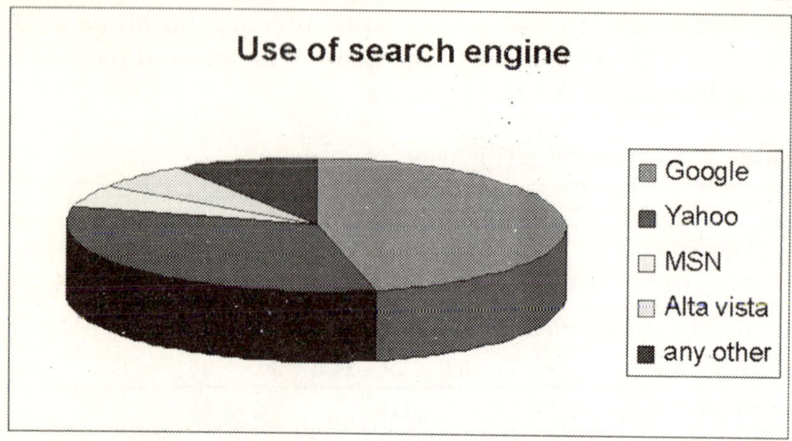

Table 8. Obstacles Faced by the Users in Accessing IT Facilities

	Obstacles	Total	S	%	T	%
1	Inadequate IT infrastructure	166	106	53	60	50
2	Lack of training and Knowledge	150	40	20	110	91.66
3	Lack of timing	144	94	47	50	41.66
4	Low speed of Internet	260	160	80	100	83.33
	Total		400		320	

Pearson Chi-square = 64.613a df=3 P = .000

Respondents were asked to indicate the problems they face while accessing IT tools. The variables provided in the questionnaire are given in the above table. Out of 200 respondents, the majority of the users 160(80%) have cited reason for not using IT is slow speed of Internet, slow downloading, non-availability of connectivity and 106 (53%) have indicated inadequate IT infrastructure. 94 (47%) respondents indicate that lack of time due to the pre-occupied with workload of teaching as the main reason for not accessing IT tools. 40 (20%) users have revealed the lack of training and knowledge in information technology. It has been observed that social science and humanities users access internet and IT products less compared to science and technology users.

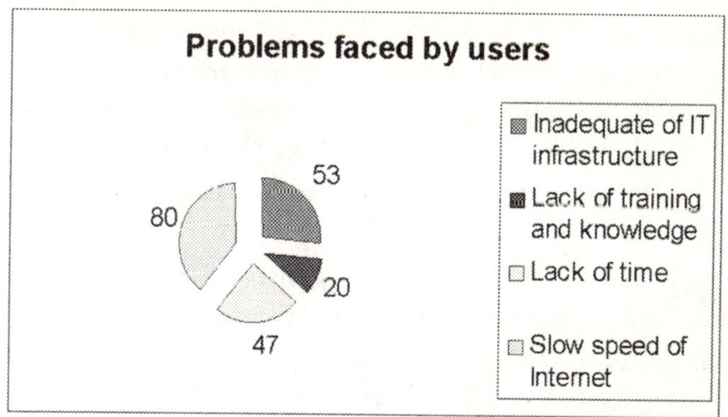

Table 9. Information Literacy Programme (IL) Received by the Users

	Total	S	%	T	%
If 'yes' whether IL programme is useful?	34	14	7	20	16.66
If 'no' whether IL programme shall be useful?	213	123	61.5	90	75
Total		137		110	

Pearson Chi-square = 3.259a df=1 P = 0.071

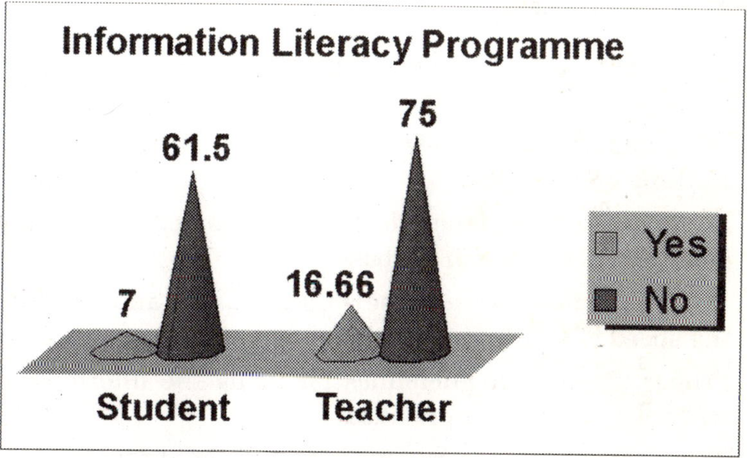

Users should be conversant with right techniques with right tools for getting the right information. They are not aware of the potential of the information technology, but without proper IL training, no one can explore the full

potentiality of ICT services. The results reveal that 75% teachers and 61.5% students have not received training in the use of ICT in library. Only 16.66% teachers and seven percent students have received orientation program. This is a serious handicap and need to be imparted adequate training in the use of IT tools.

The Banasthali University Library held the following two one-day seminars for the benefit of teachers and research scholars to improve their IT skills. However there is an imperative need to hold such programmes frequently to help the faculty and scholars.

- In November 2005, with the help of INFLIBNET staff a one day seminar was organized by the Central Library. This was attended by the faculty, M.Phill and PhD scholars as well as library staff of the Banasthali University.
- J-Gate providers also organized a one-day seminar in 2006 to familiarize with J-Gate databases.

5. SUGGESTIONS

The users have offered few suggestions :-

1. Internet speed should be improved and a new technology be implemented as servers usually go down while working on computer.
2. IT services should be implemented so as to make library more useful for search purpose.
3. There is a need to increase PCs for users and improve the speed of Internet.
4. Proper training or guidelines for using the information technology should be provided.
5. User education programmes should be organised to make the users aware of the library collection as well as its services. Users should also be given training so that they can handle the computer systems independently. This will increase the use of library by the readers.

Regarding suggestions offered by the users, it has been noticed that their suggestions are not clear. For example they suggested that number of PCs be increased, but generally it has been found that even the existing PCs remain unoccupied.

CONCLUSION

Most of the readers know little about the technology. Those who know about information resources, and those who do not know, account for a small percentage. It is observed that undergraduates usually obtain documents through the traditional holdings of the library. Thus paper documents still play an important role and electronic books and virtual accessing cannot replace the traditional print material in near future. 75% users are satisfied with the availability of electronic resources in the library. The readers who have not joined any information literacy programme account for 61.5% students and 75% teachers. Only 7% students and 16.7% teachers are willing to join the Information Literacy programme. It is also observed that though users do complain of more facility, but surprisingly existing facilities provided are hardly used by users. There is need of technology skills to be developed among the users (students and teachers). This is possible if academic libraries hold library orientation programmes regularly in the beginning of the academic session. Libraries should also invite commercial vendors who launch information products so that users come to know about the information products. It is necessary to make our academic campuses Wi-Fi compatible so that students may access virtual electronic databases through their laptops from any where in the campus.

Notes and references

1. Bhatt, Chris (1994). Information Technology in Public Libraries. 5th ed. Library Association Publication.

2. Collste, Goran. Ed. (1998). Ethics and Information Technology. New Academic Publisher, New Delhi.
3. Collin, S.M.H. (1996). Dictionary of Information Technology. Peter Collins Publication, London.
4. Satyanarayana, B, Ed. (1998) Information Technology: Issue and Trends: Cosmo Publication, New Delhi.
5. Touminen, Kirsti (1997) Children, Libraries and Information Technology: Results of User need Analyses. Helsinki: Association of Finnish Local and Regional Authorities.

BIBLIOGRAPHY

1. Ali, Naushad (2005). The Use of Electronic Resources at IIT Delhi Library: a Study of Search Behaviours. *The Electronic Library*. 23.6: 691-700.
2. Haneefa, Mohamed (2007). Application of Information and Communication Technologies in Special Libraries in Kerela (India). *Library Review*. 56.7: 603-620.
3. Shuling, Wu. (2007). Investigation and Analysis of Current use of Electronic Resources in University Libraries. *Library Management*. 28.1/2 : 72-88.
4. Singh, S.P. (2001) Computer Applications in Indian Institutes of Technology libraries. *The Electronic Library*. 19.2 : 92-101.
5. Thappa, Neelam and Sahoo, K.C. (2005) Problems and Prospects of Automation : a survey of Special Libraries in Bhopal. *Library Progress*. 25.1 : 70-83.
6. Vyas, S.D. (2005) Application of Information Technology (IT) in University Libraries of Rajasthan: A Survey. *RLA Bulletin*. 9.1-4 : 12-42.

RFID System for Libraries in Present I.T. Era

Deep Singh

Librarian, Malaviya National Institute of Technology (MNIT), Jaipur-302 017 (Raj.)

ABSTRACT

This paper describes about the main features of RFID System and its use in the modern libraries. It includes the usefulness of the RFID System in providing better library services and to install a Security System or as a device for theft control. Limitations of the system have also been mentioned in the paper. In the last the financial implications for a library having a collection of about 50,000 holdings has been given to take an idea for its application.

INTRODUCTION

RFID (Radio Frequency Identification) is an innovative technology, which is used for the Theft Detection in the modern libraries. During last several years Electro-Mechanical (EM) system and RFID (Radio Frequency Identification) systems are being used in the libraries of developed countries. In the present I.T. era this system is being used not only for the control on theft of the library materials or holdings, but for Charging/Discharging (borrowing/returning) of books etc. and Self-Charging and Discharging system also. By the use of this technology library services becomes very smooth. In fact RFID is a combination of 'Radio-Frequency-based Technology' and 'Microchip Technology'. By using Radio Frequency Technology the information given on Microchip of the Tag affixed on the library book/document is read. With the help of sensor, scanner or interrogator and antenna of the tags, the information is retrieved from the microchips EM or RF theft detection barcodes and targets can be replaced through the tags used in the RFID system. Although Hybrid system introduced 3M in 2000 replaced only Barcodes but retained the EM strips in the belief that EM is superior to RFID for security. 3M did introduce a comprehensive RFID product that replaces both EM and barcodes in 2004.

In short RFID System may be understood in following few sentences:

"RFID tags replace both the EM security strips and Barcode, simplify patron self check-out/ check-in, ability to handle material without exception for video and audio tapes. Radio Frequency anti-theft detection is innovative and safe. High-speed inventory and identify items which are out of proper order and long-term development guarantee when using Open Standard"

ADVANTAGES OF RFID SYSTEM

Though there are many features of the RFID system, some main advantages are mentioned here which are generally useful for the libraries-

1. RAPID CHARGING/DISCHARGING (Circulation)

RFID system is very useful in saving the time of Circulation Operations. This technology is faster than the Barcode Technology, as the information can be read from the tags faster than the barcode sticker. That is due to the fact that the tags can be read regardless of item orientation or alignment (i.e., the technology does not require line-of-sight or a fixed plane to read tags as do older technologies) and that several items in a stack can be read at the same time.

While initially unreliable, the anti-collision algorithm that allows an entire stack to be charged or discharged now appears to be working well. Finally, RFID tags can be read from distances of up to 24 inches far greater than the use of light pens and barcode wands used with EM technology. That is what makes RFID systems not only faster, but also make it able to support electronic inventorying with handheld devices.

2. SELF CHARGING/ DISCHARGING BECOMES SIMPLIFIED

In the self-charging used by the users , there is a marked improvement because they do not have to carefully place documents within a designated template and they can charge several documents/holdings at the same time. User self-discharging services, which can be achieved by installing readers in book drops or with self-discharge stations, shifts work from staff to patrons.

Dimensions of various components of self check In/ Out work station

- **Cabinet Only**: 26" d x 36" h x 44" w, (660 mm x 914 mm x 1118 mm)
- **Monitor**: 22.75" h (57.8 mm) above counter, High resolution, 15" (381 mm) diagonal LCD touch screen, flat panel display
- **Printer:** 8.5" d x 5.9" h x 6.25" w, (216 **mm** x 149 mm x 159 mm), Thermal, built into kiosk or standalone, 280 Printer
- **Energy Profile:** 100–120 or 200–240 VAC; 50–60 Hz; 3.0/1.5 A

3. READERS ARE HIGHLY RELIABLE

The readers are highly reliable. Several vendors of RFID library systems claim an almost 100% detection rate using RFID tags. If the reader is within the range of 18 inches, it works properly. As per the experiences of the libraries using RFID and EM system, RFID is having 50 to 75% reduction in False Alarm. Some RFID systems are having interface connectivity between circulation reader and the exit sensor (reader) for identifying the moving out activity of the library.

In case any document is stolen or taken out without getting it charged properly by the user, the system can indentify that who has done this activity, if the user's card is also having RFID tag. In other RFID system, the circulation status is encoded on the tag. This is done by designating a bit as the "theft" bit and turning it off at time of charge and discharge. If the document/ book that has not been properly charged is taken an immediate alarm is raised. In another option "theft" bit and the online interface to an integrated library system can be used to raise an immediate alarm and the second to identify the stolen document/book.

High-Speed Electronic Stock Verification/ Inventorying and proper Shelving

RFID system is having a specific feature that by moving a Hand–held inventory reader rapidly, the books kept in the shelves can be checked with a distance of about six inches. Also it is useful in shelving the books properly. By using this system, stock verification of the books has become very easy and fast.

Interfaces with Document/Book Handling Systems

Another application of RFID technology is an interface with a document or book handling system, a system that consists of conveyors and sorting equipment that can move library documents/books and sort them mechanically by category into separate boxes or onto separate carts. This activity significantly reduces a very good amount of time of working manpower required to prepare documents/books for re shelving or rearranging in the stacks. This application is not used widely, as it is very costly.

Tag Life is Longer than Barcode

The RFID Tags are having long life instead of Barcodes Labels, as nothing comes into contact with them. Generally about 100,000 times transactions can be done with one tag and after that it is replaced, while Barcode labels may be damaged using frequently or by the users also.

Demerits of RFID System

As any technology or application has its limitation, RFID system is also having some demerits and these are as mentioned below :

High Cost

The components being used in RFID Technology are very expensive. The readers used to read the information of the document or book are comparable in cost of an EM or RF. Theft detection system, approx. Rs. 1,25,000/- to Rs. 3,75,000/-. The cost of the RFID tag varies from one make to another. On Internet the cost of the Tags can be obtained from the websites of the companies or from their agencies. It may vary from approximately Rs. 250/- to Rs. 2000/-, which is higher than Barcodes, EM strips or RF targets.

Compromise Vulnerablly

RFID system can be compromised by using two to three folds/layers of household foil around the document/book, as it blocks the radio signals. So, by using the foil by the users the documents/books can be stolen from the library. In EM technology a magnet can make the system failure and visitor can bring the book or document out of the library without raising the alarm at the exit of the library. One more thing is that if two books/documents are placed against one another, one tag exactly overlays another. This act will cancel out the signals. For this kind of activity some one should have knowledge of Technology.

Removal of exposed Tags

According to a study involved making the libraries automated, EM strips are concealed in the spine or gutter of the book, which is very difficult to find and to remove, while in RFID system the tags are pasted just inside the back cover of the book/document , which can be removed easily. If users are more familiar with the role of tags, it may be removed or damaged. Now a days the technology has been developed to make little thinner tags, which are difficult to detect.

Earlier the tags were based on the 'Solder and Bond' technology, under which a detectable bump remains there and the circuit attached to the chip remains raised. A later method known as 'Flip Chip' fuses the chip onto the antenna in which the bump is reduced and tag remains thinner so that it conceals with a bookplate with a much less noticeable bump.

Sensor Problems at Exit

One side the short range readers are having 100% accuracy for charging and discharging performance, but the other side the gate sensors are more problematic. Their reading capacity should be more than double of the readers' capacity and should be able to catch the range of antennae of the book/document. But it works only when the tags are larger or the exit lanes are of 36 to 42 inches, rather than 48 inches, as some libraries are having such lanes.

Perceived Invasion of User's Privacy

There is a perception among some that RFID is a threat to patron privacy. Also it is argued that after getting the book/document charged at the reader, the information of the tags can be read from a distance of two feet or less because the tags reflect a signal that comes from a reader or sensor and the readers that are available for the frequency range used in library tags are limited in their power to ten watts. The range/ power of the tags and the reader can also be increased. It is known that the information about borrower and borrowed books are maintained in the "Circulation or Charging /Discharging Module" of the Library Management Software/ system. In this system the information about the book being and the borrower are easily visible while processing, but in RFID tag only limited information like Call Number, location etc. are maintained and other information like title, author etc. are stored rarely.

DEVICES REQUIRED FOR AN RFID SYSTEM

Components of an RFID System

A comprehensive RFID system has five major components which are as below:

i. RFID tags that are electronically programmed with unique information.

ii. Readers or Sensors to interrogate the tags.

iii. Sensors(including Antenna) at the exit.

iv. Server/ Docking station.

v. Self Check out/ in system.

i . TAGS

RFID tags let us accurately identify and track our library materials. Information about the book/ document is stored in a tiny memory chip, and the tags are rewriteable, so we don't need to buy new ones when you change the information. RFID tags eliminate **"line of sight"** needed to process books/ documents. Each tag is guaranteed for the life of the book or document it identifies. The tags should have all the ISO standards. The paper- thin tag has an antenna and a microchip, which generally contains at least **64 bits**. There are three types of tags and that are- **'Read only', 'WORM' and 'Read/ Write'.**

In the libraries 'Read only' tags are used where barcodes are not being used for the books/ documents. For this kind of tags not more than **96 bits** are required. These tags are not rewritable. Another tags WORM (Write-Once –Read –Many) are used where Barcodes are already being used in the library and a retrospective conversion work of the holdings is undertaken. The main advantage of this tag is that additional information can also be added to the existing identification number. Such information contains author, title etc. Generally these tags have a capacity of at least **256 bits**. 'Read / Write tags' are used by most of the libraries, because any information related to the document can be added or changed. Some of the libraries add subject or branch name. In case of location of the any document/book is changeable, the location can be changed accordingly. When a vendor includes a "theft" bit that can be turned on and off, the RFID tag can function much like an EM or RF tag. Such tags usually have a capacity of at least 1024 bits. A minimum capacity of 1024 bits is essential if the tags are to be used in electronic inventorying and/ or with a materials handling system.

All the RFID tags being used in the libraries are **'Passive'**, as the power required for reading the tags comes either from reader or from exit sensor not from the tag itself. The tags used by most vendors of library RFID are not compatible even when they conform to the same standards because the current standards only seek electronic compatibility between tags and readers. The pattern of encoding information and the software that processes the information differs from vendor to vendor. Therefore, a change from one vendor's system to another would require certain modifications in the library management software. Here a picture of RFID Tag is given just for an idea. It is being pasted/fitted on the books/documents/materials etc.

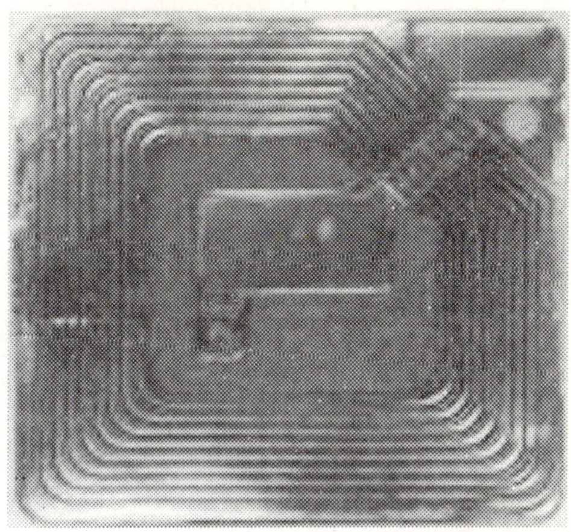

Figure 1. RFID Tag

i.i. Tagging material

Libraries can involve volunteers in addition to their regular staff for RFID tagging in the books / materials. This planning will reduce not only time but also cost of tagging. By giving limited training, the staff can be trained in tagging work. The tags should be fitted/pasted at the consistent location on the books. The inside of the back cover of the book is the recommended location because right hand installer can reach this place faster. Most libraries are not able to tag their entire collections at one time. It is difficult to tag the entire collection of the library at a time. Therefore, a phased implementation should be planned. The retrospective conversion of existing bar coded books etc., including affixing the tags to other materials, takes 15-30 seconds per holding depending on the amount of information added to the tag and the skill of the person doing the tagging. Tags, which are pre-programmed are used for new acquisitions in libraries that want only identification numbers on the tags. Such tagging work takes even less time, because they do not involve scanning of existing barcodes.

This picture shows about internal parts of a Tag and how does a tag work:

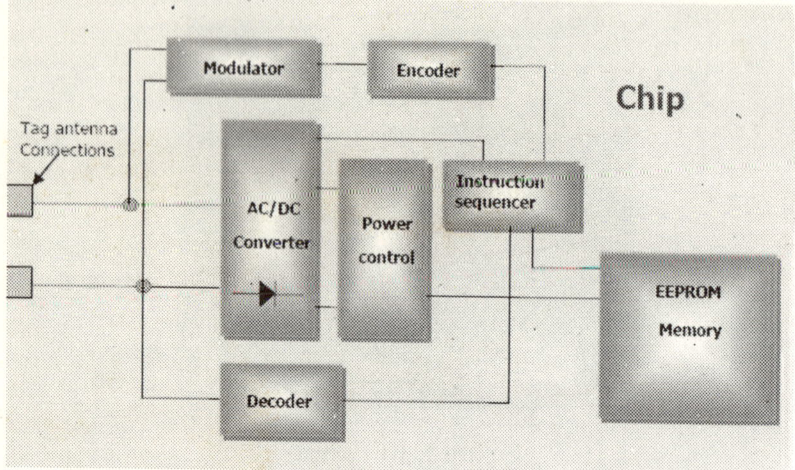

Figure 2: Basic Tag IC Architecture

ii. Readers/Staff Workstation for Circulation

A typical system includes several different kinds of readers, also known as sensors when installed at library exits. These are radio frequency devices being designed to detect and read tags to obtain the information stored thereon. The reader powers an antenna to generate an RF field. When a book or document having tag passes through the field, the information stored on the chip in the tag is decoded by the reader and stored and sent to a server or communicated to an integrated library management software, which is interfaced with RFID system. The types of readers include Conversion Stations, staff workstations for Circulation Desk charging and discharging, patron self-charging and discharging stations, book drop readers, and longer-range walk-through exit sensors to detect and read an RFID tag for the purposes of determining whether the book or document is charged or discharged. If the book is not charged through the reader, the system antenna will raise the alarm at the exit of the library.

One portable device 'Hand held scanner' or gun also remains there in the library, which is used for scanning and recording the data of the holdings from shelves. This helps in stock verification and for proper shelving of the books/ documents.

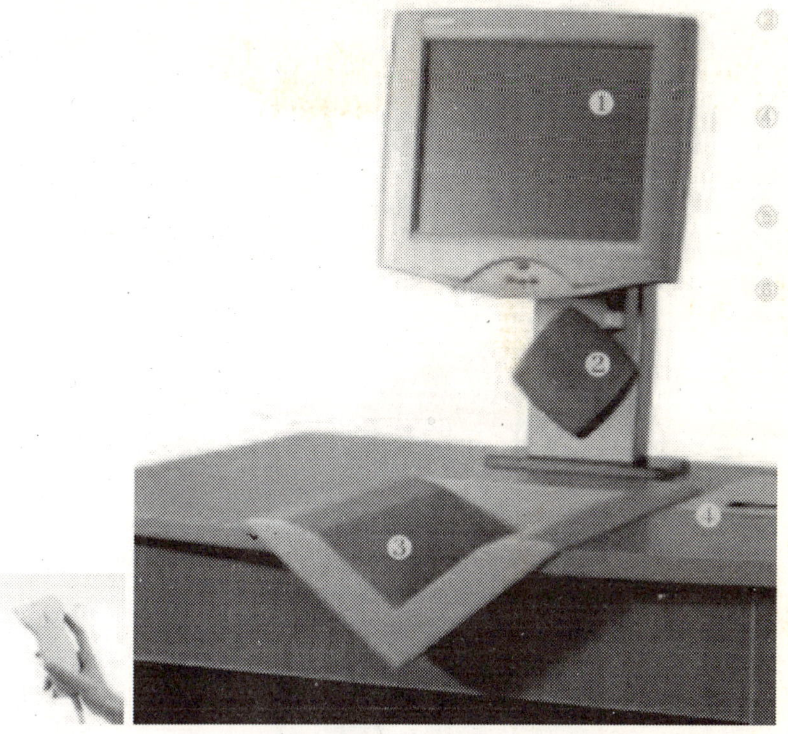

Figure 3 : Circulation System with Hand held Scanner

iii. Sensors (Including Antennae) at Exit

As it's name, the Exit Sensors and Antennae are installed just at the exit of the library. The sensors are fitted parallel both side of the exit gate .The main role and feature of the sensors are to detect and control the theft of the books or documents from the library. The sensor and antenna produce radio signals to activate the tag and read and write data to it. Sensors and Antennae are the channels between the tag and the reader, which manage the system's data acquisitions and communication. The electromagnetic field produced by an antenna can constantly present when multiple tags are expected continually. Antennae can be built into a doorframe to receive tag data from book/ document passing through the door. While a user crosses the exit gate without getting the book issued or processed at the reader, the sensors and antennae installed there become activated and start raising the alarm. That means one has to get the book processed at the reader machine available at the Circulation Counter, the reader decodes the tag fitted in the book and makes the book allowable to take it out of the exit. If this procedure is not followed and book is taken out of the exit, the sensors and antennae will raise the alarm and the person concerned will be caught presuming that the book was being stolen.

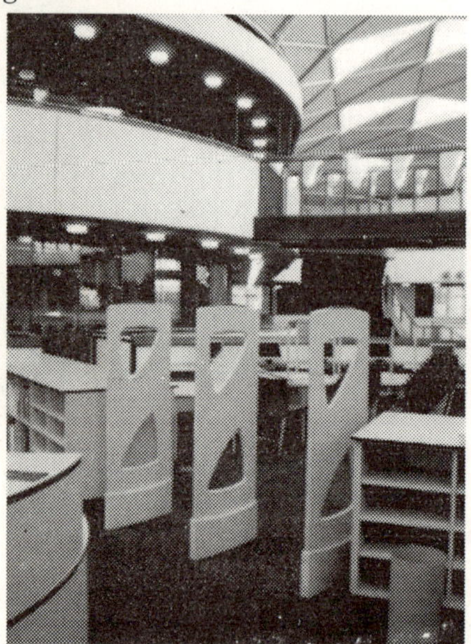

Figure 4 : Sensors/ Exit Gate with Reader

iv. Server/ Docking Station

It is well known that Server is the heart of a comprehensive RFID System. It plays the role of a Gateway for communicating among different components of the system, as it receives the information from the reader(s) and exchanges information with the 'Circulation Database'. API (Applications Programming Interface) is the necessary part of the software to interface it with the automated library system. The server typically includes a transaction database so that reports can be produced.

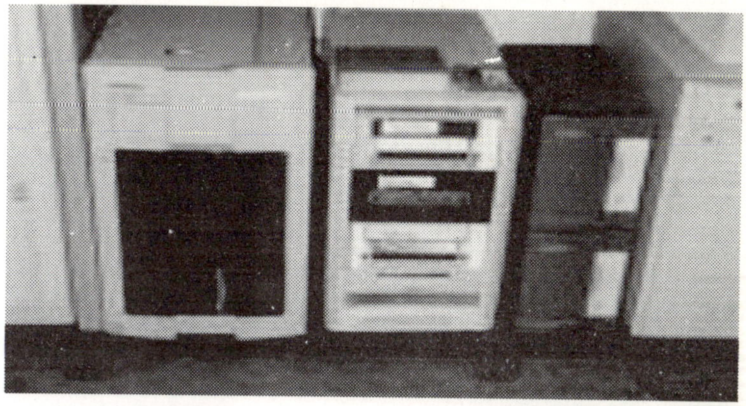

Figure 5.1. Server for Data Storage

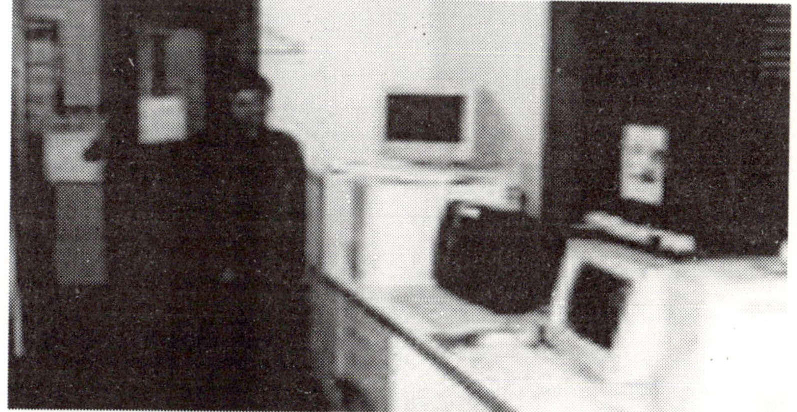

Figure 5.2. Server Room

v. Self Check in / Check out

Self Check out/ in is also an another feature of RFID system. User can check out the books/ materials himself/ herself without any assistance from library. User can check out more than one book at one tme and all the books being checking out will be read by the device of the system. This system is a fast, versatile checkout solution that is so intuitive it virtually assures first-time success. A touch screen is also part of it, which is easy- to- use and all the instructions are given on it. Similarly user can self check in the books etc. back in the library.

v.i. Dimensions of Self Check out/ in system

- **Cabinet Only:** 26" d x 36" h x 44" w, (660 mm x 914 mm x 1118 mm)
- **Monitor**: 22.75" h (57.8mm) above counter, High resolution, 15" (381 mm) diagonal, LCD touch screen flat panel display
- **Printer**: 8.5" d x 5.9" h x 6.25" w, (216 mm x 149 mm x 159 mm), Thermal, built into kiosk or standalone

Energy Profile: 100–120 or 200–240 VAC, 50–60 Hz, 3.0/1.5 A

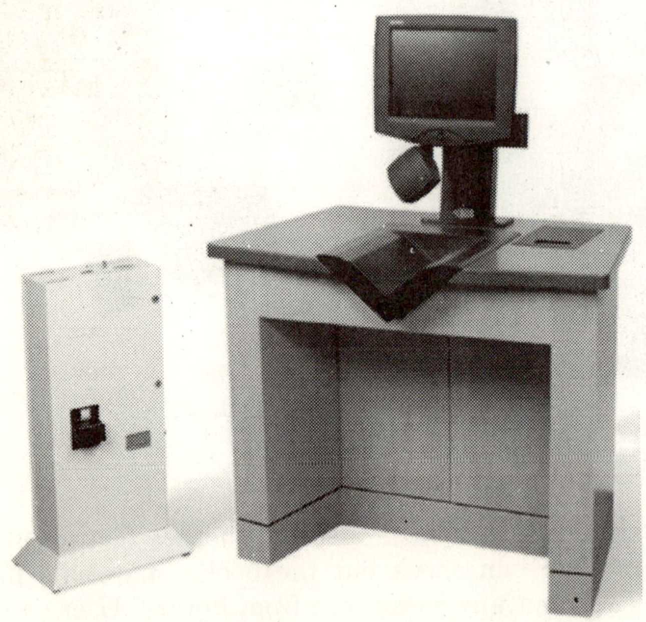

Figure 6.1. Self Check Out/ In System

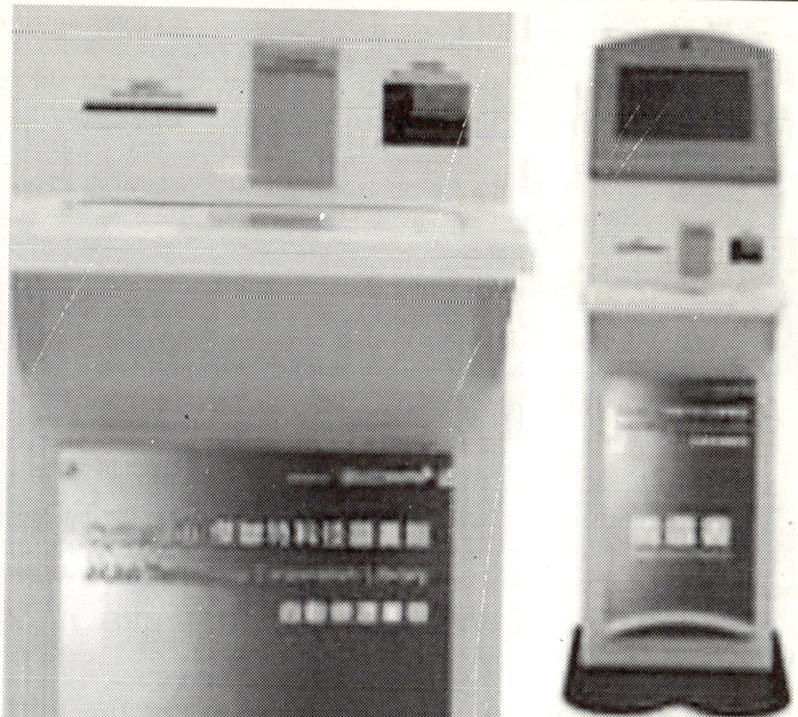

Figure 6.2. Another Model of Self Check Out/ In System

BUDGET FOR RFID SYSTEM

For a library having a collection of 50,000 documents/ books/ other materials , at least the budget mentioned below would be required for the complete RFID system installation in the library :

S.No.	Items required	Quantity	Rate in Rs.	Total Budget in Rs.
01	Tags	50,000	35.00	17,50,000.00
02	Staff Station/Readers	02	1,25,000.00	2,50,000.00
03	Wireless Portable Scanner	01	2,00,000.00	2,00,000.00
04	Server with latest Features	01	6,00,000.00	6,00,000.00
05	Exit Sensors/ Antennae	02	1,50,000.00	3,00,000.00

06	Labour for tagging work (3 tags in one minute)	278 hours	300.00	8.34.000.00
07	Carpentry and Electrical work	--------	---------	1,00,000.00
08	Hand held scanner (in case of Barcodes are also used)	02	10,000.00	20,000.00
09	Books Drop Unit	01	1,75,000.00	1,75,000.00
10	Installation, Training, stationery and other expenses	----------	----------------	1,50,000.00
11	Self Check In/ Check Out Unit	01	1,25,000.00	1,25,000.00
			Total	**45,04,000.00**

Prices are quite tentative. Actual rates are considered according to the firm's invoicing.

LIST OF MANUFACTURERS AND SUPPLIERS OF RFID SYSTEM

Though there are many manufacturers of the RFID system in India, some of them are mentioned below. The components of the RFID system are manufactured by different manufacturers. Before purchasing, the specifications/ configurations and features of the RFID system should be taken care of. Many manufacturers supply the system directly and some of them supply through their agencies.

1. IBM India
   External Relations Manager
   Landline: +91 80 2678 8015
   E-mail: pbalaram@in.ibm.com
2. **ASTER MICRO ELECTRONICS**

   RFID READ/ WRITE UNITS, RFID TAGS, GPS & GSM UNITS, AUTOMATIC VEHICLE LOCATOR, VEHICLE TRACKING SYSTEM RFID TAGS, GPS & GSM UNITS, AUTOMATIC VEHICLE LOCATOR, VEHICLE TRACKING SYSTEM

Products/Services: tags, tracking system, locator, gsm units, ...

Address: 95/6, PUTTENAHALLI, 3RD MAIN ROAD, BANK OF BARODA COLONY, JP NAGAR, 7TH PHASE,BANGALORE560078,KARNATAKA

Phone: 91-80-32949190 **Fax:** +919844116927, Fax :+91-80-4068 4225

Website: http://www.trademart.in/astere2409.htm

3. **ORIZIN TECHNOLOGIES PRIVATE LIMITED**

Manufacturers of all kinds of RFID Readers, Antennas, Hand-held Readers etc
Products/Services : readers, rfid readers, readers etc, antennas, ...

Address: NO.8, OPPOSITE HIGH TENSION LINE NORTH GOKULAM, MYSORE - 570 002, INDIA,
Phone: +(91)-(821)-4258452
Website:http://www.trademart.in/orizintechnologiesprivatelimited.htm

4. **CHIP SILICON PRIVATE LIMITED**

Exporters of auto id products like rfid, smart labels, rf card readers, id card system, barcode, smart cards, proximity cards, mifare cards, magnetic swipe, rf remotes and related accessories. **Products/Services:** related accessories, mifare cards, labels, rfid, ...

Address: C4/1,RAKSHA LEKHA SOCIETY, KOREGAON PARK, PUNE-411001,
Phone: +(91)-(98)-50555711, **Fax:** +(91)-(20)-26141659
Website:
http://www.trademart.in/chipsiliconprivatelimited1.htm

5. **RAPID RADIO SOLUTIONS PRIVATE LIMITED**

RFID READER, RFID TAGS, RFID ANTENNAS, RFID HARDWARE SOLUTIONS RFID READER, RFID TAGS RFID ANTENNAS, RFID HARDWARE SOLUTIONS

Address: B-404, SATYAMEV I, OPP. GUJARAT HIGH COURT, S.G. HIGHWAY, AHMEDABAD, Phone: 917927412256 , Fax: 917927412256
Website: http://www.trademart.in/rapide7383.htm, http://www.trademart.in/rapide7383.htm

6. **KENT SMART CONTROL**

Manufacturers and exporters of rfid card & miare card.

Products/Services: miarecar,

Address: C- 15, SECTOR - 07, NOIDA - 201 301 (UP), Phone: +(91)-(120)-2423191

Fax: +(91)-(120)-2423654, Website: http://www.trademart.in/kentsmartcontrol.htm

7. **SENERGY INTELLUTION PVT. LTD.**

RFID READER,REAL TIMES SYSTEM SOFTWARE EMBEDED ELECTRONICS

Address:112, DAULAT IND. ESTATE, WADHAVALI, CHEMBUR (E), MUMBAI

Phone 912266240969/25558798 **Fax:** 912225558798
Website: http://www.trademart.in/senergye9484.htm

8. **BARTRONICS**

Access Control System+ Bi metrics + Barcode Printers Scanners+ AIDC+ RFID+ Smart

Cards Manufacturing + Solutions with Application And Services

Address: SALTLAKE,KOLKATA (WB)

Phone: 09748314743,**Website:**http://www.trademart.in / bartronics.htm

9. **VALUE ADD SOLUTIONS**

Barcode/RFID Solutions Mobile Computing solutions Wi-Fi Solutions Software development and integration

Address:#8/1, 8TH CROSS ST, LENIN NAGAR, AMBATTUR, CHENNAI- 600053(TN)

Phone: 9840395517,**Website:**http://www.trademart.in/valueaddsolutions.htm

10. **SOFTTECH SOLUTION**

    Zebra Technologies is world leading Barcode & RFID printers manufacturer, SoftTech Solution is authorized Zebra reseller and promoter with authorized Zebra certified & trained engineers. Soft Tech So ...

    Address:174/E, REGENT COLONY, KOLKATA-40 (WB), **Phone:** 9830738263

    Website:http://www.trademart.in/mfiquebal.htm

11.1. M/s 3M India Limited, Concorde Block, UB City, 24, Vittal Mallya Road, Bangalore - 560001 **Tel No** : 0091-80-22231414 / 66595759, **Fax No** : 0091-80-22231450

11.2. M/s 3M India Limited, 2F, M6, Uppal Tower, Jasola District Center, New Delhi - 110076 **Tel No** : 011 405762 01/02/03/04, **Fax No** : 011 4057 6203

11.3. M/s 3M India Limited, Makhija Chambers, 3rd floor, 196 Turner Road, Bandra, Mumbai - 400 050. **Tel No** : 022 - 2655 1883 / 2655 1884, **Fax No** : 022 - 2655 1881

In addition to these Manufacturers/Suppliers, many Suppliers and Vendors are available in the market who are involved in supplying the RFID systems directly or indirectly. Some Library Management Software Suppliers also supply the RFID system. With the help of Internet facilities, one can trace out the supplier as per their requirement.

CONCLUSION

In present IT era, it has become necessary to equip the libraries well with all the latest technologies and electronic equipments, which are helpful in providing updated Library and Information Services to the society. RFID system has given a new dimension to the libraries to cater their users with all the latest tools and equipments. It has changed the entire library system and developed a fully automated system.

The libraries which are progressing towards automation, should install the RFID system in their libraries. With the help of the system, libraries can automate not only the Circulation (Issue/ Return) system of the books etc., but also can save the time of the Library staff and the users. It is also useful in proper shelving of the books and Stock Verification of the holdings. Though the RFID system is costier than the Bar Code Technology and other systems, but it is more reliable and effective. It is a **powerful tool** to control the theft of the holdings.

In India some libraries are using this technology. IIT Madras (Chennai), IIT Mumbai and many more institutes are using this system in their libraries successfully. The cost of the RFID system varies from one company to another. Therefore, it is suggested that before purchasing the system, a comparative statement of latest configurations and cost of the RFID system should be prepared.

REFERENCES

Berkeley Public Library (ND). Berkeley Public Library: Best practices for RFID technology. 2004.

Boss, Richard W. "*RFID Technology for Libraries*" *ALA Tech Notes*, 2004.

Brown, Dennis E. *RFID Implementation.* New Delhi : T.M.H. 2006. Cavoukian, A. Guidelines for using RFID tags in Ontario Public Libraries. Toronto, Ontario: Information and Privacy Commissioner. 2004.

Finkenzeller, Klaus. ***RFID** handbook: Radio-frequency identification fundamentals and Applications* : Chechester: John Wiley. 2000.

Flagg, G. *Should libraries play tag with RFID?* American Libraries, *34(11): 69-71,* Chicago: American Libraries. 2003.

Glover, Bill and Bhatt, Himanshu. *RFID Essentials*. New York: O'Reilly Media, 2006.

Garfinkel, Simon and Rosenberg, Beth. *RFID: Applications, Security, and Privacy.* New Jersy: Pearson Education, Inc. 2005.

Jones, Erick C. and Chung Christopher A. *RFID in Logistics : a practical introduction.* Boca Raton: CRC Press (Taylor and Francis Group). 2007.

Thornton, Frank; Haines Brad and Das, Anand M. ***RFID*** *security.* Mumbai : Shroff Publishers and Distributors Pvt. Ltd. 2006.

Taming e-Resources through Academic Repositories for Knowledge Management

Madan Singh Rana

University Librarian, Banasthali University,
Bansthali-304022 (Rajasthan)
E-mail: msrana_2007@yahoo.co.in

INTRODUCTION

During the last three decades, there have been a lot of changes in library and information activities in the world. The changes in the late 90s and thereafter, have been very fast. Basically, two fundamental changes have been observed by the library: (i) The abundance of thc digital resources and (ii) development of ICTs. The developments in ICTs have forced global information system to settle into new pattern. The major impact of such developments is that the information is now being considered as a 'commodity'. Besides, the world's digital resources are possible to be harnessed by sophisticated search and retrieval mechanism. The old information delivery and seeking methods are being replaced by applying new modified technology-based methods. Now information no longer has a physical existence and it is moving into the cloud.

The tremendous growth of Internet and WWW, high resolution capture devices, highly capable digital storage media, multi-faceted search engines, fast processing power of computer, dropping computer cost and increased band-width network have forced librarians and information professionals to integrate them and develop new methods of archiving and delivery like open access, digital publishing and self archiving and academic digital repositories. Most of the academic and research institutions have signed-up *en masse* the concept of digital library and archive. Institutional repositories are an emerging trend among institutions of higher education as tool to make knowledge bank of an institution's intellectual output to the global community *via* the Internet. By this way, the academic institutions are performing their social obligations to disseminate their research output to a larger clientele. An institutional repository (IR) is a digital collection of a university's scholarly and creative output. Institutional repositories collect, preserve, and make accessible the knowledge, generated by academic institutions. IR is a part of larger global information system of repositories. Therefore, these are indexed in a standardized way and searchable using one interface, providing the foundation for a new model of scholarly publishing.

Taming e-Resources

A diffusion of communication and computational capacity has been increasingly used into a growing part of research, learning and social activities. The diffused network has changed, how we co-ordinate our resources to achieve goals in order to utilize time and space. Most of the users, especially students of 'generation Y' are results-oriented and value convenience. As a result of this, socialization, personalization and location awareness become increasingly very important. Libraries have been working to develop network-ready services and as recent communication technology intensifies this activity, adds new challenges, promotes and needs to get relevance quickly.

Further, due to open source software and open access movement like institutional repositories, gateways, portals, etc., a plethora of information, more precisely e-information is available to the patrons. Such electronic information can be categorized into e-resources based on print resources like e-books, e-journals etc. and non-print e-resources like e-portals, subject gateways, Wikis, Search engines, etc. The e-resources are mushrooming day by day to such an extent that their proper organization would not only be a priority but also a basic requirement of library professionals for their survival in the present era of machine-engineering model of information handling. Many information providers and developers think that technology has sufficient capabilities to handle information in terms of its organization and access. Actually, they consider information as a 'data' which can be easily structured, captured and stored on machine. But the fact is that as we know, there is a difference between data and information. Since the information is being created by human so it is essential to be handled by human as an intermediary with the help of machine. So the term 'information explosion' can be replaced by 'information abundance'. Because an explosion is not due to information '*per se*' but it is due to unorganized or badly organized information.

In the present era, information professionals must be equipped with tools necessary to manage information resources on the internet. Open source software offers a wide spectrum of such tools and enables us to organize and manage the e-resources properly. Such software and tools provide cost-effective and technically feasible solution for creating high quality subject gateways, portals and institutional repositories, etc. The role of library professionals has been becoming very important as being trained in knowledge organization, faceted way of classification, cataloguing, using control vocabularies etc. So they can organize these resources keeping in view of user-centric approach. For proper information advocacy and marketing of e-resources, there are so many new and interactive tools available now on the internet like weblog, RSS feeds, e-mails, etc.

Davenport (1997) in his book 'Information Ecology', rightly said that information should be organized and handled through in view of ecological approach where the external environment keep on influencing to internal environment. They should be considered as complementary and supplementary to each other. The proper information strategy, communication among the staff (top to bottom and vise versa) and more importantly, the user-centric view of information architecture are the key factors in the present e-environment. Besides, the library professionals are not only intermediary where good knowledge of sources and understanding the requirements are important, but also their role as trainer, evaluator, negotiator, project manager; innovator, fund raiser etc. are inevitable. Further, a role of team player working with colleagues in the library, computer centres, academics and other information providers and aggregators would be increasingly important. Such collaboration and building partnership would be in the interest of the libraries and also certainly helpful in enhancing the visibility and credibility of librarianship. The direct outcomes of such collaborations would be helpful in enhancing the quality of services, buying power of libraries, improvement in quality of collection and collaboration among the staff to work as a team. Such a multi-dimensional collaboration will definitely provide an impetus to enhance to maturity of librarianship as a profession and gain serious professional discipline.

Present scenario is of e-resources and India is not far beyond so far as technical advancement is concerned. LIS professional should be ready with technological application in their work environment more especially with Internet and its attributes. As our role is defined we work as information intermediary. We must track the roots of information generation, distribution and dissemination. Virtually internet has become the only source of information store house, data mining and cultivation of information in the 21st century. We all the librarians hold the ethical responsibility how quick we reach to our patrons. The time factor plays a vital role as it elevates our societal responsibility or it can down grade our image. By looking at the above gamut of issues defined and redefined our responsibilities. E-resou-rces, the buzz word has made more prompt, smarter to satisfy the users. At the other hand, the patrons also take the path of technical advancement and well equipped with latest laptop to palmtop with hi-fi connectivity. The local area network has become a common phenomenon in every higher learning institute.

Gradually, we have overcome the possibilities of availing e-resources at our end-user point as e-products are of foreign origin. Now it is the time of open sources. The open sources have got its momentum by virtue of its more and more democratic features. The slogan 'more information to more people' has reached its point of zenith. Now, the digital device is no more. Paying heavy and exorbitant for buying the e-products has vanished. So we are overload with galaxy of e-products freely at our door-step. The question is how to store, orga-nize, administer, filter and reaching with accuracy to our users. More solution to these problems is the success story of the contemporary librarians.

Solution: finding solution to this problem is neither easy and nor even feasible. The professional compulsion, ethical responsibilities and working along with technological develo-pment has become real threats before us. There are few possible solutions:

1. *Self archive:* Self archive is a term which is defined in a way every information producer more simply who prod-uces academic research papers, articles or any other write-ups should collect his/her own publications on the net. It is simply the one-line version of maintaining the files and folders in our personal computers. Certain tags or keywords can be given for indexing these archives. Mostly the name of scholar and his affiliation with the institutions e.g. M.S. Rana and Banasthali University

can be two major keywords for if M.S. Rana is self archivist. Other users can gradually come to know by any work and institution. Same way others will be maintaining their own archives.

2. *Institutional repositories:* As we have discussed above, self-archive solution method that it would be cumbersome to maintain a large self-archivist. To reduce the problem why can't as the individual archivist join together under the same banner may be the name of the institutions e.g. Banasthali University. If this process continues all the institutions in that case universities and colleges will be ready with their own institutional repositories. Again some indexing term can represent the respective institutional repositories so that control over e-resources explosion can be temped to some extent.

Institutional Repository (IR)

Repository means formally organized and managed collection of digital content generated by faculty, staff and students at an institution. The main purpose of institutional repositories is to bring together and preserve the intellectual output of a laboratory, department and academic community.

IR is a set of services that an institute offers to the members of its community for the management and dissemination of digital materials created by the institution and its community. IR may contain the intellectual works of faculty and students – both research and teaching material and also documentation of the activities of the institution itself in the form of records of events and performance and of the ongoing intellectual life of the institution. IR may also contain experimental and observational data captured by members that supports scholarly activities and to preserve them and make them available to the members of their communities and to the public.

According to the SPAR, an IR is `a digital archive of the research output of faculty, researchers, and students of an institution and usually accessible freely to end user both within and outside of the institution'. It is supported by a set of information technologies, but an important part is services that comprise the management of technological changes, and the migration of digital content from one set of technologies to the next as part of the organizational commitment for providing repository services.

Institutional Repository (IR) has emerged as a new model for Scholarly Publishing and Communication. IR is becoming popular in institutions of higher education as it has potential to bring significant benefits to institutions (e.g. imposed visibility, status and public value, and effective knowledge management) and also individual researchers (e.g. impact of research). In India, however, it still depends on the more traditional information sources. Though a lot of good work is being carried out by the institutes but never reaches to the user community, simply has not been published. The classified reports containing valuable data or information are lost forever due to the security reasons. But, it is well known fact that the development of nations now depends upon their ability to compete in the knowledge society.

Essential elements of IR

A digital institutional repository could be any collection of digital material hosted, owned or controlled, or disseminated by an institute. So, the content of an institutional repository is:

- Institutionally defined - IR represent an historical and tangible embodiment of the intellectual life and output of an institution;
- Scholarly content - This may include pre-prints and other works-in-progress, peer reviewed articles,

monographs, conference papers, theses and dissertations, etc.

- Cumulative and perpetual - IR aims to preserve and make accessible digital content on a long-term basis; and
- Open and interoperable - IR systems must be able to support interoperability in order to provide access via multiple search engines and other discovery tools.

Contents of an Institutional Repository

- Pre-prints of articles or research reports submitted for publication.
- The text of articles accepted for publication in journal.
- Revision of published work with comments for academic readers.
- Conference paper.
- Teaching materials.
- Students projects.
- Doctorial thesis and dissertations.
- Databases resulting for research projects.
- Committee paper.
- Computer software.
- Works of art.
- Photographs and video recordings.

Setting-up an IR requires infrastructural resources, like:

- Repository server with support for fault tolerant operation and adequate network bandwidth.
- Human resources– Appropriate manpower for installation, configuration and administration of the

repository software and server, and manpower for content management and collection development.

- Management commitment and long term funding support.
- Development of policies, metadata and cataloguing.
- Selection of repository software system.
- Advocacy for getting content by encouraging researches and faculty members to participate in IR.
- Dissemination and extension of services.

"Library is a growing organism", as one of S.R. Ranganathan's five laws of library science were written in 1931. This indicates that the library must be willing to adapt new conditions (changing social and technological conditions as well as changing needs among its clientele), if it is to meet its goal of maximizing accessibility and exposure while minimizing the user's time and effort. Moreover, now information is considered as one of the natural resource. So, developing digital repositories system would be an essential to make information resource more accessible. It would be a collaborative effort of major stake–holders, who can play an important role in developing IR, such as– Librarian and Library staff, IT personnel, faculty, researchers, students, administration & Finance, etc.

Key issues related to IR

- Proper policies related to types and formats of documents to be considered for IR, along with issues, like user permissions and rights, peer-review and quality assessment of open access material. It is suggested that for perpetual license, the author should be asked to grant the right to the institution to preserve and distribute the research and others work through IR.
- Organization of content : It is a well known fact that finding information on the Internet is only half job done. Researchers and scientists spend more time in

analyzing information than finding it. Therefore, organization of content, cataloguing, meta-data and assigning subjects may be properly planned and implemented. Otherwise, we may require human search engine for analyzing information for researchers and scientists.

- Selection of IR software and other related requirements would be clear and fully identified.
- Administration and maintenance of IR : Identify a suitable person as an in-charge who would be responsible for collection development, promotion and dissemination of services

The libraries have primarily been engaged in developing, organizing and managing scholarly contents as one of the most important responsibilities in their job card. LIS professionals are being considered as one of the front line professionals accepting new technology got improving their library management and services. They, with such a bent of mind, can play vital role in developing IRs for scholarly publications rather than any other. Therefore, they can treat these challenges as the opportunities to make their presence in the society.

There are number of softwares available in market for Institutional Repository. Some of them are on payment basis and some are freely downloaded software for example: D-Space, GNU E-prints, CD-Sware, Fedora, and Greenstone. Among them D-Space, Greenstone and E-print are free software.

CONCLUSION

ICT has changed the whole library and information landscape in the world. However, in the developing countries in general and India in particular, the situation is not much encouraging expect some national institutions and well reputed universities which have started to work in developing which digital repositories. But, the trend towards in the direction shows that very soon a large number of the academic institutions will join their hands in the movement and get their visibility of academic importance published and make the research output available to the worldwide. Time has come to make it not only mandatory but also compulsory for universities.

In the present context knowledge is considered one of the important primary production resource for the development of nation. It is only possible when India's indigenous achievements in the field of Science and Technology are available in electronic format and disseminated to researchers and information professionals in both India and to the wider scientific world. An effort needs to be done collectively to preserve and share our invaluable knowledge globally and over come a serious barrier of digital divide. According to R.N. Mashelkar, if India plays its card right it can become by 2020 the world's number one knowledge production centre. So, IRs can play an important role to accelerate the use of electronic information resources in Indian libraries and research centres to become the centre of excellence for knowledge workers, innovators of the future, and hub of global R & D activities.

REFERENCES

1. Bhogle, Srinivas, Ed (2005). Turning Pages; reflections in Infotimes. Bangalore.
2. Centre for Science & Environment (2005). Basics of Digital Library (course material).
3. Crow, Raym (2002). The case for Institutional repositories: A SPARC position paper.
4. Davenport, Thomas H. (1997). Information ecology: mastering the information and knowledge environment. Oxford University Press, New York, 255p.
5. Perera (Kamini). E-resources: One stop shopping of big shopping mall for scholarly communication. In Kataria (Sanjay), Nigam (B S) and Shukla (Rama Kant), Ed. Emerging

trends and technologies in libraries and information services. KBD Publications; New Delhi, 2009. 576-582 p.

6. Rajashekar, T.B. (2004). Institutional repositories: Improving preservation, organization and dissemination of institutional research (tutorial). ICDL 2004, TERI: (New Delhi).
7. Rajashekar, T.B. (2004). Institutional repositories. U & I (January issue).

Digital Revolution and Indian Academic Libraries in the 21st Century : Need for Innovative Services

S.S. Pawar & Monika Sharma***

*Deputy Librarian, CAS in Geology, Panjab University, Chandigarh - (INDIA).

**Librarian, UIET, Panjab University, Chandigarh (INDIA)

ABSTRACT

The information era with its electronic facilities emerged with many challenges in all sectors. Business, education, training, researches-indeed, all aspects of life-are increasingly affected by electronic networks and multimedia technologies, which are opening up new vistas, like digital libraries (DLS), knowledge management (KM), E-learning (EL), and E-archiving (EA). All these and many such initiatives may help libraries realizing the vision of anytime, anywhere access to the best and latest of human thought and information. Hence libraries are emerging as crucial components of global information infrastructure.

The world is embossed with the new technological era that the library professional is confronted today with the technology. Myriad kind of technology is available now and technological innovations are bound to occur in future. These innovations and innovative ideas including, artificial intelligence, robotics, speech synthesis, electronic mail, CD-

Rom, CD networking, barcode system, electronic publishing, hypermedia, multimedia, tale facsimile, radio data paging, networks, etc. are sharing common technology revolving around electronics, computers, telecommunication, printing and reprography, popularly known as Information and Communication Technology (ICT). Technology is driving change across the entire range of library responsibilities. Today, University libraries are emerging as information services centers, providing electronic cataloguing (OPAC), electronic acquisition, serial control, electronic inter-library loan and electronic circulation functions.

INTRODUCTION

Academic libraries are considered as hub of the academic institutions and are supporting teaching, research, and other academic programmes. With the advent of Information and Communication Technology (ICT), the nature of libraries has dramatically changed. Computers are being used in libraries to process, store, retrieve and disseminate information. Majority of the university libraries offer internet facilities to their users and some are having their web site and providing web-based library and information services.

The pace of technology innovation in libraries has steadily accelerated over the past decade. Now library work itself is changing, with technological innovation leading to design of new services for users. As a result, new roles for librarians have also emerged in facilitating access to, and navigation of electronic collections and other resour-ces. The modern electronic library has much more to offer in terms of service modalities and options for users.

The Indian university libraries are in the process of restructuring their facilities and work processes, remodeling their factions and re-engineering their services to facilitate their enhanced role in the new information environment. A number of libraries are digitizing their uniquely held collections. To facilitate compact storage of information, they are even converting their print archives of information to CD-ROMs and DVD. Development of databases, application of expert systems, mobile computing and more focused flow of specific information through intranets is likely to have further impact on the way services are offered to information user communities. Besides INFLIBNET, several library and information networks have been developed in view of the importance and need of sharing of available resources. The existing ones include, NICNET (National Informatics Center's Network), INDONET, ERNET (Education and Research Network), DELNET (Developing Library Network), etc. A number of educational institutions are members of such networks.

The Traditional Knowledge Digital Library (TKDL), a project of NISCAIR (CSIR) INDEST (Indian digital library in Engineering Services Technology) is being planned to provide access to electronic resources in Science and Technology; Engineering and Management in India. CSIR is engaged in a project to provide access to e-journals in the country. The Prime Minister on Feb. 8.2004 launched National Mission for Manuscripts by Department of Culture, Government of India.

The Govt. of India and University Grants Commission (UGC) have given prime importance for upgrading the university libraries to meet the changing needs of their users. In this Context, the prime minister of India constituted National Knowledge Commission (NKC) in 2005, which is focused on - access to knowledge, knowledge concepts, knowledge creation, knowledge application and development of better knowledge services. This includes a variety of subject areas such as language, translations, libraries-networks, portals, affirmative action, distance e-learning, intellectual property, e-governance etc. One of the key to this effort is to build a national broadband gigabite of networks of 500 nodes to connect universities, Libraries, to share resources to meet the challenges of the knowledge economy in the 21st Century and increase India's competitive advantage in the global market.

2. CHANGING SCENARIO

Library services have been tremendously influenced by rapid technological innovations over the years. The Internet has virtually provided a new dimension to every area of the library services and operations.

2.1 Change of information needs : The users need more precise current and factual information and they need it fast.

2.2 Change of information habits : The users especially younger users are more comfortable with digital resources than printed bibliographies or traditional catalogues.

2.3 Open to all: The ``library without walls is not just a term. Via Open Public Access Catalogue (OPAC) and home-pages, libraries become more visible and accessible than ever before.

2.4 Networking : It is no longer important what a library has but more important to what sources a library can provide access.

In the electronic environment, a library researcher has the control of browsing the information in whatever direction they choose. The 24/7 availability of the Web provides patrons with the opportunity to conduct library research anytime. This has resulted in library patrons expecting 24/7 accesses to not only the library electronic collections, but also online help or other forms of mediation as and when needed.

About ten years ago, libraries had a collection `Just in case'; should someone ask for a certain subject, there would be a stock of carefully chosen books, bibliographies and other materials readily available. Five years ago, libraries began to work `just in since then, upon request, the best and most up-to-date materials are gathered to answer the demand. Today, we are heading towards service `Just foe you'; knowing the customer and his or her information needs, libraries will provide tailor-made services.

During 90s with pc revolution, development of high speed LAN, growth of Internet and Internet base services the professional started thinking of news services.

Changes experienced in libraries.

80s	90s	2000
Print	CD Rom	web based
Library Catalogue	OPAC	Web
Manual indexing bibliographies	Index based databases	Full text databases
Closed access	Open Access	24 x 7 x 365 access from Anywhere
Reference Desk	Telephone, fax based Ref. service	On-line reference service
Inter library loan	Document Delivery	Electronic Delivery services
Manual sharing of resources	Cooperation movement	Dedicated library networks
Paper based collection	Hybrid collection	Digital library, Virtual Library

3. INTERNET AND WEB BASED SERVICES

Libraries are mainly entrusted with a host of predetermined tasks like acquiring, organizing, preserving, retrieving and disseminating information to the users. Right from ancient times to the present Internet era, the primary objective of library has always been this. However, the way this purpose has been achieved has drastically changed. Libraries are undergoing significant changes today not only in outlook but also in function, services, methods and techniques for collection development, processing and dissemination of information. Librarians are exploring ways of supporting patrons in the emerging virtual communities such as offering online and real-time reference service. This way, the user can get assistance from the reference librarian without physically coming to the library. The terms `Live reference, Virtual reference, Digital reference, Online reference, Electronic reference, and Remote reference are often used for similar services (Internet Based).

Today, the most Indian University libraries have its own web site and provide access to various resources, like :

PUNJAB UNIVERSITY LIBRARY: (http://www.library.puchd.ac.in) The University Library is fully computerized with an integrated system connected to the campus Network providing internet and e-mail facility to the university community. The reference collection of the library is continuously updated, and augmented with the acquisition of CD-ROM databases and access to on-line databases on Internet. On-line Public Access Catalogue (OPAC) facility is available at the Reference Desk on the First Floor of the library. OPAC can also be accessed through any terminal on the campus network. Library collection can also be searched through **Web OPAC.**

Electronic Journals

UGC - Infonet : E-journals Consortium : These are the periodical publications which are available online through internet or through CD-ROM. Under the e-journals consortium around 45000 full text scholarly journals from 25 publishers across the world can be accessed. It provides current as well as archival access and most of the areas of learning like Arts, Humanities, Social sciences, and Sciences etc. are covered.

INDEST Journals : University libraries are also accessing e-journals available through INDEST consortium, which is setup by the Ministry of Human Resource Development as the : Indian Digital library in Engineering science and technology Consortium. The Library subscribes to about

600 current periodicals. Its holdings of back volumes of periodicals go back to nineteenths century. Library subscribes to **MathSciNet** online comprising of current Mathematical publications & Mathematical Reviews, and has access to 225 Online full text journals as part of print journals subscription. Now University library is ready for providing INFO-RESOURCE SHARING free of cost to the students, with research journals from 23 universities from across India.

Online Books : It further provides link to the digital book index which provides links to Approximately seven lakhs records of books, periodicals and thesis is web-based and can be accessed through OPAC anywhere on 24 x 7 basis under the GUC-INFONET Consortium.

Subject Gateways : The value of website as information sources for libraries has been greatly increase with the emergence of gateways, Portals and votals These services provide structured access to other related website and save the time of the user by not wasting his time in selection process that is used to select a site. Links to PSIgate, EEVL SOSIG etc information gateways have been provided.

INFLIBNET : Information and Library Network Center : www.inflibnet.ac.in Developed by the UGC in collaboration with NISSAT. This digital library network is probably one of the most full-fledged steps towards digital libraries in India. Major activities of this association include Library Automation, Database Creation, Software Development, Human Resources Development, Information Services and Networking. They have created a software SOUL that is based on a rational database management language, which is used for cataloguing, archiving as well as online public access of resources.

DELNET Databases : Developing Library Network : DELNET is the first major operational library network in the South Asia Connecting more than 1140 libraries as its members which include 175 libraries in Delhi, 950 libraries outside Delhi in 30 States and Union Territories and 16 in overseas Countries. DELNET provides access to more than seven million bibliographic records of books, journals, articles etc.

4. FUTURE LOGISTICS

1. The need for a consortium : Access to resources is now considered more important than collection building especially, if the access is perpetual in nature. The consortium facilitates the libraries to get the benefit of wider access to electronic resources at affordable cost and at the best terms of licenses. A consortium of various institutions available to it, is in a better position to address and resolve the problems of managing, organizing and archiving the electronic resources. Moreover, the technology has changed expectations of researchers, their patience and their willingness to accept services that are available on demand. The Web-based electronic resource is an apt answer to the expectations of researchers.

2. Strategic Planning : A process to develop formal strategic and operating plans, including establishment of mission and vision statements that position the library as a central element within the academic mission of the university.

3. Staff Development Program : Keeping in view the changing scenario and new responsibilities, the existing staffing pattern, duties and qualifications of library staff in university libraries should be reviewed and altered wherever required to meet the new challenges.

A system should be set up to foster close-operation between the teaching/research faculty and librarians at all academic and research institutions, by measures such as :

i. Mobility of staff (in terms of recruitment and in terms of teaching) should be made possible.

ii. Practicing librarian and experts should be associated with the teaching faculty for offering specialized courses.

iii. Similarly, teachers could be associated with libraries may be treated consultants, for carrying out projects, and for carrying out continuing education programmes for library staff etc.

4. Know your Users and Keep them Close : If there is a common message across from all those thinking deeply about the future of libraries, it is that we need to be more deeply involved with our users to really understand how their work patterns are changing, to anticipate their future requirement and how information services can be better integrated with the increasingly digital life-style of new generations of students, researchers and knowledge workers.

5. Expand faculty Interactions : Librarians should find ways to work more closely and collaboratively with faculty (e.g. to develop program to instruct faculty in the use of new resources and technologies)

6. Develop new Approaches to Reference Services : Librarian should begin to explore the many new models for reference assistance that are being pursued at academic libraries throughout the country.

7. Involve Librarians in Curriculum Development : University curriculum committee should include librarian as ex-officio member so that the importance of library resources is always considered.

8. Improve Stack Services and Material Availability : The innovations in this include installation of phone to circulation on each floor so that clients who are unable to locate material or have other information needs can call for assistance rather than having to go down to the other floor to do so and improvement of shelf reading bar of miss-shelved items in the collections.

CONCLUSION

Indian university libraries have an important part to play in innovation agenda. University libraries have been adapting and innovating to ensure the provision of a wealth of information resources in a changing technological environment. Indian University libraries also support innovation in many other ways. Over the past decade, libraries have proven to be effective partners with the Government of India for community development like, delivery and support of a broad range of programs such as E-learning, and delivery of services to rural and remote areas. The University library plays an important role in fostering a knowledge-based society, and significantly contributes to the advancement of innovation in development of library services now and in the future. In this way, Punjab University library takes the challenge to develop strategic plans for harnessing technology to offer viable services in a cost effective manner within the dynamic technology environment.

REFERENCES

Books

Barker, Shirley K. and Jackson, Mary E, (1995). The future of resource sharing. New York, Haworth Information press.

Grosch, A.N. (1995). Library Information Technology and networks. New York, Marcel dekker.

Kaliammal, A. and Thamaraiselvi, G. (2005). Role if ICT in library and information science. Delhi.

Kaul, H.K. (1999). Library Information Sharing and Networks. Virgo publication, New Delhi.

Lee, Sul, H. (2002). Impact of Digital technology on library collection and resources sharing. New York, Haworth information press.

Journals/Proceedings/Reports/etc.

Arora, J. (2005). Managing electronic resources through consortia : an overview, in library and information Networking-NACLIN-2005; PP 145-170.

Chowdhury, Gobinda, G. (2002). Digital libraries and reference services : present and future, Journal of Documentation, vol. 58, No. 3, pp. 258-283.

Glenda, A. Thornton (2000). Impact of Electronic resources on collection development, the role of libraries and library Consortia. ``Library Trends" Vol. 48, No. 4 pp. 842-856.

Jebaraj, F. (2003). ``The Electronic Library : An Indian Scenario". Library Philosophy and Practice. V5. N2. Spring 2003.

Krishnamurthy, M. and Chan, W.S. (2005). Implementation of library portals for Information resources : A case study of the Indian Statistical Institute, Ban galore, (ISIB). International Information and Library Review, 37, No. 1, pp. 45-50.

Lynch, C. (2005). ``Where do we go from here? The next decade for digital libraries" D-lib. Magazine, Vol., 11, No. 7/8.

Moyo, Lesley, M. (2004). Electronic libraries and the emergence of new service paradigms. The Electronic Library, Vol. 22, No. 3, pp. 220-230.

Murthy, T.A.V. (2002). Resource Sharing and Consortia for India. Proceeding, Lit Seminar, Kharagpur, Feb., pp. 14-15.

Sthwartz, C. (2000). ``Digital libraries : an overview,' The Journal of Academic Librarianship. Vol. 26, No. 6, pp. 385-93.

Library Acquisition Policy of National Academy for Legal Studies and Research, Hyderabad : A Case Study

P. Radha

Assistant Librarian, NALSAR, University of Law, Shameerpet,
Hyderabad - 500 078

ABSTRACT

The article discusses acquisition policy of the NALSAR Library. Acquisition policy intends to communicate the methods through library database to all faculty members and other staff who are involved in the development of collection in the library. It clarifies library acquisition procedures followed in the library. It also explains journals acquisition policy. Describes how Virtua - a library management software helps the library in acquiring print resources systematically.

1. INTRODUCTION

NALSAR University of Law, Hyderabad, was established in 1998 under the National Academy of Legal Studies and Research University Act (Andhra Pradesh Act 34 of 1998) of the Andhra Pradesh State Legislature. It has also been recognized by the University Grants Commission under sections 2 (f) and 12 (b) of the UGC Act, 1956. It is a residential university which provides an opportunity to explore limitless options in legal profession and in setting new standards in legal education. The university has as its primary mission to create a generation of able, competent and humane lawyers who will not only enter the Bar and Bench, but will also be equipped to address effectively the imperatives of the new millennium and to engage in community services.

The NALSAR library has an independent building in the heart of the university campus. It comprises three floors spread across an area of 54.323 Sq. Ft. It is a majestic and architectural building. It has a collection of more than 26,000 documents, which includes back volumes of Journals and approximately 6000 Law Reports and Reviews. There are morethan 6000 online journals and nearly a 100 journals in print, which includes both Indian and foreign. The library also has a collection of legal materials in CD-ROM.

There is a reading space for more than 300 users. Wireless run internet facility is available on all the floors of the library. There is separate enclosure with carrels for students and faculty members. There are two Discussion Rooms and two Moot Court Rooms also on the first floor of the library.

All the house keeping activities are automated which are powered by VITRUA of VTLS Inc.; one of the best software. The library has adopted Radio Frequency Identity (RFID) based solutions for its circulation, management, inventory and security systems. Students are provided with RFID equipped identity cards.

The NALSAR library acquisition policy is ``to acquire materials in appropriate formats and in sufficient quantity, depth and diversity to support the academic needs of the faculty and students in the subject areas of the curriculum". In this process, it aims to foster an intellectual partnership with the faculty and the students to become involved in building its collection. The acquistion of library material can be divided into two phases-selection of titles for purchashing and the actual acquisition process. These reading materials may be selected in various ways; by request form faculty and students, by exchanges with other universities and institutions, and as gifts. The acquisition process consists of several stages : verification, ordering, receiving and fund accounting, after which materials move into the processing stages of cataloguing, labeling and shelving. Using a electronic database the library staff verify that the information submitted to them both accurate and complete so that the correct item is ordered.

2. OBJECTIVES

The Following are the objectives of acquisition policy :

- Acquire materials in appropriate formats and in sufficient quantity, depth, and diversity to support teaching in the subject areas of the curriculum.
- Organize collections logically, making materials available for use in a timely and efficient manner.
- Assure equitable and unbiased access for patrons of the institute to the library's collections and services.
- Provide guidance to readers in the identification, interpretation and use of library materials and information.
- Provide the expertise necessary to support the development, preservation, and security of the collections.
- House collections in surroundings conductive to their use and preservation.
- Respond to the changing stage of knowledge and the curriculum by continually evaluating collections and services, implementing change as appropriate.
- Establish and maintain cooperative agreements for resource sharing with other libraries and organizations.

3. ACQUISITION OF MONOGRAPHS

The academic staff or the students recommending books have to furnish information about the title, author, publisher, edition, number of copies and price if known or initiate dialogue with the librarian about the information and then get formal approval by the convenor of the librry committee. The committee reviews requests and recommendation from faculty and students. It will seek to acquire them unless they fail to meet the library's collection development guidelines. Not all requests can be granted, there may be an alternative to acquisition. Such as inter-library loan. The library processes the request and review it against the selection parameters. The library normally purchases books and reference materials pertaining to the subjects of the curriculum.

The suggested books should be :

- Relevant to the curriculum;
- Support for needs of students;
- Support for faculty course preparation; and
- Relationship to existing holding.

The library does not reimburse faculty who purchase a book for the library. Exceptions can be made only if pre-approval has been taken from the library. It is much more efficient and cost-effective for the library to purchase materials directly from wholesale book vendors. The library receives significant discount, does not pay for tax, shipping and handling, and has time and cost-efficient means to pay these vendors. The library receives significant discounts, does not pay tax, shipping and handling, and has time and cost-efficient means to pay these vendors. The library takes 4 to 6 weeks to acquire a foreign publications and 2 to 4 weeks for the Indian counterpart.

3.1 On Approval

The titles are selected from the new catalogues on the basis of the subject by the faculty. These are again cross checked with the existing collection in the library database for any duplication. These books are kept before the Library Committee for approval. Purchase order is prepared in the database and order is placed for the approved titles. Sometimes, when new titles appear in the publishing world, a display is arranged with booksellers in the library to facilitate the faculty to browse them before recommending to the title for its acquisition.

3.2 Ordering

Upon receiving the request from the faculty member, a purchase order is placed with the approved vendors who are identified to supply the books. The Purchase orders are generated with the information about the title, author, edition, publisher, no. of copies. Information about price if known would be mentioned. The original copy is given to the vendor.

- Only one copy of each book shall be supplied or otherwise stated.
- Only one copy of each title shall be supplied unless mentioned otherwise.
- Publisher's price should only be charged and price proof should be shown. Conversion rate shall be followed as agreed upon by UGC/GOC/Bank conversion from time to time.
- For Indian publications-percent and for foreign publication-percent discount has to be given. For sets and law reports-percent discount shall be applicable.
- If books are not supplied within 45 days, the book order shall be treated automatically cancelled. The same order shall be given to the other library supplier.
- Damaged, disfigured, broken binding of books shall not be accepted. If noticed after stamping such books shall have to be taken back at your expense.
- Please give your IT/PAN Number on the bill.

- Your printed bill should have enough space for stamping and processing as well as it should have been neatly typed.
- Dollar/Pound and Euro Dollar Currencies shall be charged for the books belonging to the countries of publications.
- The university shall not pay for any freight charges, insurance money or postal charges.

3.3 Receiving the Titles and Tallying

The invoice is to be submitted by the vendor in triplicate. The books are tallied with bill, the order list and their editions and imprints are verified. The tallying work includes the tallying of the prices of the books. The price is to be found from publishers' or bookseller's catalogues. If any discrepancies in prices are found, the bookseller is asked to supply the documentary proof in support of the price charged. The conversion rates are tallied with the latest GOC (Good Offices Committee) rates.

3.4 Accessioning

The books after being checked and tallied with bill are accessioned. A stock register is maintained in the library, which is known as Accession Register. Each book is entered with a unique number consecutively. This number is stamped on the titled page, verso of the title page of the book, on secret page and as well as on the last page of the book. The librarian certifies the bill that : books received are in good condition and have been entered in the accession register vide accession numbers. It also mentions about the quoted prices and approved rates of conversion as per GOC.

3.5 Processing of Bills

- A copy of Purchase Order issued by the library, and the proof of approval (request form bearing the signature of the authorities) are sent to the Registrar for his verification and signature.

- An original invoice along with a copy of a purchase order is sent to the Accounts Section for payment.
- Patrons can view the titles for which the order is placed and get to know its status of item in the online catalogue. However, it is not possible to notify individually to the patron upon the receipt of the title in the library.
- The Accession section maintains a separate purchase order file for checking and verification.

3.6 Technical Processing of Monographs

The following functions are performed in the acquisition and technical section by the staff.

- Circulating the publishers catalogue and other selection tools among the faculty.
- Placing purchase orders for approved titles received form the approving authority.
- Receiving, invoicing and accessioning the titles in printed register as well as the database.
- Physically processing the books by stamping, putting RFID tag, laminating, pasting various labels and due date slips.
- Keeping the track of budget spent under the each heads like NALSAR Account and UGC Account for a financial year.
- Sending reminders and keeping track of purchase orders placed or non-supply of books.
- Generate various acquisition reports like New Accession List, Order Status etc., through the library database.
- Catalogue the titles received for online public access, according to MARC21 in the library database Virtua.

4. ACQUISITION OF JOURNALS

The library subscribesd to sixty national and nine international journals. These are meant for library reference only. The table of contents of each issue is scanned and uploaded on the library portal. It also subscribes a few magazines for general interest of students and teachers.

The following procedure is involved :

- The request for subscription of journals is reviewed in the Library committee and before placing the order for subscription, a specimen copy is requested from the concerned publisher.
- The subscription of journals is entrusted to a reputed agent on behalf of the library and they update us on the received issues, missing issues and notify on the availability of online access and any change in the publication pattern of the journal during the subscription year. Some times subscription is made directly to the publisher itself also.
- The selected agency make upfront payment to the publishers which will be reimbursed by the library after the agent shows price proofs and proper documents of payment towards subscription to the publisher.

5. CONCLUSION

The acquisition policy of NALSAR Library through library database has brought tremendous benefits in collection development by controlling the collection of information by imposing rigorous book selection, effective search strategies, establishing linkages with remote databases, updating information collection, keeping users aware of new additions of information in the storage device. It has saved the time of the library users and academic staff. It has benefited the staff by reducing the workload which involves automatic generation of reminders to the vendors for the missing issues of journals and cancellation of purchase orders after the stipulated time. The users or patrons can view the OPAC termination from any where in the world for the status of the books, journals and electronic resources. So, it would be best practice in libraries to acquire books through library database and achieve better results.

REFERENCES

Brophy, Peter, "*The Academic Library*"; London : Facet, 2005.

NALSAR Library Information brochure, 2009. Hyderabad, NALSAR.

Thomas, Philip A., "How to Use a Law Library : an Introduction to Legal Skills", London : Sweet & Maxwell, 2001.

Indian Agricultural Research Institute Library : A Profile

Sunita Gupta* and Praveen Mahajan**

*Technical Officer (T-7/8) and ** Technical Officer (T-5)
IARI Library, Pusa, New Delhi - 110012

ABSTRACT

The paper traces the success story of IARI library since its birth in 1905 at Pusa, Bihar. Provides brief information about its unique and rare collection comprising of books, serials, series publications, report literature, theses, rare books and non-book material. It highlights the linkages of IARI library at national and international level. Presently the library has been computerized and offers its services through - OPAC, CD-ROM workstation and CD-ROM data-bases, Online journl subscription, E-mail, internet browsing, website access facilities to research scholars and scientists of IARI. Discusses its role in education, training services, and library publications. The paper also regrets to mention the pathos of libraries which is a black spot shining on great agricultural system in the country. Authors have made a few suggestions for improvement of library services, collection development and status of library staff.

1. HISTORIC LOOK

The Indian Agricultural Research Institute (IARI) is a premier and the oldest agricultural institute in the country. Its Central Library works as the nerve center of research, education and extension activities of the institute. The library provides classic as well as latest literature to fulfill information needs of research managers, policy-makers, scientists, teachers, technical staff, students, research scholars, extension workers and educated farmers.

The Library as an organ of the institute was established at Pusa (Bihar) with a small collection of 5000 publications donated by the Secretry, Department of Agriculture, Government of India in 1905 (IARI Report, 1907-09). In 1934a devasting earthquake damaged the main building known as Phipps Laboratory, then the Govt. of India decided to shift the institute along with the Library to its present campus in New Delhi.

The institute comprising of library and some more buildings was inaugurated on November 7, 1936 by the then Viceroy Lord Linlithgo and the library was named after him as Linlithgo Library with 70,000 volumes shifted from PUSA (Bihar). The inauguration stone mounted on a podium may still be seen kept in the library, which was laid down on April 1, 1905 by Nithniel Curzon. The Viceroy and Governor General of India. The main building of then Agricultural Research Institute at PUSA was also known as Naulakha having 5 major divisions (i) Agronomy (ii) Soil Chemistry (iii) Botany (iv) Entomology (v) Mycology. Library building at PUSA campus in New Delhi is the icon of IARI (IARI Report, 1937). In 1947 the name of Imperial Agricultural Research Institute was changed to Indian Agricultural Research Institute. IARI was accorded the status of a deemed to be university in 1958 under the UGC Act of 1956 and since 1958 it started Ph.D. degree programme along with M.Sc. courses. At present the institute library works as a part of and under PG school providing information support to the clientele of IARI, users from different parts of India and abroad.

The Indian Agricultural Research Institute Library has been keeping pace for the lst over 100 years with the ever growing needs of the scientific community and has asumed *the de facto* status of National Agricultural Library of India and has been regarded as one of the 10 best agro-biological libraries of the world as well as the finest and the richest agricultural library in the South-East Asia. Library reading halls and Council Room were enriched by a collection of the finest paintings of Russian Painter Nicholas Roerich, and Mr. Brewster, Mr. Bireeswar Sen and other artists, generously presented by Dr. M.S. Randhawa, Deputy Commissioner of Delhi in 1947 (IARI Report, 1947). The country witnessed ``Green Revolution" during 1967-1968 to which this library played a significant role as a Think-Tank. Smt. Indira Gandhi, the then Prime Minister of India released a postal stamp in 1968 commemorating the ``Wheat Revolution" depicting IARI Library clock-tower-Icon of IARI (IARI Report, 1968).

2. UNIQUE COLLECTION OF THE LIBRARY

2.1 Book Collection

Indian Agricultural Research Institute Library today has a specialized research collection of over 6,00,000 publications consisting of books, mono-graphs, reference books, journals, advances and annual reviews, abstracting and indexing journals, conference proceedings, statistical publications, research bulletins (series publications), reports, reprints, post graduate theses of IARI and ICAR research fellowship theses and non book material, etc. in agricultural and biological sciences. The collection gets enriched annually at the rate of 3,000 to 5,000 documents. Library has nearly 1,30,000 accessioned books, monographs and textbooks.

Rare Collection : The library has no parallel in the country so far as its old literature is concerned. It has large number of rare and valuable publications such as :- (i) J. Gerrd's Herbal - ``*A General History of Plants*'' (1957), Norton Co., London in original. It is the first book ever published in the discipline of agriculture. (ii) ``*Philosophical Transactions of the Royal Society*'', London Vol. 1 April 1665-66. The first ever published English language scientific journal. The library gets this series of proceedings till date since beginning. The reference books collection (3500 volumes) comprises of bibliographies, handbooks, manuals, dictionaries, encyclopedias, glossaries, directories, year-books, gazetteers, atlses, statisticl data publications, etc.

2.2 Serial Collection

The total files of scientific serials in the library is about 11,000 and the number of current serials subscription has come down to about 250 in the year 2002 from 5,100 from 90 countries in 40 languages in 1972 and earlier. The unique feature of serial acquisition programme is the procurement of the maximum number of publications through exchange and gift by maintaining excellent exchange relations with nearly 300 organizations in the world. The library offers in exchange Annual Report of IARI (149 No.) and (20 No.), journals published by the ICAR (4 No.) and Scientific Societies (11 No.) housed in IARI Campus. The library has a comprehensive collection of Abstracting, Indexing, Advances and Reviewing journals, comprising all CABI journals in the field of Agriculture, Bibliography of Agriculture (USA), Agrindex (FAO), Biological Abstracts (USA) and Chemical Index (1907-1993), and Science Citation Index (1964-1992), which form a large collection of old and current titles to about 7,000 volumes. There were about 35 cover to cover translated journals mostly from Russian language and about 30 reserch newsletters which are of great interest to highly specialized research programmes. Now, most of the translated titles have been stopped. Collection of about 1500 series files of research bulletins mostly field reports from agricultural experiment stations of USA and other foreign countries. Tody, the library has over 4,54,000 accessioned documents in this category of micro literature and currently procuring 500 titles. Retrieval of bulletins is supported by a location list and guide lists. Pamphlets and Reprints Collection contains nearly 5000 documents. Scientific reports, mostly published as annual reports, form a collection of about 20,000 documents arranged on shelves in classified order geographically, supported by catalogue as well as location list placed in stack room itself.

2.3 Theses Collection

IARI library has two groups of P.G. theses, namely, IARI Theses (collection marked T-number) and ICAR Research Fellowship theses (marked RFT-number). Library has a total collection of 16,000 theses (7500 IARI and 9000 RFT). Research fellowship theses are those which are submitted in different Indian Universities against fellowships granted to researchers of ICAR, New Delhi.

2.4 Non-Book Material

The library has large number of non-print material in the form of Microfiches, Microfilms, cassettes, slides, CDs of books and video cassettes, agricultural databases and online search databases i.e. Web of Science, Current Contents Connect etc.

2.5 Organization of the collection

The first scholarly Librarian of the Institute Mr. K.K. Guha Roy in 1930's adopted different methods for organizing various categories of documents on different lines contrary to traditional method of classification. Series publications (Bulletins) were organized according to country, state and institute-wise in alphabetical (series title) order. Journals were organized alphabetically under broad subject groupings. Annual Reports are organized geographically in classified order, P.G. theses by Accession (Serial) number given to IARI theses and Research Fellowship Theses. Books are arranged in traditional classified order. Since the library contains a large number of old collection for four countries, the book collection has been divided into post 1976 and Pre 1975. All pre 1975 books and journals are housed in 4-storied Annexe building with proper arrangement of guides and location lists. The growth of agricultural literature in the library has been as following :

1907	1937	1947	1987	2007
5,000	60,000	1,60,000	6,00,000	5,80,000

Unaccessioned worn-out documents have been weeded out under the weeding process before the digitization and with the result the number has gone down in 2007.

3. LINKAGES OF IARI LIBRARY

3.1 National

(i) IARI Library is a member of Developing Library Network (DELNET) and has access to the holdings of 965 Indian Libraries and 14 libraries outside India. Readers can access library's OPAC, Catalogue of DELNET, through IARI library Password in which Delhi-based required material/ information is available.

(ii) The Library has also access to the holdings of member libraries of INFLIBNET (Information and Library Network) - a network of university libraries in India sponsored by the University Grants Commission with its Headquarters at Ahmedabad (Gujarat).

(iii) Being a lead center of National Agricultural Technology Project (NATP) supported by World Bank, IARI library is having linkages with Libraries of ICAR institutes and State Agricultural Universities (SAUs). A researcher can know about the holdings of those library and may know about its library services.

3.2 International Linkages and Depository Library

(i) IARI Library is the member of FAO's Agricultural Library Network (AGLINET) since 1993. It is the first library in India under ICAR-SAU system becoming member of AGLINET and fulfills the dream of Dr. M.S. Randhawa, Chairman, Review Committee of ICAR Institutes and SAUs (1979).

(ii) Library has been functioning as the National Focal Center for CGIAR, ISNAR publications and thus, works as a Depository of 16 CGIAR international research institutes publications and provides information on CGIAR literature at national level since 1989.

(iii) The library plays its role on international level and so far, the library works as depository of FAO, World Bank, AVRDC, IDRC, CGIAR publications.

(iv) The library cooperates with SAARC Agricultural Information Center (SAIC, Dhaka) for the exchange of Information.

(v) IARI library worked for sometime as the Center for Agricultural Libraries in North India under ASTINFO Project of Australian National Library for providing photocopying and inter-library loan services (Chhotey Lal, 1998).

4. AUTOMATION OF LIBRARY & ELECTRONIC INFORMATION SERVICES

IARI established a fiber-optic backbone based 100 Mbps structured LAN in 1996. The library has connectivity to 17 major buildings, 48 nodes spread through out the buildings. It has a CD-ROM workstation, ERL Server accessible to campus LAN 24-hours throughout the year. Library has 41PCs, 10 printers, LibSys software and Color Digital Photo copier. It started electronic circulation of Bar-coded publications and bar-coded Library ID cards since 2005. The data in digital form comprises of Foreign Journals (88) 2006; E-Journals (40) 2006; CD-ROM Bibliographic Databases, namely AGRIS, AGRICOLA, CABI, BIOTECHNOLOGY ABSTRACTS, FOOD SCIENCE TECHNOLOGY ABSTRACTS, WATER RESOURCES ABSTRACTS, ZOOLOGICAL RECORDS and SILVER LINKERS. Retro Conversion of bound volumes of periodicals (1,09,116), Digitization of rare books (27), References of Bibliography of Indian Agriculture database (1,39,000), IARI/RFT Theses (11782), Hindi Publications (4269); Depository Publications (34,053) and digitization of bulletins (24,787).

4.1 Online Journals/E-Journals

Library had 135 On-line journals in 2005 and 45 in 2006 which are free against subscription of print journals and were accessed through Internet On-line.

4.2 CD-Rom Workstation and E-Databases

CD-ROM publishing since 1985 has brought a worldwide revolution in the field of information storage and retrievaal. It provides instant random access to multi users to huge amount of literature. Library has adopted this technology since 1993 for the benefit of the scientific community in the field of agro-biological sciences. In the year 1993 Soil-CD, Hort-CD and Crop-CD were procured and serviced through the stand-alone model of Hitachi CD-ROM Drives. Further, in 1996, 14-Drive CD-Net workstation and subsequently 28-Drive CD-Net workstation were installed and used through ten-dummy terminals. CD-ROM Technology has been further extended to all Divisions by the Campus based 100 mbps LAN Connectivity through (11 km) Fiber Optic Cable. NATP LIS Project of the ICAR, enables the scientists and research workers of the country to have access to the latest world agricultural literature.

Eight highly important international databases are subscribed i.e. *CABI, AGRIS, AGRICOLA, DERWENT BIOTEHCNOLOGY ABSTRACT, ZOOLOGICAL RECORD, FOOD SCIENCE AND TECHNOLOGY ABSTRACT, WATER RESOURCES ABSTRACT, AGRICULTURE AND NATURAL RESOURCES.* The access to CD-ROM databases is given through LAN using Mirror-Server. CD-Net Towers have been replaced by Mirror-Server in the year 2000 to provide better services. At present Literature Search Services are extended to P.G. students and scientists of IARI and the research scholars from all over India. The following data (Table 1) speaks the volume of electronic information search and retrieval by the outside users visiting IARI Library (IARI Report, 2006).

Table 1 CD-ROM Database Searches

Year	Number of users	Number of References Searched
1997	5040	2,83,850
1999	6880	3,30,949
2001	6330	6,72,056
2003	6824	3,35,090
2005	4468	1,99,8512
2007	3000+	89,048

However, students and scientists of IARI generally access databases through Intranet (LAN) from their Divisions.

A unique database of Science Citation Index has been acquired since 1989 with the financial support from NATP grant which can be accessed on INTERNET and IARI INTRANET through URL:httl://access.isiproducts.com/IARI through which ICAR institutes and SAU's can be benifitted to the maximum extent. Current Contents Connect has proved to be a worthwhile database for nascent timely information. This facility was available upto 31st December 2005 and renewal subject to payment.

4.3 Internet/E-mail Facilities

Library has a well-equipped Facility Management Unit with 10 PCs (personal computers) for M.Sc. and Ph.D. students for Internet and E-mail facilities and remains open from morning till 8.00 p.m. in the evening.

4.4 IARI Website

Outside users can have the connectivity with the IARI website on IP Address : 203/97.227.226 and the library's web page can be accessed on www.iari.res.in/~Library. On the library web page itself 42 major libraries of the ICAR System - (35 Agricultural Universities and 7 ICAR Institutes) have been provided interlinks through which connectivity can be established.

4.5 AGRIS/FAO Database Input Centre

IARI Library has been sharing AGRIS database input activities for NARD (National Agricultural Research Database) in ISO format using AGRIN methodology. This library scans 10 core Indian Journals starting from the year 2000. It includes scanning of each article by conceptual and depth analysis of the contents of the articles, assigning of AGROVOC Descriptors up to 10 numbers as well as the primary and secondary subjects up to 2 levels for indexing purpose. The compiled data for AGRIS Project is submitted to National Agris Input Center at ICAR Headquarters.

5. ROLE IN EDUCATION AND TRAINING

5.1 User Education

AIS (Agricultural Information System) one credit course on Agricultural Information search and retrieval/ is compulsory, for M.Sc. and Ph.D. students and was started in 1982-83. The aim of the course is to acquaint students with the role of library in society, organization of library resources, searching of literature and information services rendered by the library, technical report writing, search and information retrieval techniques. In an academic year, in three trimesters the course is conducted, having about 120 students of M.Sc. and Ph.D. In each trimester five faculty members take 10-12 classes and Head Library Services is the Coordinator of this course. In routine orientation a guidance and training is given to new visitors (Chhotey Lal, 1998).

5.2 Training of ICAR Librarians under NATP-LIS Project

IARI Library as a national lead center for NATP activities during 2000-2007 identified 161 professionals from different ICAR institutes and SAU's and arranged training in 9 batches at INFLIBNET CENTRE (Ahmedabad) for the creation of digital library, On-line access, e-journal, creation of Web Pages for the library, Internet access, sharing of resources from different websites, library software applications, forming of consortia, sharing of resources, etc. In addition to these, 21 senior librarians from different ICAR institutes/SAU's were given training at INFLIBNET (Ahmedabad) in two batches. The ICAR through NATP support was given the job of providing trained manpower to the libraries with the most sophisticated technology and appropriate infrastructure, which is expected to bring about a sea change in the efficiency of the libraries during the 21st century. Towards this, the IARI library identifies various professionals from different ICAR institutes/SAU's requiring training at INFLIBNET, Ahemedabad.

5.3 Training Cell of IARI Library

Library is having a well-equipped computer Lab with 24 terminals with Internet connectivity. Time to time training is given to scientists and students of IARI for CD-ROM literature search, Web of Science, Current Contents Connect, Digital Resources, E-Journals, On-line information retrieval, etc.

6. SERVICES OFFERED

IARI library offers following library and information services :

- CD-ROM Database search and Retrieval Services.
- Current Awareness Services.
- Bibliographical Services.
- Selective Dissemination of Information Service.
- News Clipping Service.
- Reference and Book Loan.
- Document Delivery Services.
- Resource Sharing.
- Inter Library Loan.

7. REPROGRAPHY AND DOCUMENT DELIVERY

From 1953 the Reprography Section of IARI LIbrary was equipped with Kodak overhead microfilm camera, photo state machine with prism lens, and Rank Xerox Floor copying machines. Upto 1984 the Reprography section was equipped with manually operated xerox photocopying machines with a speed of 5 copies per minute. Thereafter, in 1985 Photocopier machine having 10 cpm was purchased. At present the section is equipped with machines like Digital Analog PPC (plain paper copier), Monocolor duplicating machine, and full color PPC machine. The speed of photocopier machines presently available in the section is 35 to 120 cpm. A Risograph machine GR17 installed in 1996-97 produces print quality copies in colour with a faster speed of 130 cpm. It is very much cost effective.

Reprography section provides the facility of photocopying of research articles to research scholars and scientists of the institute, universities, and international organizations. Microfilming and Color Photocopying facility is also available in the section. Scientists of IARI are provided the facility of photocopies as free of cost for official purposes.

A MOU was signed between IARI and C-DAC (Noida) for scanning of old and rare documents, not covered under copyright Act. Till date more than 6250 publications have been digitized containing 42,38,997 pages. The oldest publication digitized belongs to 1597.

8. LIBRARY PUBLICATIONS

For bibliographic control, IARI library has compiled so far the following publications :

(i) Catalogue of publications in the library since 1907 to 1933 in different volumes in print format for different periods.

(ii) Catalogue of Serials, in IARI Library (1905-1967).

(iii) Catalogue of serials, supplemnt (1967-1987).

(iv) Highlights of research-a supplement catalogue of theses (1961-1980).

(v) Bibliography of IARI publications (1905-1963).

(vi) Bibliography of Theses in IARI library (1939-1969).

(vii) Bibliolography of IARI Theses, supplement (1980-2000)

(viii) Bibliography of Indian Agriculture (1944-2000) (on cards as well as CD-ROM).

(ix) Agriculture Press Bulletin (Discontinued).

(x) Current Contents in Agriculture (In four disciplines) (available on-line at Intranet).

(xi) Monthly List of Additions. (now available on-line).

(xii) Guide to Information Sources in IARI Library (1985).

Dr. S.S. Johl, Chairman, Quinquennial Team (QRT) on IARI (1983-90) remarked that ``IARI Library had done greatest and highest quality work under its documentation activities as compared to any other agricultural library in the country" (Chhotey Lal, 1998).

9. LIBRARIANS AS FACULTY OF P.G. SCHOOL (IARI)

The senior librarians of IARI are faculty members and teaching one credit compulsory course named as Agricultural Information System (AIS) to the post-graduate students of IARI in each trimester. The AIS Course was introduced in Post Graduate School curriculum in 1982-83 academic year. It is also recorded in *Universitites Handbook* published by the Association of Indian Universities, New Delhi and *World of Learning (Europa)*.

9.1 Ironical Situation

ICAR has classified its employees into four categories namely, (1) Scientists, (2) Technical (3) Adminstrative and (4) Supporting Staff. Librarians, documentalists, information specialties have been classified as Technical and put along with field men, drivers, butchers, editorial and book production staff. Librarians throughout the country in general university as well as State Agricultural Universities have been equated with or designated as teachers on par with university teachers/faculties and have been awarded UGC pay scales acquiring other benefits thereof.

It is unfortunate and pathetic to record that the pay scales of librarians of National Agricultural Library and other ICAR deemed universities and institutes have been brought down to a far lower ranking as compared to the same functional fraternity of SAU's.

ICAR sponsored joint Indo-American Library Survey and Study Team known as Dr. Dorothy Parker Committee (1967) and Dr. Ramaiah Committee (1969) recommended on par status of the head of National Agricultural Library with that of professors of a university and UGC pay scales.

QRT (Quinquennial Review Team) of ICAR (1983-90) headed by Dr. A.B. Joshi and Dr. S.S. Johl stated that librarians are academic staff and they should be governed by the UGC pay scales. Librarians in SAU's as well as in

General Universities have already been equated with academic staff and awarded UGC pay scales whereas librarians in IARI are full-fledged faculties teaching P.G. School course for the last 25 years are depriving of this status.

10. RESEARCH REPORTS ON IARI LIBRARY

It has been reported by Dr. K.P. Singh (2007) that journals are the most used source (83.2%) ranked I, followed by books/monographs (72.8%) and the majority scientists (84.6%) approached for them to the National Agricultural Library, IARI, New Delhi. The use of photocopy service was preferred most when online search was found to be the least used. Anita Singh (2004) and Prashar (1991) made suggestions for the improvement of documentation services, reprography service and collection development. Chhotey Lal (1998) reported a few pathos concerning staff of National Agricultural Library.

11. SUGGESTIONS

National Agricultural Library (IARI) New Delhi, for playing its role in true sense, needs following improvement :

(i) Journals subscription which has been facing axe due to financial cut, need to be increased following a balanced acquisition policy for all subject fields. Policy for online journals be reviewed.

(ii) Indigenous agricultural knowledge databases and union catalogues for online information exchange need to be developed and linked through a National Agricultural Information Network to fulfill information needs of agricultural scientists of the country.

(iii) In view of very thin attendance of library users in NAL, Documentation, CAS, ADONIS and Alert Services should be initiated and disseminated. Reprographic services should be improved.

(iv) For the safety and conservation of rare documents, they need to be preserved through scientific methods and technologies since rare is gold. Weeding policy be devised for the removal of obsolete and unused publications.

(v) To stop theft and mutilation close circuit cameras and remote sensing electronic device should be installed for better surveillance.

(vi) NAL can not be better managed and provide better services without adequate, qualified and experienced professionals, hence, sanctioned vacant positions be filled up or outsourced.

(vii) It is suggested that librarian of NAL must be given status equal to faculty and UGC pay scales on par with SAU's Libr-arians as per UGC norms, terms and conditions. ICAR must equate them with teachers/scientists being P.G. School Faculty and remove their Technical Category-III bar for the purpose from Asstt. Librarian and above level. NAL must regain its past glory and its Librarians a respectful place in professional community.

(viii) NAL be given official status *de jure*/through adminstrative order like National Science Library (NISCAIR) and National Medical Library (ICMR).

CONCLUSION

IARI Librry has been renovated in 1996 assuming world class standard in terms of physical facilities, digital catalogue and electronic information services. ICAR and IARI authorities together can take measures to raise the status of IARI Library on par with National Agricultural Libraries in other parts of the world and restore its past glory and honour.

REFERENCES

Chhotey Lal, Growth of Agricultural Libraries in the Post-Independence Era. *DESIDOC Bulletin of Information and Technology* 18 (2) 1998, p. 13-20.

IARI Annual Report, 1907-09, 1937, 1947, 1968, 2006.

ICAR, Joint Indo American Library Survey and Study Team-1967 (Dr. Dorothy Parker Committee) Final Report. New Delhi ICAR 1968. 182p.

ICAR, Quinquennial Review Team. Report 1983-90 (Chairman: Dr. A.B. Joshi & Dr. S.S. Johl). New Delhi, ICAR.

ICAR, Ramiah Committee Report, 1969.

Prashar, R.G. Managing University Libraries. New Delhi, Today & Tomorrow's Printers & Publishers, 1991. 350 p.

Singh, Anita. Information needs and user satisfaction of agricultural research scholars in the libraries of Allahabad Agriculture Institute (Deemed University) and National Agricultural Library, IARI (New Delhi) - A Comparative Study. Ph.D. Thesis 2004.

Singh, K.P. Information Seeking Behaviour of Agriculture Scientists working in the select ICAR Institutes in Delhi & the Punjab Agricultural University, Ludhiana : A Study. *Library Herald* 45 (4) Dec. 2007. pp. 370-81.

Government Knowledge Centre, Gandhinagar: A model for State Public Library

Geeta G. Gadhavi

Sr. Lecturer & Head, Dept. of Library & Information Science, Gujarat University, Ahmedabad – 380 009
e-mail: geetmin@yahoo.co.in

ABSTRACT

Paper discusses about the transformation of State Central Library, Gandhinagar in to Knowledge Centre. Discusses about the process and progress of knowledge centre in respect of manpower, infrastructure, resources and services. For the renovation of building's floor plan has been prepared by NID, Ahmedabad which is attached herewith.

INTRODUCTION

"Knowledge is one of the core missions of the library". Knowledge has been placed in the spotlight of the international arena. Developed world is entering in new knowledge based economy or Knowledge economy which is known as "Knowledge Revolution". The Knowledge Revolution is the process of paradigm shift on the way to knowledge economy, which includes infrastructure like educated people, knowledge institutions, knowledge networks and telecommunication. So, library should be, by nature an essential part of the knowledge infrastructure. It has significant impact upon developing and developed countries. "Knowledge Revolution" can be another renaissance for the library community. Public libraries can be an integral part of the information highway, allowing people to access the untold wealth of knowledge available in any sources. At the same time, the library can serve as a human and people-centered place for rest and relaxation. As per vision statement of the Library of Congress, "The library is in the unique position to be both Catalyst and Participant in the intellectual process that transforms information into knowledge and knowledge into wisdom.

Unesco and Public Library Manifesto

The UNESCO Public Library Manifesto has also designated public library, "The local gateway to knowledge". Public Library converge social knowledge, adds value to it, produces new knowledge and diffuses it as requested. The Library building can be a place for gathering of educated people to communicate and create tacit knowledge, and interpret tacit knowledge in to codified knowledge. At the same time public library can be a "server" as it provide access, it can act as an offline relay, by downloading and sending network available information and knowledge to those out of the network reach, or by attracting people to the nearby libraries to access internet. Additionally with the global networking of Library Community and other information servers, local libraries became globally accessible libraries. Modern Public libraries became globally accessible libraries. Modern public libraries are widespread, popular and of enduring importance to social justice and the maintenance of the democratic society. Now, it becomes a multipurpose agency with multiple roles covering the areas of information and lifelong learning, recreation and leisure, culture and research. The ICT do not threaten the existence of public libraries but offers an opportunity to provide increasing valuable and effective services for user, and librarians of public libraries will have to grow as specialist in each discipline and make the selection of knowledge easy and more effective distribution. To empowered people; National Knowledge Commission was set up in 2005, which explicit India's recognition of the importance of knowledge in a globalized world. Its mandate is to suggest steps which would give India the knowledge edge in today's competitive times. Its objective is to make India a leader in the creation, application and dissemination of knowledge.

Importance of Knowledge in Society

The Gujarat has a great historical and cultural heritage in the past. Its literacy ratio is about 70%, which leads great scope for introducing measures that reduce illiteracy and increase better employment opportunities for the people. These measures can be taken only if people have access to appropriate knowledge and skills. Knowledge which is available in libraries and being created so rapidly now is beyond the reach of every individual. Everybody should have access to the desired knowledge. Measures therefore needed to be taken to overcome this problem. It would be important to understand the role of knowledge played for the transformation of the society.

We all know that the internet has emerged as a major tool for churning out information and producing new knowledge, which created information overload and as a result knowledge is getting lost in information. Before three to four decades the speed of generation of information was within manageable limits of library and information professionals. A professional could disseminate information about every important work or article. Where as today's situation is quite difficult to manage. As per a estimated study, the online information doubles in every six months, where as unstructured information doubles every three months. Same is with the corporate information; it doubles in every 18 months. In the case of medical information it gets doubled in every five years. In the process of knowledge revolution, study has identified some facts regarding know-ledge generation, i.e. the sum total of human knowledge doubles every two to three years. The world's knowledge doubles every six months. Printed knowledge gets double in every five years, and Medical knowledge will take three and half years to be doubled. Due to the use of ICT, we can access world's know-ledge resources. If the users donot update themselves accordingly the use of knowledge and the development of nation will leg behind. Considering these factors the Govern-ment of Gujarat has decided to convert the State Central Library in to Knowledge Centre, the first state in India to accomplish this work.

Towards Knowledge Society

A knowledge Society can grow only if knowledge is accessible freely to people, or otherwise even the literate will become uneducated. Mark Twain says "The man who does not read books has no advantage over the man who cannot read". We have therefore to transform our society into a Knowledge Society which is equitable in nature. In it every person can contribute at the local level in terms of experience, initiatives or needs and this can result in local and national development with the use of practical knowledge. The need for gaining access to appropriate knowledge and the skills associated with it can also grow faster. Every skilled person, creating or marketing a product becomes a contributing member of the Knowledge Society. As their competencies grow, innovative changes in the products take place and the economy flourishes.

The knowledge Centre which will collect information on Indian and foreign R&D results, as far as possible, will help the public with the required information about patents and unused R&D results of government managed laboratories. As the State Knowledge Centre is established as a one-stop window not only will the time of professionals be saved but the duplication in the creation of similar products or R&D efforts will be minimized. We will find that people will begin to specialize in interested disciplines. Nowadays, knowledge about a discovery can be made available to a large number of users at a very low cost around the world and its application can result in economic development. It can support a poor economy. A poor economy can be transformed into a knowledge-driven economy. Small-scale individual enterprises can grow extensively as knowledge becomes available to the public freely and unemployment levels can decline drastically. The economic implications of knowledge give rise to knowledge economy. Obsolescence of technology and its replacement by improved technology gives rise to new products at less cost. This environment gives rise to competition and expansion of the market activities. That who have access to precise knowledge, creates new and better products, market them well, attract finance, and use raw materials effectively among other benefits. They in turn become part of the growing knowledge economy. Knowledge is the key to the economic development of the State. While the rich will use it for wealth generation, the poor will use it for poverty alleviation using the State Knowledge Centre.

Transforming traditional Library to Knowledge Centre

A knowledge centre is an extended version of a public library. Its main objective is to impart appropriate knowledge to every user and provide useful information to the public that triggers transformation in the society. One fine and foremost question arise in our minds that how do we get it? It is as simple as anything. By collecting, organizing and disseminating both knowledge and information one can visualize knowledge centre. Knowledge will be pooled systematically for wider use in various context. Knowledge will be available locally with the help of ICT, traditional services will get benefited. As ICT does not merely help in matching users' needs with knowledge resources, but also assists in taking decisions in global and futuristic perspectives. Every day new development occurs in the knowledge sector. These have to be captured on each subject which will preserve and presented in digital form. Knowledge centre will cull knowledge from every source of information and will adopt various methods to collect information on the issues of local interest. Public Library of Gandhinagar is going to turn its face to knowledge centre (GKC), transformation in all and every sector is required. It includes personnel sector, service sector, physical condition and resources.

Personnel Sector

To provide sophisticated service with traditional mind set is not possible. Trained and skilled manpower will grasp up changes in all walk of library services. Gujarat Knowledge Centre has to work with the coordination of National Knowledge Centre in respect of international standards. Staff will be selected on the basis of various activities, size of their operations and the efficiency of the staff with whom the work has to be done. GKC will have Manager, Knowledge Centre, Consultant for Content Creation Centre and for Digital Library Unit, RTI queries, State Archives and for Extension Activities GKC will have Knowledge Associates and Knowledge Assistants. For existing staff GKC will provide intensive training about their new jobs. Personnel with IT and ICT skills will get priorities. Suitable communication skills, managerial skills and office etiquettes will be the criterion for key posts. Recently GKC employed 53 surplus employees from government. More than 10 IT professionals will be recruited after one month for GKC. Government of Gujarat State has decided to promote existing staff after their intensive training. State librarians in class I and II cadre will be recruited directly. Other professionals will be appointed on fixed pay as per State Government rules.

Infrastructure

Building: GKC will be the new name, face and identity of State Central Library, Gandhinagar. Existing building will get modern look. It will have renovated auditorium, rare books and manuscripts section, children library, women library, senior citizen section, braille section, text book section, fumigation unit, maintenance unit, reprography unit, unprocessed books and record room, exhibition gallery, canteen and reception/personal belongings/counter. NID, Ahmedabad has designed the floor plan (Enclosed as annexure 1-3). Government of Gujarat has sanctioned Rs. 2.5 crore for modernization of building and infrastructure. GKC will spent Rs. 2 crore for renovation of building and Rs. 50 lakhs for furniture. Adequate furniture has been planned for the centre. Suitable tables and chairs for staff as well as for computer terminal's utility have been selected. Good quality waiting lounge is being developed. In order to maintain office documents and records filing racks and storage units have been purchased for CDs, DVDs and computer related stationery. GKC will equip with centrally A.C. system in near future.

To maintain building, infrastructure facilities, cleaning and security will be out sourced.

Technology

Sixty computers have been purchased from RRRLF Grants. All the computers will be equipped with internet accessibility. Intranet connectivity will be provided to staff members of GKC. To create digital contents using international standards adequate plotters, printers and related hardware and software are planned to be procured. GKC has planned out time to time upgradation for technology change. It has been decided that GKC will have access to books and other documents available in India and outside India by using Library Networks like DELNET. State central library has its own website which will be shortly converted in GKC's website, online renewing books and reserving book request facilities will be provided in near future. Telephones with STD connections for senior officers will be provided. One or two coin system public telephone lines will be provided for users and other than staff members. In order to provide suitable facilities to physically challenged people, dedicated elevator facility will be provided. For auto check in/out, Book drop facility, controlling loss of books, use of smart card, to maintain patron records, usage tracking - RFID system will implemented in GKC within reasonable period.

Resources

GKC has Rs. Six crore as fixed deposits and earns Rs. 54 lakhs rupees of interest. To serve their clientele, GKC will purchase books from the interest amount. Books will be purchased from the grants released by R.R.R.L.F. There will be a separate collection of books those received under the copyright Act. To identify core subjects, need survey of surroundings of Gujarat State will be planned out. Books and Journals will be purchased by innovative ideas of generating income. Through request and advertisement manuscripts laying with or available to any one will be procured and will be preserved for next generation. The rare books will be identified from the collection. E-books, E-journals, E-newspapers, and E-theses with other web-based resources will be subscribe by GKC and will be provided access to its clientele. To create an automated and user-friendly environment GKC will enrich its collection and accessible services; resource mobility is required to be managed. GKC's chief source of income is Government grants, subscription amount, grants from RRRLF, donations in terms of books, cash, land and building. Each and every sectors of service have to generate their finance by offering value added services and from some paid services also. One of the ways of generating revenue through innovative ideas like utilizing the space of building which is lying unused, making use of that place by pasting advertising / hoardings.

State Central Library implemented this idea only for Rajkot city's libraries and earned Rs. 12 lakhs. They utilized this money to purchase books/resources. Now, Junagadh, Jamnagar, Baroda and Mahesana District's library's place will also be utilized gradually.

Services

With all traditional library services GKC requires some new service provider, with IT based knowledge. Online renewal and reserving books services, document delivery service, Ask the Librarian (Reference desk), alerting services, reprography services, resource Web form, FAQs and many more nontraditional services will be offered by GKC. To furnish these services qualified staff with ample experience will be required.

Objectives of GKC

1. To make the GKC inter - sectoral in due course of time so that it becomes a one-stop centre for accessing knowledge on different subjects or topics of interest to users in Gujarat.
2. To capture knowledge from projects, assignments, grey literature, case studies, experts, etc. on identified subjects and make them accessible in database form.
3. To develop collections on important subjects.
4. To connect each component of knowledge with a set of experts and develop an active database of such experts.
5. To create databases, develop an intranet and maintain information on important knowledge repositories.
6. To develop catalogues and indexes in machine readable form using international standards of physical and electronic resources.

7. To develop links with resources which are both physical; such as institutions and individuals, and electronic resources available through the internet.
8. To furnish as much information to the users as the users' need to complete their assignments.
9. To give knowledge and information support to the adult population and to see how they are benefitted from new technology and avenues.
10. To offer knowledge inputs to deprived sections of the society who come from rural and urban sectors so that they upgrade their standards of living.
11. To distribute knowledge on health and family welfare.
12. To train every user in accessing information and guide the users to the appropriate resource.
13. To give integrated access to information available with DELNET on the subjects and collect relevant information on the subjects from other sources.
14. To coordinate with National Knowledge Centre at DELNET in order to:
    - Collect useful knowledge resources from India and International sources for the benefit of users in Gujarat;
    - Promote awareness about the resources of Gujarat in India and outside India specially among those users who use knowledge for development; and
    - Seek support and collaboration for projects to be established in Gujarat

Functions of GKC

GKC will occupy resources based on the result of local surveys and will accordingly disseminate appropriate knowledge to its clientele.

As per Dr. H. K. Kaul's report the GKC will:

1. Make surveys of people living around, at least 5 kms. in radius, and find out:
    a. The number of unemployed youth and their interests and specializations;
    b. The number of women who have time to learn skills and are interested in making a living by using those skills;
    c. The number of physically challenged people who need support of knowledge and skills; and
    d. Identify all skills in which the public is interested in adopting or developing it further.
2. Offer knowledge support to public.
3. Identify the languages in which content will be serviced and the relative content in English.
4. Coordinate with other Departments of the knowledge centre and will be linked up with knowledge Gateway of DELNET for giving knowledge support to the users, with the support of Dept. of Learning Skills, Dept. of Web resources/Development, Dept. of Training and Surveys and Dept. of Administration and Publicity.

CONCLUSION

Gujarat has the credit of having Government Knowledge Centre (GKC) first of its kind. Information Technology is used for effective collection, storage and dissemination of information and knowledge. There is an urgent need to use all library material for disseminating knowledge to the public. Like GKC, all other libraries can be modernized in phases using information and communication technologies. Promotion of quality in services and creation of products could be introduced gradually by the knowledge centre among the industrial community. It can introduce E-commerce applications and serve the business community too. Government of Gujarat has taken praise worthy initiative to have knowledge centre for dissemination of knowledge and information which people of Gujarat have and which they deserve. This knowledge centre will be the role model for other State Public Libraries.

REFERENCES

Kaul, H. K. Public Libraries as knowledge centres, *in* Kaul, H.K. and Malhan, I.V., *ed.* Knowledge, Library and Information Networking – NACLIN 2006, New Delhi : DELNET-Developing Library Network, 2007, pp 1-18

Satija, M.P. Democracy and knowledge society in India, *in* Kaul, H.K. and Malhan, I.V. (ed). Knowledge, Library and Information Networking – NACLIN 2006, New Delhi: DELNET-Developing Library Network, 2007, pp 19-31

The Library of Congress in the year 2000: A Vision Management and Planning Committee, The Library of Congress, Washington DC, June 29, 1988: VIII

UNESCO Public Library Manifesto, November, 1994

Kaul, H.K. Report of the modernisation of State Central Library, Gandhinagar, 2006.

Ground Floor Plan

Appendix - 1

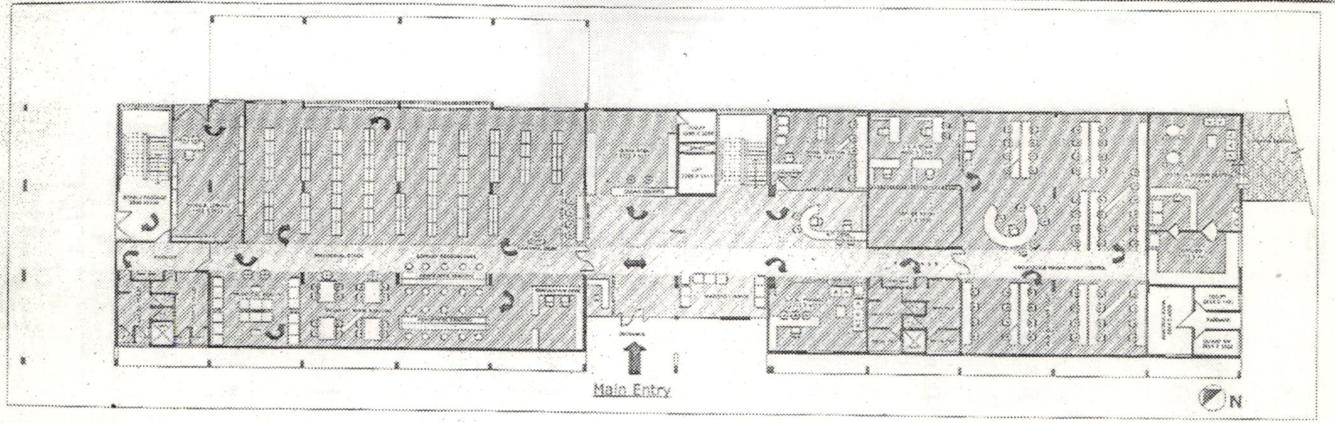

Main Entry

N

LEGEND

- Foyer, Waiting Lounge, RTI Desk
- Passage
- Cloak Counter
- Brail Section
- G.K.G Manager & Staff Cabins
- Information & Control Desk, I.T. Area With Server Room (Knowledge Management Center)
- Free Internet Zone (Knowledge Management Center)
- Cafeteria with Kitchen
- Gujarati Book Stacks & Digital Cataloguing
- Library Reading Hall with Periodical Stacks & Newspaper Reading
- Mobile Library
- General Toilets (facility provided for Handicaps)

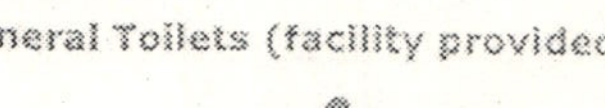

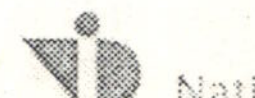

National Institute of Design, Ahmedabad

Appendix - 2

First Floor Plan

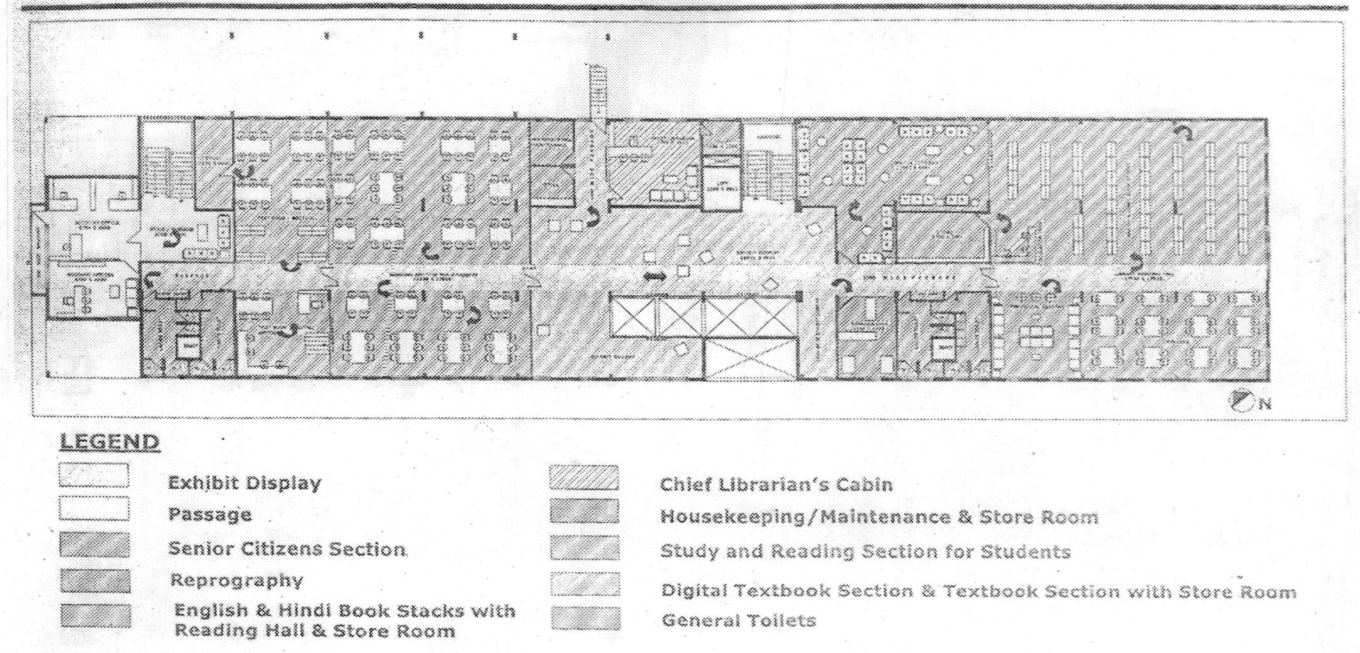

Appendix - 3

Second Floor Plan

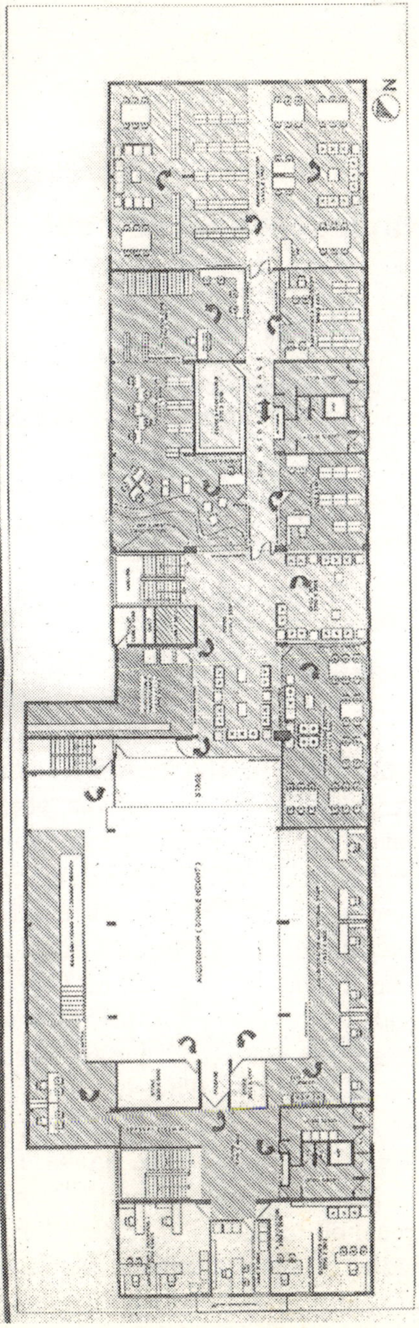

LEGEND

- Foyer, Lounge & Chill zone
- Passage & Store
- Children's Section
- Archival
- Multimedia Zone
- Rare Books & Manuscripts
- Reference Section
- Foyer, Lounge & Administrative and Technical Staff
- Fumigation & Maintenance
- General Toilets
- Women's Reading Section

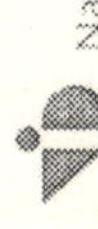

National Institute of Design, Ahmedabad

Digital Libraries : An Overview

Tirth Das

Librarian, Dr. Raheja Library,
Central Arid Zone Research Institute, Jodhpur - 342 003.

INTRODUCTION

Digital library means to exploit the facilities of Information Technology (IT) with the object to share resources available globally so as to render right information to the right user at right time. In the present scenario, where in though the world has become too narrow, yet, it is very difficult to retrieve desired information without wasting reader's precious time. Prof. Finagle has rightly observed, `the information we have is not we need, the information we want is not we need and the information we need is not available'. The impact of IT such as CD-ROM, Multimedia, CD-Net, Local Area Network, Internet, various Web Sites, etc. are dragging the traditional libraries, towards Virtual or Digital libraries. The libraries have completed their progress circle. They started their growth in the ``Paperless" form i.e. (Clay tablets Tree Barks, Inscriptions, Copper plates etc.) and after completing their growth circle they have again reached in the ``Paperless" form i.e. computers, CDs. Multimedia, Internet. E-books, E-Journals.

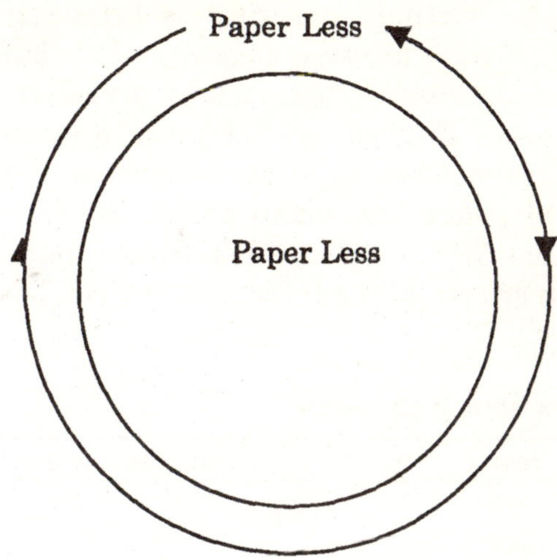

Fig. 1. Growth and Development of Libraries

The traditional libraries earlier used to work in isolations due to one or the other reasons are now stepping in a positive way and seem to be ready to share their resources and are also prepared to opt newer IT to convert library resources in digital form. Use of Internet for search of any kind of information has become a common phenomenon now a day. The World Wide Web (WWW) has become an important tool for searching and dissemination of information. To cope up with the emerging trends in IT, prehaps none can afford to ignore digitization in libraries. IT in the field of library and Information Science is emerging and changing every day and the information needs of users and especially the way of getting them is also changing. For librarians it has become almost essential to adopt newer technology and to make aware themselves with the digital information system, electronic publishing, Internet and Intranet, multimedia, CD-ROM. The basic purpose of digital library/e-library is to provide instant service to the readers from the remotest corner using World Wide Webs.

Use of Internet has tremendously increased in the recent past. There are severaal Directories, Search engines and Meta-Search engines available. The concept of ``Digital libraries" and ``Virtual libraries" is becoming more and more popular. These libraries involve a distributed team of librarins and databases that can be searched across the world. However, English is the most popular language (57.7%) for Internet search at the same time United States where 46% of population make use of the Internet. According to gender 59% male and 41% female make use of the Internet. The growth of the Internet users can be seen in the Table 1 below :

Table 1. Growth of Web Users

Year	Internet users in million
1996	70
1997	117
1998	151
1999	206
2000	322
2001	574
2002	625
2003	700 Approx.

DIGITAL LIBRARIES

The concept of digital libraries is becoming popular because it facilitates end users needs and which has the capability to handle vast amount of complex data. The term virtual library, electronic library or digital library is more or less synonymous. All such libraries would largely contain digitized information along with print based publications. In broad sense it is a computerized system that allows user to access information and data from electronically stored repository. The information/data in such libraries is available in digital, and analog form. One of the much-desired advantages of the digital library is that is accessible twenty fours hours of a day, seven days a week, 30 days of the month and 365 days of the year. It is more accessible for larger hours than the traditional library. Another advantage of the digital library is that it goes beyond a single collection and provides access to resources not held by the host library.

1.1 History

Though the concept of digital library is growing very fast, yet its progress is nearly 30 years old. Way back to early 1970, the digital libraries started functioning using computers and communication technology available at that time. In 1967, Air Force Department in US Govt. started digitizing their legal documents followed by scientific communication. Several character-coded software packages were released during mid 1970 and late 1970 for storage, indexing and retrievaal of documents. By the end of 1980 many mainframe, microcomputers and Local Area Network (LAN) were available for storage and retrieval of text. During this period several sophisticated information storage and retrieval systems were built. Online hosts like DIALOG and STN came forward and started providing not only online data based service but also the full text online journals. However, their files did not contain pictures and graphics. The use of CD-ROMs started in 1980"s with heavy storage capacity, long lasting, easy in transportation and requiring minimum storage space. The real digital era started in between late 1980's and early 1990 with the beginning of full text online databases. Use of scanner and camera for digitizing documents was a step ahead in the formation of digital libraries. At present several document imaging software packages are available in the market. In India ommiDoc (Newgen) and Data scan document imaging software are available. The work of digitization started with the help of using client systems such as MS Window, MS-DOS, Apple and UNIX. These systems in those days had several problems mainly the maintenance and up keeping. Every after one or two years they needed upgradation for creating new facilities invented during that period. The development of World Wide Web (WWW) brought a revolution in true sense and offered several facilities which includes Graphical Web Browser and other ready to use technologies. Netscape Navigator and Internet Explorer are being improved regularly for proper functioning of e-mail, JAVA and to view stored information without using plug in systems. These innovations solved all earlier problems of maintenance and up gradation allowing user to work in friendly environment not requiring any specific training.

1.2 Definition

The definition formulated by Digital Library Foundation (DFL) and cited by Waters (1998) is in broad sense :

``Digital libraries are organizations that provide the resources, including the specialized staff to select structure, offer intellectual access to interpret, distribute and preserve the integrity of and ensure the persistence over time of collection of digital works so that they are readily and economically available for use by a defined community or set of communities."

It is interesting to note here that if we remove the word ``digital" from this definition, it becomes a good definition of a library. It is not a single entity requires technologies to link the resources, digital libraries and information services with the end user. A digital library is a group of distributed repositories that users see as a single repository in digital from. UCLA-NSF Social aspect of Digital Libraries Workshop, 1996 defined the digital library in following words :

``Digital libraries are a set of electronic resources and associated technical capabilities for creating, searching and using information. In this sense they are on extension and enhancement of information storage and retrieval systems that manipulate digital data in any medium (text, image, sounds, static or dynamic images) and exist in distributed networks. The content of digital libraries include data, metadata that describes various aspects of the data (e.g. Representation, creator, owner, reproduction rights), and metadata thaat consist of links or relationship to other data or meta data, whether internal or external to the digital library". Michel Lesk (1997), a well known promoter of digital libraries predicts that by the early 21st century, half of the material being accessed in major academic and research libraries will be in digital, offered the following definition :

``Digital libraries are organized collection of digital information. They combine the structuring and gathering of information, which libraries and archives have always done, with the digital representation the computers have mode possible. Digital information can be accessed rapidly around the world, copies for preservation without error, stored compactly and searched very quickly. . . .A true digital library also provides principles governing what is included and how the collection is organized."

Clifford Lynch (1995) renowned personality on digital libraries defines digital libraries as, ``System providing a community of users with coherent access to a large organized repository of information and knowledge. The digital library is not just one entity, but multiple sources seamlessly integrated."

Like traditional libraries, digital libraries also need to have resources. As a major function they are suppose to collect, store, analyze, arrange, manipulate information and to make it available on web. The role of the librarian will be entirely different and they will be named as ``Cybrarian" `E-Librarian", ``Digital librarian". ``Knowledge librarian". ``Virtual librarian", ``Internet librarian and Web librarian etc. Both, library managers and library users will be required to have proper training for making information available and to make use of the available information collection and selection of digital material will involve two processes-one selecting digital material to include in the collection and secondly selecting material which needs be digitized. It is already clear that all printed documents cannot be digitized because of several problems mainly of copyright act. The digital libraries provide user-friendly interface, network accessibility, need based services and retrospective searches. The life span of digital documents is said to be longer but the statement is yet to be examined. In case of printed documents the books published/printed in AD 700/800 can be read without any additional equipment.

In real sense, the formation of a digital library, involves a number of processes starting from selection policies, managing information resources, deciding hardware and software, policies for conservation, dissemination and preservation of digital information resources. A developing country like India, need to take a policy decision for procurement of two important components of digital library i.e. e-books and e-journals. The number os online journals, cyber books, magazines and use of CD-ROM is increasing tremendously day by day. Looking to the fast growing concept of digital libraries, the planners and policy makers are engaged in evolving a system which is suppose to be most user friendly.

2. E-BOOKS

E-books, an acronym of electronic-book, now refers to the electronic or digital version of a printed book requiring an equipment, hardware and software to read the book may be termed as e-book. By this advent, an attempt has been made to overcome the limitations of paper books by adding a series of useful features that are made possible through the nature of an electronic environment. The main features of the electronic books are that they are dynamic, reactive and can be made available in different formats and editions in short time. These are as comfortable to read as a printed book and yet these offer more opportunities, the prime among them that it requires minimum space. A reader can store his whole library in a drawer. E-books, once downloaded on computers hard disc, can be red offline or in print form. The e-books are cheaper, portable, early searchable free from maintenance cost etc. But still it will not be appropriate to convert all books into electronic format.

2.1 Browsing e-Book

For browsing e-books, now days several options are available, the popular among them are Personal Digital Assistant (PDA), Pocket Personal Computer (PPC) and Personal Computer (PC) using Microsoft or Adobe software. At present e-publications as well as readers are facing problems because of various formats opted by the publishers. Thus an e-publisher is compelled to connect their contents of e-books in multiple formats. A reader also feels handicapped when the content bought by the reader/ customer compatible with one device/format doesn't matches with any other device or format. Large number of e-publishers putting their publicity and other related material in Hyper Text Markup Language (HTML) format, which can be accessed or read using any popular Web Browser Software (WBS). Adobe System International has recently developed Portable Document Format (PDF), which is compatible and is widely used for electronic editions of publications. However, it is very difficult to say that any single format will serve all the purposes and will match with the e-publishers requirements. A new concept called open e-book format (OEB) is developing where in leading e-publishers of the world are interested to have a standard format and are thinking for a common platform to digitize the contents of e-books/documents once only and then multiply it as and when needed.

2.2 E-book Reading

For reading an e-book similar to paper book perhaps, a dedicated reading gadget is the best option. In these gadgets a touch sensitive LCD screen is fitted in an e-book. Simple feather touch button monitors the book to move forward and backward. The gadget users hâve to purchase specially formatted content either from online bookstores through their PCs or directly from the device maker via built in MODEM.

2.3 Types of e-Books

A variety of e-books are available in the market. The academicians/e-publishers have classified them in the following manners :

1. Easy to carry books (Portable)
2. Page turner book
3. Multimedia book
4. Scroll metaphor book
5. Cyber book

2.3.1 Easy to carry books

These books are becoming more and more popular because of their portability from one place to another. Appropriate hardwares and softwares are the pre-requisites of the portable books. The hardware provides tools to read these books and the software used for the purpose makes it convenient to browse the books. The software also provides extra functionalities such as annotations, bookmarks, different fonts and colours to help the reader in reading and scanning process. The Microsoft has given a great boost in the year 2001 in the use of easy to carry books. The Microsoft allows user in browsing e-books using various platforms from Desktop to Palmtop computers.

2.3.2 Page-turner book

A Mercury Project has covered page-turner book device. It is based on the idea of a full text electronic library and has been developed by Arms and Michalak (1990) at Carnegie Mellon University. The major objectives of the project were to demonstrate that current technology and the techniques for processing electronic documents and help in building e-libraries. Various techniques for acquiring and storing information are being evaluated by Mercury.

2.3.3 Multimedia book

Multimedia book is a step ahead from the paper or printed book. Such books are no longer only the electronic texts or pictures/graphics but it is mixture of different works such as Video, Sound, Animation, Text and Pictures. There is no point in hiding such valuable information in the form of paper or in audio-visual form from its end users. For such types of classic works, perhaps, the electronic medias are the best source for preservation and making them available as and when required. They still borrow essential features from the book metaphor by either imitating its physical appearance or keeping the same logical structure.

2.3.4 Scroll metaphor books

In such types of books the text is presented in the scroll form. The page as logical and physical unit, no longer exists, nor does any reference to page number or to the page sequence. The text scrolls almost without any physcial limitation. Thus we can say that electronic scrolling book is portable on different platforms and does not have any dependency on serene dimensions. Another important matter is that information in this class of electronic book is made of text and graphics. It is still a very traditional way of interpreting the concept of a book in electronic terms and for this reason it is closely related to the paper book. In scrolling books, the system has capability to import text automatically available electronically in different formats.

2.3.5 Cyber books

This is actually the real property of virtual or wall free library. These books don't have any concern with paper/ press because they are fully electronic. These are known as books only in their broader sense otherwisely they don't have any textual basis. They can be defined as digital or active books with which the reader can approach from any corner of the world and at any time using their PCs and Internet.

For e-books, Personal Digital Assistant (PDA) is the most common way, people like to use it. Since it is known as Palm Computer, the size of the screen is just 5.7 cm and approximately it accommodates 15-20 lines of one column of any standard newspaper. The draw back with the system is that it requires frequent page flipping. However the cost factor is the major issue in the use of e-book. This is mainly due to the high manufacturing cost of LCD screens, which accounts for a major portion of the total cost. Of course PDAs are most popular by virtue of their portability yet they have tiny and hard to read screens. The engineers from Microsoft and Adobe are working hard to supplement this device of PDA. An average e-book should ideally be in the screen size of 4" x 6" and should have the capacity to store/ accommodate 5,20,000 pages on FBK ebooks memory chips. The battery attached to the system last upto 10,000/- pages turns.

2.4 Indian Scenario

Ashtel group of London based at Pune (Ashtel India), launched an e-book reader for first time in India. This e-book reader is in Palm size and has capacity to store 15,000 to 20,000 printed pages. The device uses very little battery. It is interesting to state that no power is utilized when a page is displayed on the screen and the battery power is consumed only when the user turns the pages. The Pune based Ashtel India is engaged in further research for transforming printed books into e-books and setup an assembly plant for the e-book readers. Recently, the Banglore based Indian Science Academy has made a tie up with this company (Ashtel India) for digitizing its valuable collection of scientific journals published prior to 1935 of more than 1,00,000 pages.

3. ELECTRONIC JOURNALS

Electronic journals are those journls which are available in electronic form through an online host are known as e-journals. Of course the idea of e-journals conceived in late 1970s, however, its real progress could be noticed during mid 1990 especially with the progress of INTERNET and World Wide Web (WWW). The major benefit of this advent is that it can be accessed from the remotest place of the country/region or world. Secondly, it allows a reader to search the derived article/paper without having being searched a paritcular volume of issue or page number. Thus e-journals form a major part of digital library. Increasing number of e-publishers are now using the internet as a global way to alter their publications to the international community.

3.1 E-Journals Service Provides

It is a well known fact that at one side many e-journals are available online/Internet/www at the same time many e-Journals service providers have emerged in India. The important among them are J-Gate and INGENTA. Since readers are moving towards on-line access of e-Journals, the libraries also need to play a significant role n selecting, evaluating, describing, annotating and providing prompt access to electronic information available on web.

3.1:1 J-Gate service

J-Gate is the first major e-jorunal service provider agency established in India by Informatics India Pvt. Ltd., Banglore to bridge the gap between information generation and information provider. It is an e-journal portal and access gateway. This service has specially been customized for agricultural Information with the following specil features :

- Bibliographic database of 2.5 Lacs records in Agriculture, Environment and Life Science from more than 1200+ journals available online.
- Table of contents of more that 1200 + journals.
- Access to more than 2200 free journals on web.
- Weekly update of database.
- E-Journals directory of more than 10,000 + e-journals.

For more details about J-Gate Services visit the Site : http://gate.informindia.co.in

3.1.2 Ingenta

Ingenta provides on line access to professionals and researchers. It has got the following important features :

- Ingenta offers access to nearly 6,000 electronic full text journals and millions of articles from world's leading scholarly and professional publications.
- Ingenta offers access to nearly 6,000 electronic full text journals and millions of articles from world's leading scholarly and professional publications.
- It allows searching for more than 27,000 publications including more than 5400 electronic journals from more than 190 publishers. Publications and articles are available in downloadable format.
- It doesn't require any investment in software/ hardware.
- Ingenta is hosted on world leading platforms and guarantees assured uptime and robust infrastructure to support it.
- Assured availability of over 99.5% over a calendar month.
- Services of Ingenta are independent. They do not depend on intranet.
- Service is weekly updated.

- Search through key word, Author, Title is possible. The search can also be limited to period, volume and issue, subject alphabetical directory, by world in title, publisher.

3.1.3 Other agencies

Besides above, there are numerous publishers and other agencies offering e-journals services to large number of reading community through out the world. The popular among them are :

- Elsevier Science Publisher, Netherlands.
- American Physical Society (APS), New York.
- American Institute of Physics, New York.
- University of Chicago Press, Chicago and Cambridge University Press, Cambridge.

The progress and habit of accesing information through net particularly in India is slow because of several reasons among which the most particular and prominent is limitation of band width and with the result the path remains busy particularly during peak period. Due to the advaancement of e-media, particularly the e-journals, now more and more people want to make use of e-journals, not only of current issues but also the back files. However, in practice, the soon we stop subscription of particular journals we are deprived to make use of those back files also to whom we have subscribed. It is unlike the print version and this state of affair restrict librarian/user to subscribe e-journals. The difficultty, which a reader may feel is non or partial availability of page-to-page version and at the same time the quality of diagrams, photographs, graphs, tables etc. deteriorates as compared to print media.

CONCLUSION

It is being said that within 20 years or so from now the paper will die and will be kept in the museum for our future generation. In a short span of time all printed materials may it be book, journals or newspaper will be available in electronic form only. E-publishers will swallow the traditional publishers. Mr. Dick Brass, Vice President, Micro Soft Technology Department, predicted that by 2003, one to five million e-books will be sold out and in the following year i.e. 2004, e-titles sales will surpass an incredible one billion. By 2006, the e-newspaper and e-magazines will be available on newsstands. He boldly predicted that between 2008 to 2010, there will be a flood of cyber books and print version of books, journals and newspapers will start disappearing.

REFERENCES

ARORA (J) Building Digital Libraries : An overview. INFLIBNET courseware, Ahmedabad, INFLIBNET Centre, IUC of UGC; 2003, pp. 262-321.

BAMAN (P) Digital Library Collection Management in India in Planned-2003 edited by T.A.V. Murthy. Ahmedabad, INFLIBNET Centre 2003, pp. 23-29.

DAS (N) Electronic Journals : Problems and Prospects *in Planner - 2003* edited by T.A.V. Murthy Ahmedabad, INFLIBNET Centre, 2003 : 365-370.

e-books - All set to Replace Paperbooks : Report Electronics For You 2003, pp. 30-34

FEATHER (J) and STURGES (P) International Encyclopedia of Information and Library Science. 2nd ed. London, Routledge - Taylar & Francis Group 2003, pp. 136-179.

KUNY (T) and CLEVELAND (G) The Digital Library : Myths and Challenges. IFLA Journals 1998 : 24 (2). pp. 107-113.

PATEL (DR) and SHARMA (RS) Digital Library : A Need of Tomorrow *in Planner-2003* edited by T.A.V. Murthy. Ahmedabad, INFLIBNET Centre, 2003, pp. 365-370.

ROGERS (SA) Electronic Journal Usage at Ohio State University. College and Research Libraries. 2001. 62 (1), pp. 25-34.

WILSON (R) Designing a Readable E-book Information. Today and Tomorrow 2001. 20(3), pp. 7-8.

Library 2.0 : Technology Based Services

Vinod. D

Asst. Librarian, National Law University, Jodhpur

1. INTRODUCTION

Information technology has brought tremendous changes in libraries. Traditional methods of library services are giving way to innovative changes in libraries. Funding limits and changing user demands are transforming the library and information services like never before. Librry administrators and users are seeking more efficient ways of providing services to achieve greater returns on financial investments. Libraries are under increasing pressure to provide services that both compliment and diverge from amazon, google, yahoo, other search engines and online book services. Here lies the importance of library 2.0. Library 2.0 is user oriented virtual community. The role of librarian in library 2.0 is not only as a facilitator but also as to provide support, unlike the traditional libraries he is not merely a collection superviser, instead, librarian acts as a link between user community and library in virtual world. In some ways it is a virtual reality for libraries, a web manifestation of the library as place.

2. NEED FOR LIBRARY 2.0

2.1 Interlibrary co operation

Library 2.0 requires the co-operation between libraries to achieve its goals. Resources of various libraries can be utilized for providing better customer services. In turn, it enables the libraries to share its resources between each other. Unlike the traditional interlibrary programme, library 2.0 based library resource sharing programmes will be faster, elaborative and technology driven. Library 2.0 opens up new frontiers in library services by incorporating better and efficient user service programmes. In order to face the challenges by various search engine services the future librarians will have to adopt better collection management and recourse sharing methods. Library 2.0 concepts assist 'the librarian to implement better service techniques in libraries.

2.2 Library as Search Engine

The aim of severl search engines in a web based environment is to provide information services to its users. Google has declared that its aim is to make available the information sources scattered in different ways on a single platform. In the highly competitive environment search engine services are in a tough competition to ensure better services to its customers. Google book search is one example where search engines are employing innovative services to expand its user coverage. Google has entered into an agreement between several of worlds leading libraries where they will be digitalizing the collection of libraries and will provide the content in online on either subscription based services or free services. Here lies the importance of library portals. It is very clear that unlike good old times libraries also will have to compete with search engines to ensure better services. Future users of library will be looking towards faster and effective user services. Also library users of technological era will be relying on the accuracy and authenticity of the information providing by the libraries. In this context libraries will have to utilize its web content for reaching out to more users. Library 2.0 will act as a channel for this transformation of libraries.

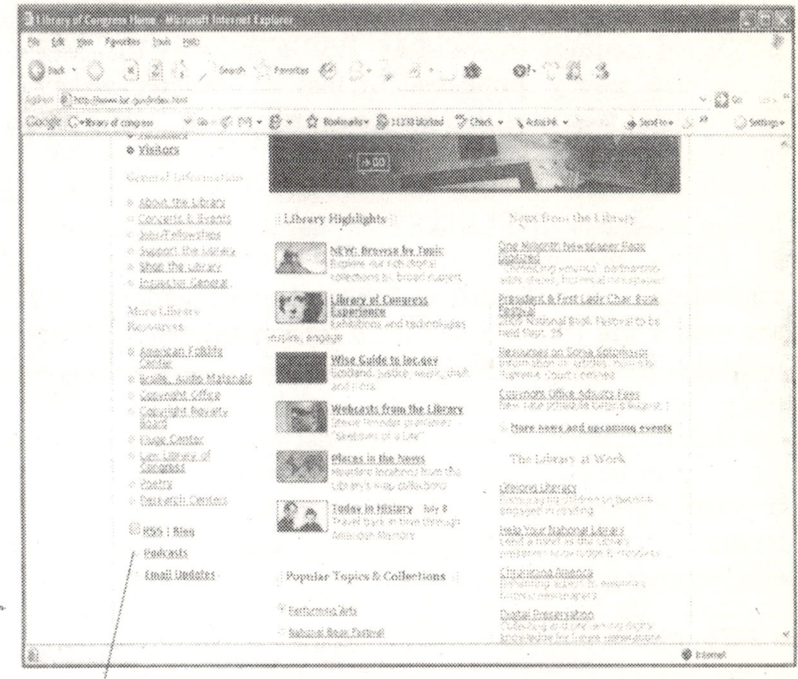

Fig. 1. Library of Congress web portal showing its various library 2.0 services.

3. DEFINITION

The term library 2.0 was coined by Michel Casey on his library crunch blog. Casey argued that libraries have to incorporate the elements of web 2.0 so as to increase the value of technology driven user services. He further argued that libraries have to reach out new users, better service environments and user oriented services. Library 2.0 points out the better usage of technology in the overall functioning of library in a web based environment.

4. TECHNOLOGICAL CONCEPTS BEHIND LIBRARY 2.0

4.1 RSS feeds

RSS stand for Real Simple Syndication or rich site summary. This technology is using for enlisting the newly published updates in websites. RSS also helps the user to track the newly published items in various websites. Commercial websites like google is using this technology to provide latest information published in websites to its registered users through its RSS based alert services. In Indian scenario INFLIBNET is using this technological service to its subscribers of UGC infonet digital library consortium. Several other websites like newspaper websites are also using this technology to inform the users of latest updates. In libraries this technology is slowly taking the place of Selective Dissemination of Information (SDI). Several U.S. and European libraries, which are using RSS, e.g. Library of congress, Cornell university library, Harward university library etc. feeds for users to subscribe updates including collection, new services, and new content in subscription databases.

4.2 Synchronous Messaging

Also known as Instant Messaging (IM) allows the users real time text communication. Libraries are using IM for real time chat reference services. Under these services users can communicate with librarians. INFLIBNET soul support services are an excellent example for the enormous opportunity of this service in libraries. Chat reference service can be a value added service in libraries since it enhances the image of the libraries in a virtual web environment.

4.3 Streaming Media

Streaming audio and video presentation with interactive facilities provides users a platform to interact with library. These can be effectively used for library orientation and similar services, where a librarian's physical presence is not required. With the application of streaming media library resources are not confined within the walls of library. By using the streaming media technology libraries can reach its users beyond space and time. Another facet for streaming media in libraries is about the collection management. As a regulator of streaming media services libraries will be responsible for archiving and providing to the media collection. It opens up new challenges to the library since they cannot confine the streaming media within the four walls of the library. Libraries will have to employ better digital management technology where users can interact with the libraries to enhance the accessibility of streaming media.

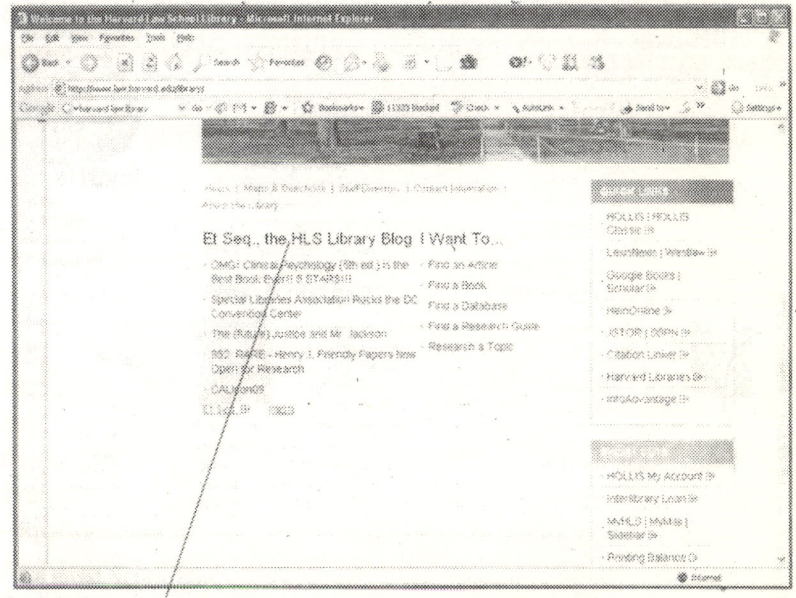

Fig. 2. Harvard law Library Blog Service

4.4 Blogs

The term blog is derived from web log. Blogs are created greater inroads in the services of libraries. It enables the rapid production and consumption of web based publications. Blogs allow the users to publish in the web spectrum. Blogs are now becoming the essential part of the libraries. Librarians can write blog services for dissemination notification of new arrivals and other events for library. Blogs can also act as a platform for users to discuss library matters. Eventhough blogs lack editorial governance, in modern libraries it is an essential service component due to its many advantages.

4.5 Wikis

Wikis are basically open web page where any one can register, publish, amend, and change the contents. Wikipedia is an example for the wiki services. Wikis as items in a collection of library can be very useful to library user. However users should be informed about its lack of peer review and editorship.

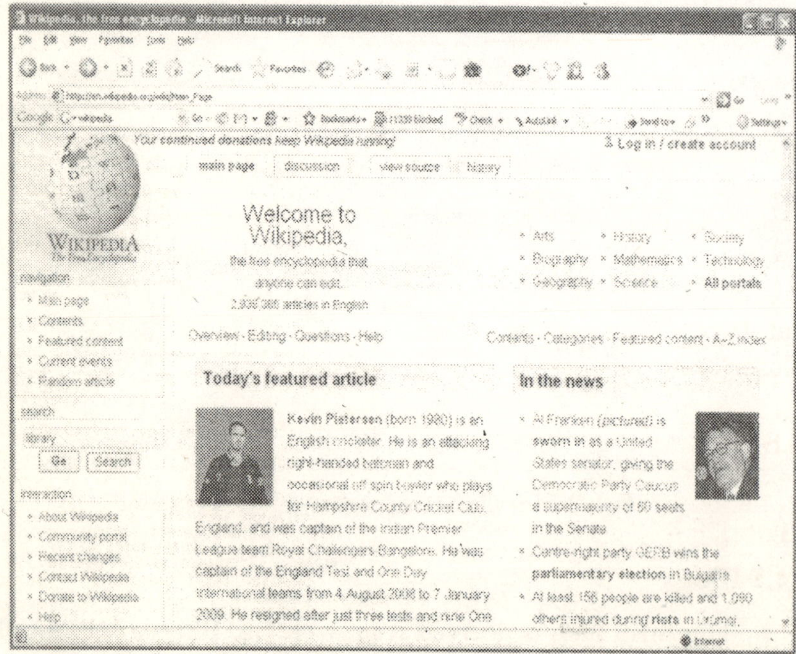

Fig. 3. Wikipedia, the free encyclopedia.

4.6 Social Networks

Social netwroks are the most promising and important technology under library 2.0 concept. It enables blogging, messaging, streaming media and other services discussed earlier. My space, Orkut. Facebook, Flicker etc. are some of the most popular social networking sites. Social net works helps the user to connect each other beyond the barriers of time and space. Library Thing is one of the library oriented social network, which facilitates the user to catalogue their books and view what other users share those books. Shelfari empowers the user to display his favorite books online and enables the users community to discuss about their books in various discussion group forums. The face of the libraries web presence in the future may look very much like a social network interface.

4.7 Tagging

Tagging is a keyword or subject heading. It is using to describe information posted in web. Ex a video or audio clip in Orkut. It is a form of metadata. Various website users use different methods to tag the information, which they post. In flicker users tag pictures to describe the information which they posted. In library users can tag books. In library 2.0 users can use the library catalogue and in turn it becomes a customized, user-friendly catalogue. Tagging of library catalogue makes the library user community to become closer to library and its operations.

4.8 Pod-casting

Pod casting is defined as ``process of capturing audio digital media files that can be distributed over the internet using RSS feeds for playing back on portable media players as well as computers. Users can subscribe to such feeds and automatically download these files into an audio management file programme on their personal computers. When a user sunchronizes their portable audio device with their personal computer the pod casts are automatically transferred to that device to be listened (Wikipedia, 2009). Pod casting is using by libraries to deliver library orientation programme.

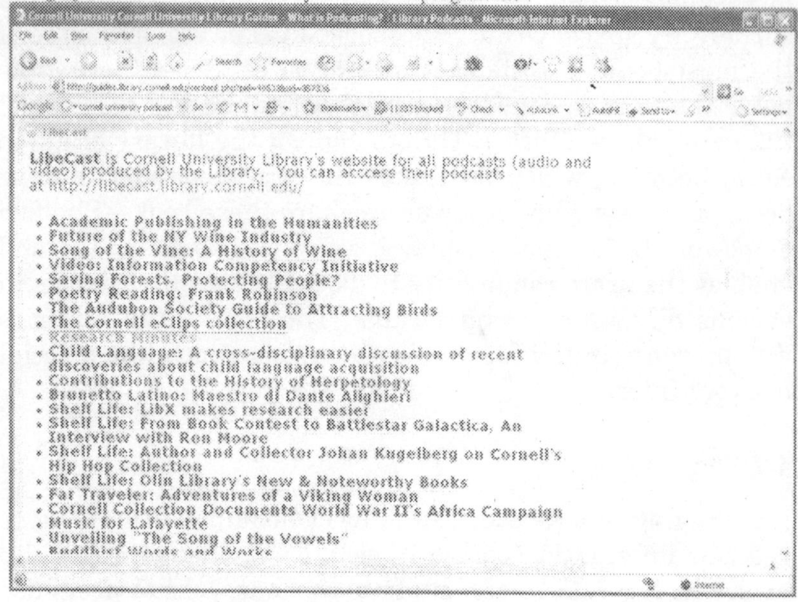

Fig. 4. Cornell university library - Pod-casts and vod-casts.

4.9 Vod casting

Vod casting stand for Video On demand. Vod casting is used for streaming video content. Vod coasting can be value added service if libraries use the enormous opportunities of it.

CONCLUSION

Clearly each one of the technologies listed above RSS, wikis, blogs podcasting, streaming media, social networks could be very useful in an institutional research, or community environment and could be introduced by these libraries. Library 2.0 enables the integration of the library to users through the library portal or local intranet. The success of the library 2.0 services are depending on adding the various services to its content. Many libraries have encouraging advances in their electronic offerings by providing access to top quality websites, downloadable books instant messaging chatting reference services. In the era of information technology diversification of library services with the help of technology will determine the success of library as a service oriented mechanism.

User participation will be the key to determine the success of the library 2.0 concept. In order to ensure the user participation libraries will have to tap the enormous opportunities providing by web 2.0 world. Providing access to e-books. Digitalized library archival collection, customization and personalization of library WebPages, Pod casting and Vod casting etc., like technologies can help the librarians to expand the horizons of library services. It makes enormous changes from the present library world where users are depending on library to provide services. In library 2.0 users may create content in the library portal with the proper authorization of library authorities. In India Indian institute of Technology, Kahragpur is already giving the opportunity to its users to publish blogs in their library web page. One thing is clear that libraries are slowly shedding its centuries old concept of collection supervisors, instead libraries of the future will work as a mediator between user and content in digitalized environment.

REFERENCES

Arora, Jagdish, Library 2.0 : Innovative technologies for libraries of tomorrow, proceedings of the national seminar on open access to textual and multimedia. January 29-30, 2009.

Casey, M. (2006). Library crunch : bringing you a library 2.0 perspective, Accessioned june 27 2009 from http:// www.library crunch.com

Casey, Michel, savastimuk laura C, Library Journal.

Multimedia contributors, library 2.0, Wikipedia Http:// www.wikipedia.org/w/index/php/title-20801d (accessioned june 27, 2009)

Web 2.0 library 2.0 and librarian 2.0, preparing for the 2.0 world, proceedings of the online information 2007.

www.inflibnet.org.

Building Digital Library Collections in Academic Libraries

Rajpal Singh Rajpurohit

Librarian, Lachoo Memorial College of Science & Technology, Jodhpur

1. INTRODUCTION

The education system provides an opportunity to the learners to build/improve the knowledge. The teacher is main source of sharing/imparting the knowledge to the learner. In addition to the teacher, the libraries are important source to supplement and complement the class room teaching. The libraries play an important role in education system, where in they procure useful and relevant information resources and provide access to these resources. Over a period of time the mode and methods of education has been changed to suit the needs of the learners by using ever changing techniques, methods and technology. We can find the changes from Gurukuls to the present system of e-learning by using the Information and Communication Technology (ICT). During the process of change, it had passed several stages, such as traditional class room teaching and learning; private study; correspondence education; distance (open) education and online learning. Even though the teacher and taught are part of any type of education system the libraries continuously played a supportive role in the learning process.

The education system is continuously tailored to suit the learners ambition such as life long learning, improving the competencies and quality of learning process. The changes were also mainly to provide the alternative and flexible learning environment. These changes had also influenced the libraries which were struggling to meet the information needs of ever changing educational environment.

During this period, the libraries changed their functioning and approach. However, the main objective of providing the information to its users is being retained in spite of several changes in the information storage processes, analysing and retrieval medias. Initially, libraries collected manuscripts and then invention of printing gave boost for improving the collection. During the period, the information was being brought out in different media/type of sources such as journals, standards, specifications, patents, films, audio materials and computer storage devices. The users have shifted from one type to another due to the comfort in using, transporting and storing the information. Every time the change in media was accepted as it gave effective support to the education system.

2. LIBRARY SUPPORT

The libraries are making all the efforts to cope up with the changes in the education system and learning methods. They have made all the attempts to understand the changes and expectations. Accordingly, they have devised and adopted various new techniques and methods in procurement, storage, display, organisation and dissemination of the information sources. To support the aspiration teachers and learners, the libraries have started making extensive use of the ICT, which brought transformation in their functioning. One can find a shift from document delivery to information access, irrespective of the physical media. Now the libraries are able to provide access to required and relevant information anywhere and any time. Thus, this is a major accomplishment to the libraries, which could be realized due to the developments/application of ICT.

ICT is enabling the libraries to support different learning styles such as observation and practice oriented through multimedia documents and manual. They are able to support the learner's desire of learning through alternative routes such as modular and distance education. In the process of changes in functioning of the libraries, they have changed their nomenclature as Information Centres, Knowledge Resource Centres, Learning Resource Centres etc. The academic libraries made the strategies to support the dynamic educational environment. These strategies are conceived by taking into consideratgion of the available tools and facilitiesm, especially ICT. The ICT is being used as tool to achieve the objectives of the libraries. Most of the strategies are related to ICT and some of them are :

(a) Creating digital environment;

(b) Developing digital collections;

(c) Planning for digital libraries;

(d) Provision of information literacy;

(e) Creating of physicl and virtual environment for informantion access;

(f) Resource sharing with other libraries;

(g) Introduction of new services at minimal cost and staff;

(h) Library support for curriculum development;

(i) Identification of alternative sources of information; and

(j) Involving the library staff to understand the information needs of the users.

3. LIBRARY COLLECTIONS

The modern libraries are able to make all the efforts to use ICT extensively to provide access to information. Most of the library staff are learning themselves out of self interest and used the same knowledge for the benefit of improving the library functioning. It is a fact that book form (print media) is the larger chunk of the collection in the academic libraries. In addition to the books and journals another important component of the collection is project reports, technical reports, dissertations, theses and reports. Over a period of time, these libraries procured various types of materials and now the emphasis is on digital/electronic collections. The digital collections consist of CDs, DVDs, audio tapes, video tapes etc. Some of the free CDs came as an attachment with the books. These days the libraries are subscribing online e-journals (sometimes getting CDs as backup). Since last two years, a few selected university libraries are getting Infonet online journals. Even many professional colleges, IITs, IIMs and engineering colleges are procuring the e-journals through INDEST-AICTE consort-ium. It may be worth to state that these libraries have turned more favourable to procurement of digital materials. Most of the libraries are part of the institutional networks and are able to provide access to digital information through the networks.

Looking at the benefits enjoyed with the use of ICT, many more academic libraries are taking initiation to develop the digital collections. Simultaneously, they are increasingly making all the efforts to develop necessary infrastructure to handle these digital collections.

3.1 What are Digital Collections?

In digital colleciton the information is stored in bits and bytes, which need the computers to write/store and read/ retrieve this information. In simple terms, it means that the information is stored in computer readable form. The medium stored could be any type using alternative technologies such as magnetic, optical magnetooptical and film. Even in each of these technologies, there are various types of storage devices (also known as Electronic Storage Devices). These storage devices need the drives to read and write the information. These devices may differ in size, storage capacity, speed etc. The tehcnological developments allow using the storage devices of variant technologies on the same machine.

These storage devices can store the content either any one or combination of media such as text, audio, maps, pictures, moving pictures (video). The libraries can convert these materials of various types of content into digital medium by digitizing the content. This process is known as reformating from one medium to another (digital). However, methods to handle, store, preserve and organize are different to all these storage devices.

3.2 Why Digital Collections?

Any and every change is accepted only when they are advantageous or beneficial. Changing is not an easy job as it involves redesigning and careful planning. Even one needs to invest finances amount to train the staff to enable them to adjust to the new environment. The staff may have to learn new techniques and methods relevant to digital environment. It is easy to say than to implement the change, that is why *management of change* is being dealt as one of the most important subjects in management. The libraries also accepted changes and physical medium used for information storage due to several accured benefits. This can be observed, when films (film strips, roll films, microfiche, super fiche, ultra fiche), tapes (audio, video) were accepted by every one, even though they cannot be used without aids to read and record information. Further, it is found that the electronic storage media are more convenient and comfortable to store and retrieve information; therefore there is major shift towards increased used of these materials. The major advantages are listed in the following paragraphs :

(a) The digital collections can provide wide access to the information. It could be either directly from a stand alone computer or through the networks (LAN or WAN) and Internet gateways;

(b) They support any time and any where (distance is immaterial) access;

(c) They support increased awareness about the materials/information;

(d) The digital environment provides facilities to simultaneous access by more than one user;

(e) The fragile and rare collections can be converted into digital medium, wherein the digital copy is just like original in terms of color, clarity and visibility. By using these materials the users can get access to the content which is similar to that of original and at the same time the original can be prevented or stored safely;

(f) Materials need less floor/shelf space for storage;

(g) They facilitate preservation for future generations;

(h) Resource sharing can be made possible without any hindrance to other own users;

(i) They provide best searching facility of the materials;

(j) It is easy to do packaging and repackaging of the content or bibliographical details on the basis of demand. Several services were only discussed but were never provided by academic libraries, have now become possible with least effort and time (for example - bibliography);

(k) A backup copy is stored in case of danger or damage or loss of the original;

(l) The users may have copies of the documents at no extra expenditure; and

(m) Earlier books were purchased on the basis of catalogues or bibliographies. Several libraries were also finding it difficult to assess the latest edition, the cost of the books (especially foreign books, where the price is not put on the book and are subject to change) and also use them as selection tools. It was difficult to get complete information including the review of the content. Now the digital material and networks are able to provide opportunity to overcome these limitations and in turn support judicious selections.

4. BUILDING DIGITAL COLLECTIONS

The traditional library's major collection is in print medium and now the libraries are being converted into hybrid libraries, wherein the collection also consists of both print and digital. As discussed earlier, looking at the advantages of digital collections, the libraries are building their digital collections. Various methods adopted for building digital collections are :

(a) By digitizing the existing collections;

(b) Directly creating the digital documents;

(c) Procurement of digital materials such as e-journals and e-books;

(d) Downloading the digital information from Internet;

(e) Getting the digital information through resource sharing and transfer of documents in digital medium; and

(f) Searching and downloading the information from databases and websites.

All the digital information created and received can be stored in digital storage medium and can be made available for access in network environment.

5. LIBRARY POLICY

It is one of the important management activities to prepare a policy document in the organizations. This document gives guidance to the staff and managers in taking the decisions from time to time. Such document also helps in systematically executing the proposed plans. Even the libraries need to prepare a policy document relating to building the digital library collections. The items to be considered to include in the policy document are stated in the following paragraphs.

(a) Digitization

What type and which print materials need to be digitized? What standards and formats ned to be followed? Selection of storage medium?

How long the material (categorization) needs to preserved-based on need and cost?

Availability of OCR for the languages selected for digitization.

(b) The documents could be simultaneously created both in soft and hard copy form building the digital collections. In the universities and colleges, the internal reports, project reports, dissertations, theses and class notes are being created initially as soft copies and are used the same for making hardcopies. But the storage of these soft copies is not taken seriously for access and preservation. It may be worth mentioning that the University Grants Commission had initiated creation of ETD (Electronic Theses and Dissertations) by all the universities and maintaining the same as repository for access. The plan was to create repositories at national and regional levels. It is also observed that few institutions are putting the class/teaching notes on their institutional websites for the benefit of the students.

(c) What types of physical materials should be used for storage of digital content? Further, access also needs to be provided to both original as well as digital content; and

(d) Which type of digital materials and on what subjects need to be procured/purchased? For example whether to procure e-journals, e-books, databases etc?

6. SELECTION CRITERIA FOR DIGITIZATION

The libraries cannot and need not to digitize all the print materials available with them. As stated earlier, they have to identify the materials that need to be digitized. The criteria for identification and selection of the materials need to be prepared as a part of the policy for building the digital library collections. It is not only difficult but also expensive to digitize all the materials. While material in public domain can be digitized without much problems, copyright clearance must be obtained from rights holders for digitizing such material. The criteria for selection should be based on the need and use. The criteria may change from library to library based on activities and collections. The important factor to be considered is copyright law and cost-benefit analysis. For example, digitizing the text books works out to be very expensive when the cost for digitization, management and preservation is taken into consideration; purchasing few more copies would be much cheaper option. It does not stop there as the library continuous to add new editions of the same book. This makes digitization of such books irrelevant. The broad criteria for digitization include :

(a) High demand collection;

(b) Material not readily accessible due to conservation or security considerations;

(c) Experiences show that relatively unknown materials have created demand when they are accessible through digital media; such collections also deserve to be digitized;

(d) Select costly, fragile and rare documents such as manuscripts or old but valuable books;

(e) Materials based on historical or intellectual content;

(f) Copyright clearance; and

(g) Format based (any one format such a photographs or pamphlets) or thematic/subject based (any material belonging to a particular/specific subjects) digitization.

The above criteria is only indicative and not exhaustive. However, the libraries can prepare their own criteria based on their needs, environment, finances and availability of infrastructure.

7. IMPLICATIONS FOR LIBRARY STAFF AND ORGANISATION

The libraries have to create digital learning environment, which means procurement of infrastructure including suitable furniture, designing the space for installation of computers, training the users to enable to identify, select and access the digital information. The issues and implications are :

(a) Design and development of the digital libraries;

(b) Planning access to other online materials;

(c) Planning the resource/knolwedge sharing programs with other libraries;

(d) Redesigning of the library building to suit to the digital environment;

(e) Providing information literacy programme to the users. It will facilitate exploitation of the `new library' (digital library);

(f) The face of the library changes and new environment prevails and naturally they make effect on the service. For example, the document delivery will be mainly `digital' rather than photocopy;

(g) The libraries must get ready to face increased demand for the information compared to the traditional environment;

(h) The libraries will be able to overcome the `digital divide' as the digital document facilitates access to every one. This is more relevant in Indian academic libraries as the print book once issued hardly comes back and others are denied of access; this problem can be taken care in digital environment;

(i) The libraries have to prepare plans for digitization projects. In this project, the libraries will have to take into consideration of technical information on digital formats and standards. The standards are being specified by many institutions especially national libraries such as Library of Congress and Australian National Library;

(j) The staff needs to be trained themselves to handle the digital collections including the equipment. They should also be trained to identify various sources for useful digital content both free and paid; and creating awareness and access of such content to the users. They should also be trained to maintain and preserve the digital material;

(k) The staff needs to design and develop the digital libraries and link the same digital learning environments;

(l) They also need to know the standards, how to plan and share the knowledge among the libraries, how to plane the space, and mainly how to support the educational process;

(m) In addition to above the library staff needs to keep themselves abreast of the changes in technological environment to enable them to incorporate the same in the libraries at regular intervals. Therefore, they have to participate in continuing education programs regularly both within and outside the country;

(n) Even though the libraries spend the funds for development of digital environment initially, they have also to allocate the funds for annual maintenance of the software and hardware; and

(o) Review of procedures, technology used, user satisfaction, needs to be the part of the management activity. These libraries must get themselves prepared for adoption changing environment.

With the traditional collections, the libraries were managing with or without major changes. But in the digital environment they have to be vigilant in organisation and management of the digital collections. Otherwise, it could be disastrous.

8. STORAGE MEDIUM

Once the library decides to build digital collections, one of the important decisions is to identify various storage media and select the best one, which support both management and preservation of electronic records over a long term. It is also essential that the staff need to know how to handle and take care of these media. If these materials are not handled properly there is every chance to get spoiled and information may not be retrieved. The library staff should have some idea of the technology and type of storage media that are emerging into the market. It is also essential to understand that what technologies are getting outdated and then only the necessary steps can be taken to refresh the date to suit to the new technology.

On the basis of the existing technology, the storage media can be categorised into magnetic optical, magneto-optical and solid state media. Most of the libraries use magnetic disks, magnetic tapes, cartridges and optical disks (such as CD, DVD). The solid state storage devices use flash memory for storage purpose. The examples include compact flash, smart media, PCMCIA cards (used in cameras and laptops). They do not have large storage capacity like magnetic and optical storages devices. Prior to taking the decision of choosing the media for storage, it is essential to understand their life (obsolescense), how safe they are in storing the data, how flexible in handling, to what extent they provide access to stored information, their weakness and sustainability in dynamic environment.

The major factors to be considered while finalizing the storage media are :

(a) Maximum life span, which is decided by both physical longevity and prevalent technology; at least the life span should be of 10 years for archival purpose.

(b) Validity and redundancy of supporting hardware and software, i.e, technological obsolescence should be considered.

(c) There is need for periodic refreshment of data or new copies; or the same data in new media; or new copies in the same media format. Careful selection may help in avoiding frequent refreshing.

(d) To store the information in multiple copies using more than one media i.e., different types of media supporting different technologies. If one technology gets outdated quickly, at least others can be used.

(e) If the storage needs to be made in the same media, it is better to make copies on the media manufactured by different companies.

(f) Quantity of data of storage capacity is also an important factor in selection of media.

(g) Cost of the storage may be calculated in terms of cost per GB/MB. It is also essential to take into consideration of its maintenance cost.

(h) To what extent the media can support in error detection, recovery of the data, protection mechanism, prevent loss of the data due to accidental erasure.

(i) Tolerant to a wide range of environmental changes without data loss.

(j) Low susceptibility for physical damage.

The experience in using the technology is being documented and publisheed in the form of reports. These reports are based on the evalution of the media and they provide all the necessary and useful information for the selection of the media. For example, solid state media is being discouraged. Optical storage media manufactured with gold reflective layer is being evaluated as more stable medium. One can find that today the 5" inch floppies are outdted and even the 3'/2 inch floppy drivers are not coming with the laptops. It means that these technologies or storage media have become obsolate. Now what is to be done with the data available in the floppies? It cannot be used. Therefore, during the transition of the technology or hardware there is a need to refresh the data, which means transferring or migrating the data into the new technological environment. To overcome this frequent refreshing or migrating, the selection of storage medium needs to be done carefully on the basis of evaluation and proven technology.

CONCLUSION

The publishing industry had increasingly assumed production of their documents in digital medium. They are also using state of art technology in order to take the benefits of the changes in the technology. The libraries have also accepted these documents due to increased facilities in providing access to the users by overcoming the distance and time. The academic libraries in India have also started procurring the digital materials but most of the library staff does not have the knowledge of managing these technologies. Even small problems cannot be handled by them, which is mainly due to lack of proper training and knowledge. Several times they neither know the procedures for accessing information nor have knowledge of handling them. Many libraries get the CDs along with the books and they do not know how to handle them. Further, few libraries do not have the necessary infrastructure for handling them. The UGC Infonet is providing access to e-journals to select university and college libraries. In spite of the fact that huge amount is spent for this purpose, still their uitlization is not satisfactory. The reasons could be many such as lack of infrastructure, training, awareness etc. The INFLIBNET, should act as a central agency for academic libraries and should play leadership role in educating/advising the library profes-sionals in handling/managing the digital documents. Even the library professionals have to develop their knowledge in this area for efficient management of the digital content.

Open Source Software for Library Management

R.K. Dave & Tirth Das

Dr. Raheja Library, Central Arid Zone Research Institute, Jodhpur - 342 003

INTRODUCTION

The biggest news in the software industry in recent months is open source. Every week in the technology news we can read bout IBM or Oracle or Netscape or Corel announcing plans to release flagship products as open source or a version of these products that runs on an open source operating system such as Linux. In its defense against the Department of Justice, Microsoft has pointed to Linux and its growing market share as evidence that Microsoft cannot exert unfair monopoly power over the software industry. Dozens of new open source products along with regular news of upgrades, bug fixes, and innovative new features for these products are announced every day at web sites followed by thousands.

Open Source is becoming an increasingly popular software development method for producing successful software like Linux Operating System, Apache Web Server, Perl. Open Source Software is licensed to guarantee free access to the precompiled binaries, so called the source code. This allows the user to install the software on a new platform without an additional purchase and to get support for a product whose creator no longer supports it. Those who are technically inclined can fix bugs themselves rather than waiting for someone else to do so.

A variety of licenses are used to ensure that the source code will remain available, wherever the code is actually used. Unlike freeware and public-domain software, Open Source Software is copyrighted and distributed with license terms designed to ensure that the source code will always be available. While a fee may be charged for the software's packaging, distribution, or support, the complete package needed to create files is included, not simply a portion needed to view files created elsewhere.

DEFINITION

Open source software is computer software whose source code is available under a license (or arrangement such as the public domain) that permits users to use, change, and improve the software, and to redistribute it in modified or unmodified form. It is often developed in a public, collaborative manner. It is the most prominent example of open source development and often compared to user generated content.[1]

HISTORY

The free software movement was launched in 1983. In 1998, group of individuals advocated that the term free software be replaced by Open Source Software (OSS) as an expression which is less ambiguous and more comfortable for the corporate world.[2] Software developers may want to publish their software with an Open Source Software license, so that anybody may also develop the same software or understand how it works. Open Source Software generally allows anybody to make a new version of the software, port it to new operating systems and processor architectures, share it with others or market it. The aim of open source is to let the product be more understandable, modifiable, duplicatable, reliable or simply accessible, while it is still marketable.

FREE/OPEN SOURCE CONCEPT

If asked, most computer-literate people would say that Free/Open Source Software includes the original code for the program, whatever language it is written in (C, C++, Perl, PHP, etc.) and that it also may be modified for local use and then subsequently redistributed for ``free''. However, the official definitions of ``free software'' and ``open source'' cover other aspects of software use and distribution that are important in understanding how this type of software differs from commercial or proprietary software.

`Free/Open Source' means

- Source code for software is distributed at no cost, with licensing conditions that allows users to modify it in any way they wish;
- any modifications that are subsequently re-distributed must also be available as free/open software;
- author's rights are protected, and changes are only incorporated into a distribution with the permission of the ``owner'' (but new projects sometimes ``fork'' from existing ones);
- two groups, the Free Software Foundation and the Open Source Initiative, represent different political positions about the reasons for making source code available, but have broadly similar positions on software distribution and licensing;
- each group maintains a list of licenses that meet their conditions; the GNU General Public License

(GPL), which is both free and open, is the most commonly used license; and

- a wide range of softwre is available under F/OF licenses, ranging from operating systems and other utilities (Linux, Apache, Sendmail, BIND) to programming languages (Perl, PHP) to database management systems (MySQL, PostgreSQL) to application software (Open Office, Koha, Greenstone, MyLibrary).

Open Source Software vs Free Software

Open Source Software and free software are different terms for software which comes with certain rights, or freedoms, for the user. They describe two approaches and philosophies towards free software. *Open source* and *Free software* (or software *libre*) both describe software which is free from onerous licensing restrictions. It may be used, copied, studied, modified and redistributed without restriction. Free software is not the same as freeware, software available at zero price.

The definition of Open Source Software was written to be almost identical to the free software definition. There are very few cases of software that is free software but is not Open Source Software, and vice versa. The difference in the terms is where they place the emphasis. ``Free software'' is defined in terms of giving the user freedom. This reflects the goal of the free software movement. ``Open source'' highlights that the source code is viewable to all and proponents of the term usually emphasize the quality of the software and how this is caused by the development models which are possible and popular among free and open source software projects.

Free software licenses are not written exclusively by the FSF. The FSF and the OSI both list licenses which meet their respective definitions of free software. Open Source Software and free software share an almost identical set of licenses. One exception is an early version of the Apple

Public Source License, which was accepted by the OSI but rejected by the FSF because it did not allow private modified versions; this restriction was removed in later version of the license. There are now new versions that are approved by both the OSI and the FSF.

The Open Source Initiative believes that more people will be convinced by the experience of freedom. The FSF believes that more people will be convinced by the concept of freedom. The FSF believes that knowledge of the concept is an essential requirement, insists on the use of the term *free*[1], and separates itself from the Open Source movement. The Open Source Initiative believes that *free* has three meanings : free as in beer, free as in freedom, and free as in unsellable. The problem with the term ``Open Source" is it says nothing about the freedom to modify and redistribute, so it is used by people who think that source access without freedom is a sufficient definition. This possibility for misuse is the case for most of the licences that make up Microsoft's ``shared source" initiative, and to a lesser extent with the ``licence-free" software of Daniel J. Bernstein.

F/OS software in Library and Information Management

Free/Open Source Software has had an increasingly high profile in the library and information management profe-ssion since 1999. A september 1999 meeting of 80 senior American academic library managers created three ``key-stone principles" to set a foundation for future developments of library services. One of these, ``libraries are responsible for creating innovative information systems for the dissemi-nation and preservation of information and new knowledge regardless of format" had an action item to ``create intero-perability in the systems they develop and create Open Source Software for the access, dissemination, and management of information" (Keystone Principles, 2000, p. 104).

Frumkin (2002) suggests that the F/OS movement gives librarians an opportunity to become more active in determining the future development of the software they use, rather than letting vendors keep control. As Brandt (2001) notes, librarians have long been active not only in taking advantage of technological innovations, but also in experimenting with new approaches (using Peter Scott's Hy Telnet as one example), and the F/OS approach should increase the opportunities for such activity.

Selected examples

This section of the paper will describe 6 examples of F/OS projects in more detail and others will be mentioned their respective name and their site address for more detail, to illustrate the outcomes of this approach.

Greenstone

Greenstone is a software package for constructing and implementing digital libraries that include documents in a variety of electronic formats. It was originally developed at the University of Waikato in New Zealand in 1995, and is available under the GPL. The current version is 2.42 (September 2003). Greenstone can be run under Windows, Linux, Solaris, Unix and MacOS X, and works with standard web servers such as Apache.

Greenstone features include :

- browser-based access;
- both full-text and field-specific searching;
- browasable lists of authors, titles, dates, classification numbers, etc.;
- use of Dublin Core and other metadata scheme;
- advanced data compression techniques that lower response times when searching large collections;
- a customisable interface based on a configuration file;

- multilingual interface, available in Arabic, Chinese, Dutch, French, German, Maori, Portuguese, and Spanish, as well as English;
- extensive use of plug-ins to convert documents in different formats such as MS Word, PDF, HTML, or email; and
- administrative features that support access control and user activity logs.

Greenstone uses Unicode for all documents and interfaces, making it suitable for use with materials in any language. It stores all documents in a standard XML form. The software is available for downloading from SourceForge. Documentation includes an installation manual, a user manual, a development manual, a guide to customising the Greenstone interface, a description of MGPP (the Greenstone text compression and indexing system), and an online FAQ. There are two electronic discussion lists, a general one, and one for Greenstone developers. A web-based form is available for questions which are not covered in the documentation of FAQ.

More information bout Greenstone is available at http://www.greenstone.org

Koha

Koha is an integrated library management system that was originally developed by Katipo Communications Limited of Wellington, New Zealand for the Horowhenua Library Trust (HLT), a regional library system located in Levin, some 100 kilometres north of Wellington. In 1999, HLT was looking for a new system to replace its DOS-based one, and found that commercially-available options would incur substantially increased communications charges. Katipo proposed developing a new system using open source tools (Perl, MySQL, and Apache) that would run under Linux and use Telnet to communicate with the branches. There has been a high level of interest in Koha internationally, and it is currently being used in New Zealand, Australia, Canada, the United States, India, Thailand, the United Kingdom, and France. Many of the libraries using Koha are small, medium and special libraries.

The initial Koha release was an early version, with functionally for circulation, simple cataloguing and acquisitions, and OPAC searching. New versions have been released by the Koha developers irregularly, and the system is gradually gaining enhanced functionality. In most cases, Koha users either undertake the development themselves and contribute the changes back to the project, or they commission a developer to undertake specific enhancements.

The Koha project uses a number of channels to allow members of its community to communicate with each other - there is a general mailing list, as well as separate ones for developers, Windows users, French-speaking Koha users/ developers, and German-speaking Koha users/developers.

More information about Koha is available at http://www.koha.org.

My Library

In 1998, Eric Lease Morgan, then employed at North Carolina State University Libraries developed a customisable, web-based interface to a database of information resources, called MyLibrary@NCState. It allows library users to create their own views of information resources, based on a user profile. Library staff maintain a database of descriptions of information resources that are matched to user profiles and create individual MyLibrary pages. The software is written in Perl and uses MySQL as the database engine. Source code for MyLibrary was released under the GPL in February 2000, and many libraries have since implemented it.

More information bout MyLibrary is at http:// dewey.library.nd.edu/mylibrary/.

Open Office

StarDivision, the original authors of the Star Office suite of software, was founded in Germany in the mid-1980s. It was acquired by Sun Microsystems during the summer of 1999 and StarOffice 5.2 was released in June of 2000. Future versions of StarOffice software, beginning with 6.0, have been built using the OpenOffice.org source, APIs, file formats, and reference implementation. Sun continues to sponsor development on OpenOffice.org and is the primary contributor of code to OpenOffice.org.Collabnet hosts the website infrastructure for development of the product and helps manage the project.

The OpenOffice.org source code includes the technology which Sun Microsystems has been developing for the future versions of StarOffice (TM) software. The source is written in C++ and delivers language-neutral and scriptable functionality, including Java (TM) APIs. This source technology introduces the next-stage architecture, allowing use of the suite as separate applications or as embedded components in other applications. Numerous other features are also present including XML-based file formats based on the vendor-neutral OpenDocument standard from OASIS and other resources.

The OpenOffice.org Community announces the availability of OpenOffice.org Release 2.2.1. This is a minor bug fix release - full details of the changes may be found in the Release Notes.

OpenOffice.org the product is a multi-platform office productivity suite. It includes the key desktop applications, such as a word processor, spreadsheet, presentation manager, and drawing program, with a user interface and feature set similar to other office suites. Sophisticated and flexible OpenOffice.org also works transparently with a variety of file formats, including those of Microsoft Office, and the vendor-neutral Open Document standard from OASIS.

Available in over 65 supported languages with more being constantly added by the community, OpenOffice.org runs stably and natively on Solaris, Linux (including PPC Linux), Windows, Mac OS X (X11), and numerous other plaftforms. Our porting page lists the plaftform (ports) that OpenOffice.org can run on.

Written in C++ and with documented APIs licensed under the LGPL open-source lincense, OpenOffice.org allows any knowledgeable developer to benefit from the source. And, because the native file format for OpenOffice.org is the vendor-independent OpenDocument open standard, interoperability is easy, making future development and adoption more certain.

More information about Open Office is at http://www.openoffice.org/

Avanti Library Systems

Avanti Library Systems grew out of a project started in 1998 to develop a simple low cost open source library system for small libraries. A key goal was to design the system around a general model of a library system rather than design it to the needs of a specific library or type of library. This resulted in an OPAC that is simple, very efficient and adaptable to a variety of libraries and situations.

The design philosophy of Avanti Library Systems emphasizes simplicity, usability and careful design. This results in software that is :

- **Easy to use.** User interfaces are carefully designed, consistent and simple, offering the user only what they need when they need it. This reduces costs by minimizing the need for extensive training of library staff and patrons.
- **Small, efficient and self-contained**. With carefull minimalist design the software can run effectively on very modest hoardware. By Keeping systems as self-contained as possible, external dependencies are

reduced or eliminated altogether. MicroLCS requires no third party software other than Java to run.

- **Flexible and powerful**. By building upon a simple well thought out architecture, power and flexibility are not sacrificed for simplicity. MicroLCS is a fully functional client/server library system. Although simple, it has a flexibility and ease of use that are rarely found in any other OPAC in its class.

Avanti Library Systems is dedicated to providing the library community with software products that are both simple to use and powerful, without complicated bells and whistles. When simplicity and power are brought together in design that captures basic principles well, they make tools that efficiently and elegantly solve the problems for which they are designed. Such tools not only enhance productivity but using them can be a joy.

More information about **Avanti, An open source library computing system** is at http://www. avanti-librarysystems.com/

Virtual Library : Open Source Information Broker

The Virtual Library System is a free Web-based system to build, manage and maintain efficiently medium to large collections of links and their meta information. It provides advanced full-text search capabilities as well as uniform access via categories to informtion on the Internet, reducing long paths leading to a few clicks.

Features

1. Easy to use :

- Information access via browsing categories and full-text search
- All administration with a standard Web-browser

2. Scalable :

- Supports unlimited number of independent libraries on one server
- Uses glimplse, a indexing tool that is successfully used with thousands of entries
- Automatic services like link-checking, execution of scripts, ...automate most of the time consuming tasks to keep the collection up-to-date

3. Conform with Standards :

- Security : password encryption and SSL (optional)
- Dublin Core compliance.
- Easy to combine with the OAI protocol from the Open Archive Initiative using XML.

4. Easy to expand :

- Easy step-by-step adjustment of content, and design (only basic HTML knowledge necessary)
- Powerful interface to expand functionality with Perl-Scripts.

More information about **Virtual Library : Open Source Information Broker** is at http://vu.wu-wien.ac.at/virlib/

Some other examples are as under :

PhpMyBibli

http://phpmybibli.sourceforge.net/

Research Guide

http://researchguide.sourceforge.net/

OpenOPAC

http://www.bl.fcen.uba.ar/openopac.pho

Open Source Digital Library System

http://intranet.library.arizona.edu/users/jfrumkin/osdls/about.html

Jake, metadata collective for ejournals

http://jake.med.yale.edu/

Success Factors for Adopting F/OS Software

In many ways, adopting open source software requires the same type of evaluation as purchasing commercial software, but with some modification. While the initial cost is zero, supporting the software over its lifetime may involve considerable costs, and organisations may find it difficult to estimate these costs when the software is initially adopted. To some organisations, the advantages of having more control over the software's future development will outweigh the perceived risks of using it, but others may come to the opposite conclusion.

Libraries thinking of adopting a F/OS software application need to consider the following factors.

Organisational Culture

What support is there within your library and its parent organisation for the F/OS philosophy, and at what level? Is the organisation willing to take some responsibility for the future development of the software? Is there a ``champion'' who will actively promote the project, and keep momentum going during implementation?

Technical Infrastructure

What operating system(s) does the software run on, and does your organisation support these ? Is the programming language (Perl, PHP, etc.) installed and available? Is the database application (MySQL or PostgreSQL for example) available? What additional technologies software does not require (e.g. Apache web server)? Is there adequate documentation about the requirements and installation procedures? Can you try the software without affecting your current system?

Staff Skills

Are staff familiar with the programming language and operating environment? Will the organisation support any staff training and development needed to support the F/OS application? If not, do you have access to an external organisation who can provide the necessary support?

Software Functionality

How mature is the software? How stable is it? How well does its functionality match your requirements? If it will need changes to meet your specific needs, does your staff has the skills and time to make these changes? Is there a process to have these changes incorporated into the package for future releases? What is the perceived risk of using the software? Using F/OS software to provide core functionality, such as a library management system, might be seen as too risky, while using F/OS software that provides stand-alone functionality that complements current systems might be acceptable.

Project community

How active is the project's community, and what resources are available to support new users of the software? Is there a coordinated effort to work on new releases, as in the Koha project? What would you be able to contribute back to the community? Where are community resources such as email archieves and documentation hosted?

CONCLUSION

F/OS software has much potential for libraries and information centres, and there are a number of projects, including Greenstone, Koha, and MyLibrary, that demonstrate its viability in this context. It gives library staff an option to be actively involved in development projects, and this involvement can take many forms, such as reporting bugs, suggesting enhancements, and testing new versions. Organisations adopting F/OS software will need to provide their staff with additional development and training to enable them to take on these new roles effectively, and will need to have a long-term commitment to the projects. Currently available F/OS projects cover application areas ranging from the traditional library management systems to innovations like Greenstone and MyLibrary, which complement traditional systems. F/OS software is well worth considering, particularly for stand-alone applications that complement traditional commercial library management systems. Systems librarians and library managers should watch this trend for future developments.

REFERENCES

1. Time Magazine Dec 25 2006
2. Eric S. Raymond (1998-02-08). Goodbye, ``Free software''; hello, ``open source''. Retrieved on 2007-02-14.

Promotion of Reading Habits

Prabha Sharma

Dy. Librarian, Rajashan University Library, Jaipur

ABSTRACT

An attempt is made in this paper to reveal the importance of reading for everybody and the need to encourage the reding habit among the Indian population. It highlights the factors limiting reading habits. This paper also discusses the issues relating to the role of parents, libraries and different organizations, which can immensely contribute to enhance reading habits. Finally effective methods and some successful programme for reading habits promotion such as reading groups, reading contensts, book talks, creative poetry, story telling sessions, educational games, craft activities, strong network of libraries, quiz competitions, mobile and portable library services, young reader's club and motivate and promote public to read are suggested.

INTRODUCTION

There is a growing consensus that human development must be at the core of any development process. Education - the empowerment of individuals through the provision of learning - is truly a human right and a social responsibility. Education leads to individual creativity, improved participation in the social, economical, cultural and political life of society and hence to a more effective contribution to human development. Today, the sheer quantity of information available in the world-much of it relevant to survival and basic well being is exponentially greater than that available only a few years ago, and the rate of its growth is accelerating. This includes information about obtaining more life enhancing knowledge.

Fortunately, it has been realized that of all the media of getting informed, reading stands out as the major source of acquiring information and reading provides bank of information and reduces ignorance, thus empowering and promoting literacy and communication. Effective reading promotes moral and mental development as well as aid growth and success in life. Reading helps us to de-stress ourselves. It enriches our knowledge, improves our vocabulary and helps to think and create new knowledge. Reading thus helps to broaden our horizon as far as our surrounding is concerned. Such persons can grow up to be informed and enlightened citizen. Reading is the voluntary education we give ourselves after the class-room learning. It involves the process of thinking, evaluating, judging, imagining, decision taking and problem solving. Reading culture is that which prepares the individuals and the populace towards a full and adequate participation in society activities. Reading is therefore, important for everybody in society activities. Reading is therefore, important for everybody in order to cope with new knowledge in the changing world of the technological age. There are still some people, young and old, who cannot get access to reading activities and reding programs at all. However, the number of those who know how to read but do not read enough is also increasing.

Many developing countries have been launching extensive literacy campaigns, in the sence of teaching people to read and write. But knowledge of characters and reading techniques alone are not sufficient to develop real reading societies. People should be motivated to read and be informed as to how to utilize reading materials to improve their own personality and their social environment. In this context role of nongovernmental organizations, governmental organizations, government sectors, libraries, schools and family are very important for mutual cooperation to promote reading habits to reders, espeically, the role of libraries is very important because libraries are very important institutions as information centers and life long educational agencies.

However, reading habits amongst the Indian population is at lower level than required. Many factors are said to be responsible for the low level of reading habits.

Factors limiting reading habits

* Reading is possible only when people are literate. We can increase reading habits if illiteracy is eradicated.
* In spite of rapid educational development policies and programme in the country, about 35% of our population is illiterate. This made the need for the citizens who are not literate to be provided with avenues for functional literacy education.
* We are not a reading society but a chatting society- the background of learning through culture. The cultural habit of our people prefer to listening and chatting more rather than reading. The inherited cultural habit has been transmitted from generation to another. In short, at present, our societies still depend upon their own information rather than written information.
* Economic hardship being experienced in many homes is also another factor for limited reading habits. As a result, most parents only managed to pay their ward's school fees and forget about buying books for them.
* Insufficient libraries; public libraries, school libraries or special libraries located in urban and rural areas.

    - Insufficient or shortage of collection of books and reading materials for public's use or students' use.
    - Insufficient or shortage of educated library manpower.
* The lure of electronic media.
    - TV's potential effect on children's reading performance has become an issue of growing concern among educationists and often cited as a cause for the decline in reading. If children spend their valuable time only viewing programs which entertain rather than educate, it will make our culturally vibrant Indian a nation of morons and human robots.

Once the factors limiting reading habits have been identified, we can easily highlight the roles of different organizations which can contribute immensely to enhance the reading habits amongst the Indian population.

Role of local Institutions and Organizations in helping Libraries conducting Reading Promotion

The task of encouraging positive reading interest to foster a love for reading which will promote a reading culture in society is not an easy one. Locl and National organizations should work together, to achieve the goal. Their role may be as follows :

Role of parents

The reading habit has to be inculcated from the start, that is right from an early age. Parents are the first persons with whom a child comes into contact. A child not only imitates their parents, but they are the hero of his early life. If parents do not introduce little children to books who else will? And how will they develop a love for books? The attitude of parents forms the base for promoting of reding habits. Narrating a story and reading aloud books to children by adults must be given priority as it nurtures love for reading. In America wide publicity was given by Nancy Reagan, wife of the then President, by reding books to her grandchildren. It started a movement of reading books to children. Volunteers offered to read in libraries for children. Hillary Clinton started the interlinking USA with children's libraries of developing nations.

Parents are clearly important socializing agents. Parents who spend time for reading to their children giving them the best possible start on the road to literacy. Many research studies have pointed out that the children who do best in literacy skills at school are those who come from homes where there are books, where their parents spend time reading to their children and where children see their parents and older siblings engage in reading activities.

Role of Libraries, Librarians and Library Programs

Libraries are means to stimulate and develop the reading interest. The following are some strategies which libraries and librarians may play in promotion of reading habits.

1. The librarian should help to develop among the reader's pleasant and positive attitude towards reading. The pleasant and positive attitude of the reader should be developed first before someone is able to automatically form the habit of reading and the love for books.
2. The principal function of the librarian is to serve the course of education formally or informally. When we think of the librarian's role in education, we think first of books and of what she does with books. Librarians have a responsibility and an opportunity to go out and tell the public what they have in their libraries and find out what they want to read,

improve and keep improve the set-up of the library to encourage readers to stay and browse.

3. In any effective school library program, the librarian should have definite responsibilities in certain areas of the curriculum and should have an actvie teaching role. But this role must always be coordinated with what is taking place in the classroom. With his wide knowledge of materials and techniques for using them, the librarian can make a strong partner in the planning and implementing of the educational enterprise.
4. Making the library attractive to public and schools.
5. Book weeks in which book discussion, writing a report or review of a book, meeting the author, book exhibition may be organized. These kind of book related activities benefit both authors and readers. Readers are exposed to vast number of books. Their critical and analytical faculties are developed. Authors gain as they come to know their readers.
6. School teachers can plan visit to public libraries. It will enable children to know the functioning of libraries, how to choose book in the library. It also makes them realize that a vast number and variety of books exist.

Role of Mass Media

Radio, TV, newspapers and magazines can help advertise reading projects, village libraries, seminars-training workshops, interviews of reading authorities/writers/ teachers and organizations involved in the reading activities, to promote reading.

Role of Private and Government Sectors helping Libraries in conducting Reading Society

The professional sectors or agencies play a great deal to elevate the standard of library and services through activities which aim to develop or to encourage activities of reading and writing. These are mainly *National Book Trust, Library Associations, Writer's Associations and Women's Associations. etc.* Reading habit programmes should be embarked upon by policy makers at different levels of operation such as schools, tertiary institutions, government agencies and Non-government organizations. They should also find means of sustaining such laudable progrmmes. The government can help by providing a favourable climate in terms of tax structures, book distribution, recognition of publishing industry, loan availability and availability of machineries and other inputs necessary for the trade. This will invariably encourage publishers as well as authors to write more books. This transcends to more books in circulation and eventually reduces the prices of book which in turn will make people to buy more books and read, thereby increasing and improving the habit of reading.

The roles of different segments of the society as mentioned can be wholly fulfilled provided certain methods and programs are implemented in the society.

Effective Methods and some Successful Programs for Reading habit Promotion in Libraries

The starting point for good programme for promotion of reading habits is to have an accurate idea of the information seeking patterns of the community members. It is important to understand the patterns of use of reading materials available in the library. The information seeking patterns of various groups in society differ. Library professionals must be aware of these differences and why they exist, in order to promote and develop reading habits for the whole community. The main groups that need special attention are, semi literate and neo-literate community members, children, young and adult community members. Programmes of activities are broadly categorized into three main groups : Those are bringing book to public, book base programming and motivate and promote public to read.

Bringing Books to Public

Various methods may be employed to attract towards reading materials. Some of them are as follow :

a. Preparation and exhibition of book authors characteristics in novels or concepts retrieved from literature and/or display of maps of book shops and libraries in the community.

b. Promote the production and distribution of easy-to-read pamphlet and low-priced printed materials. These material inform what the public interests e.g. : health or rural issues, agriculture or animal breeding and encourage subscribing.

c. Collect oral and unprinted literature.

d. Set up book reader's group in villages of community. Organize reading activities. Use books as a fundamental documents when news in newspaper, radio and T.V. has been reported.

e. Encourage public to know about books and book sources (both reading and non reading group).

Book Based Programs

Reading Programs

Easy accessibility is the key to the promotion of reading habits. The following are successful programs which may be undertaken by libraries to enhance the reading habits:

a. Reading groups : Reading group help the semi-literate people increase and strengthen their reading skills. They will involve reading newspapers, literacy primers, and novels. The reading groups should also include sharing new ideas and holding discussion forums to discuss social issues. The library may invite a speaker to talk about a topic that the group members have read about. In this way, group members can share and contribute their own thinking on the topic and inspire for further readings. This program might be aimed at exposing the readers to the various skills vis speed reading, information handling skill etc. Various activities with local writers and film shows, slides show may be carried out.

b. *Reading contest* : The aim of reading contest would be to accelerate reading habit among young generation by the use of libraries. It is considered as a potential step in nation building. The contest materials could be a number of books on literature : prose and poetry, selected by the National Committees for promotions of books. The contest participants are required to develop and deliver some book abstracts.

c. *Arrange book talks* : A low cost-effective strategy with ability to reach as wide as audience, a possible way is book talk. The schools may hold book talks and the book reporting sessions by the librarian's cooperation. The talk may be made through talk-cum-slide by librarians for the new upcoming books or orientation in the library; book talk contest, or book abstract contest after book talk session.

e. *Creative poetry* : The rules for development of love for poetry within children are: read it aloud; read it often; keep it simple; keep it joyous or spooky (ghostly) or exciting. Poetry sets an excellent medium for training the disciplines for listening and reading that are such integral parts of reading aloud program. It must be read word to word because it is bound by meter and rhythm; every word and every syllable counts.

g. *Arrange story telling sessions* : Story-telling is one of the easiest activities for the library to organize. Traditional tales or short stories of the same type and picture book are the easiest to use. Apart from these myths, legends, fairy tales, stories about animals, things which appeal to the sense of wonder and the sense of humor that stimulate the imagination of spirits of adventure are the most suitble.

Performance

a. Dramatic activities : Drama groups need careful organizing. The approach is to outline a theme, based on a story or part of a book, which can then, by the cooperation of the children and the person in change, be demonstrated in a dramatic form. Each child should be given a chance to participate.

b. Puppets show : Dramatic activity and craftwork can be combined in the making of puppets by the children, and their presentation of a performance based on a story or episode from a book. For both, the puppeteers and audience of other children, it will extend the awareness of the story and the book on which it has been based.

Craft Activities

Craft activities can use both local traditional skill and a wide range of materials, many of which can be improvised from waste materials such as newspaper, disused packagings, cardboards and so on. The link with books can be two fold; the choice of themes from books, such as giants, prehistoric animals, or other features, and the use of books for instruction in methods and techniques.

Quiz Competition

Quiz could be aimed at encouraging students to read beyond their textbooks in school, promotion of books as a source of information and promoting books themselves. Therefore, it is necessary to decide precisely what the purpose of the quiz is in each competition. Book quiz can be done just for fun. They may be set at various level for under eight to eleven and over.

Educational Games

Few libraries can provide a wider range of educational games. However, where there is suitable accommodation, jigsaws, games (particularly those linked to children's books and featuring book titles and characters and board games) may provide an additional attraction.

``Cognitive Games" are thinking game. It includes language games which need no equipment or props only imagination and words. Some language games promote memory skill, some for listening and some guessing games.

Strong Network of Libraries

A strong network of libraries is needed. The successful project may be revived by providing finances. It will promote reading habits and book culture. All schools including `*anganwadis*' in villages must be provided libraries. Panchayats should be encouraged and allowed to raise resources through cess for libraries.

Provide Mobile or Portable Library Services

Mobile or portable libraries on bicycles as in Thailand and Chennai; camel cart, bullock cart or even library on *thela* as in rural Maharashtra can be made books to reach readers. Libraries may involve young readers and their parents in running of these libraries. Once they feel it is their library, they will ensure its smooth running.

Young reader's Club

Young Readers Clubs should be organised. A book of the month can be selected on the basis of readers choice. Parents, teachers, publishers can join together and with the help of newspapers and magazine can form the club. Publishers can be requested to give discount on selected books for these readers club. This will encourage keen competition among publishers to get their book selected.

Motivate and promote Public to Read

Films and TV programme based on good books motivate public to read, i.e. demand for *Mahabharata, Ramayana etc* when they were telecasted. Book talks, interviews, quiz programmes, story telling and other books related programmes on TV inspire public to read. No such programmes are produced as they do not get sponsors. The corporate sector can help in this. They should sponsor such programmes. In Germany, a famous shoe manufacture is active in sponsoring, and film production. NGOs and voluntary organisations like Association of Writers and Illustrations for Children, Bal Kumar Sahitya Parished and others in different states should link readers and books. With their crusading spirit they can act as conscious keeper of the society.

CONCLUSION

Electronic media may create the excitement and adventures of tomorrow but there is no substitute for books. People should be motivated to read and be informed as to how to utilize reading materials to improve their own personality and their social environment. The whole network of actvities related to promotion of reading habits as cited above is a great task. Through these activities we aim to instill the love for books amongst the Indian population and to develop the reading habits. It requires the cooperation of all concerned; but with all eyes focused on the same goal and imbued with the high spirit of service, success will not be that far. The journey may be long and difficult but the first step has to be made. This is a challenge, we should be committed to accept.

REFERENCES

Cole, John Y : Promoting Book Culture and Reading Activities. Herald of Library Science. Vol. 42, No. 1-2, Jan-April, 2003, p. 78-83.

Iyiade, A K and Adekunmist, S.R. Towards the Promotion of a credible reading culture : A case study of some south western states in Nigeria. Library herald, Vol. 42, No. 3, Sep. 2004, p. 167-178.

Makenzi, Margaret and others. Nurturing readership skills in the digital age : contributions of the reading tent project in Njoro, Kenya SRELS Journal of information Management Vol. 40, No. 3, Sep. 2003, p. 211-226.

Martha Dallman and others. Teaching of Reading. Wrinston, New York, 1985.

National Library of Singapore. Promoting Reading in An Urban Environment. Singapore, 1994.

Nikam, Khaiser and N. Rajashekara. Reading Haibts of Public Library Users : A Survey. SRELS Journal of Information Management V. 40, No. 4, Dec. 2003, p. 337-363.

Ray, Sheila. Children's Librarianship, Outline of Modern Librarianship. London, Clive Bingley, 1979.

Wisconsin Department of Public Instruction. Reading and School library. 2002. http://www.dpi.state.wi.us/dpi/dlel/imt/rdgslmp.html.

Librarianship in Digital Era

M.R. Rawtani and Kamal Kant Gupta***

*Associate Professor & Head, Deptt. of Library and Information Science, University of Rajasthan, Jaipur

**Technical Assistant, University Rajasthan College, Jaipur

ABSTRACT

With the information and technological changes, library scenario is rapidly changing towards information centers. In this electronic age the librarian of the future must be equipped with a wide range of personal and transferable skills in order to manage the changing environment in which he works. Information professionals within libraries are playing a vital role in dealing with information in electronic formats by creating Web pages to promote their services to external customers/readers and choosing automated library management systems.

1 INTRODUCTION

The library in our country was originally conceived as *Pustakalya* or *Granthalaya* i.e., a storehouse of books and literature meant for dissemination of knowledge to its users. The libraries were expected to store in a systematic manner the literature, records, books and encyclopedias so as to facilitate their users to have an access to the knowledge contained in these publications. A librarian was supposed to maintain the records of the library through well defined accession and an issue and return system.

In 21st Century Information Technology is bringing revolutionary changes across all sector of society. The IT is impacting library management and information handling which again is demanding reorientation of LIS professionals to keep themselves up-to-date as per digital scenario.

2 TECHNOLOGICAL CHALLENGES

The four major developments which have changed the role of enabling technologies are:

1. The introduction of high bandwidth wide area network, which provide high speed linkage.
2. A change of electronic model towards annual subscription, which enabled unlimited access.
3. The development of wide range of data services delivered on CD-ROM.
4. Availability of network station which enabled end users to gain direct access to the data available across the world.

3 NEW ROLE OF LIBRARIAN

In addition to the professional skills, the librarian of the future must be equipped with a wide range of personal and transferable skills in order to manage the changing environment in which he or she works. Management and interpersonal skills will make librarian more effective manager of networked resources and services. As Hastings says "it is more important that digital librarians possess particular personal qualities rather than specific technical expertise."

It is needless to say that in modern times the library professionals are not to stick their heads in the sand. The information professionals must change and adapt to the new electronic information environment. He or she must learn about new technologies and be aware of the strengths and weaknesses of them. Librarians should not feel threatened by computers and technical developments but should move forward with the new technology and take a pivotal role within organisations.

Information professionals within libraries are playing an increasing role in dealing with information in electronic formats by creating Web pages to promote their services to external customers and choosing automated library management systems. Skills in information organisation are more necessary in this age of information explosion. Library and information professionals have a key role to play in this era. For example, librarians are well equipped to take intranet projects through the various stages of design and maintenance, as they understand their users and their organisations' information needs and have the range of skills to manage the knowledge effectively.

The role of the librarian in this context is to help users to find the information they require then provide them with the tools to assess and use the resources for their individual needs. Creth suggests that librarians achieve this by "actively seeking out users in a variety of settings" and by making "full use of information and multimedia technology" by offering instruction in a variety of formats (including Web based instruction and online tutorials).

4 USER EDUCATION ON THE INTERNET

As the Web is increasingly becoming the first place that students will look for materials the role of information professional, as intermediary, will also grow in importance. As librarians working with this medium, it is up to us to introduce the strengths and weaknesses of the internet as any other library resource during our user education programme. Just as a traditional academic library offers a programme of "user education" to students and teachers to maximise the benefit they receive from the library. Indian libraries working in the Internet environment in conjunction with the developing networked user education help people to get more from this very rich information service. It is our experience that many users do not realise how rich a source, the Internet, can be used to find many research and teaching materials. Traditional library user education in a university, college or school offers users:

- Library tours - to become familiar with the layout of sections of the library,
- Library induction sessions - to learn about the services available and to learn how to use them,
- Subject guides - to identify the key information resources for a particular discipline,
- Support from subject librarians - to get specialised help, and
- Information skill development - to learn transferable skills in information handling,

By applying a traditional library role such as user education and the knowledge of the best resources available for their subjects in the Internet environment, an internet librarian is well placed to provide a comprehensive internet information seeking skills.

5 ROLE AS INTERMEDIARY

The librarian acting as an intermediary will have greater access to library and external files than before, with the ability to add and manipulate them. These will include the order and receipt files as well as information databases. The technical support staff will oversee the data on the system to achieve overall efficiency and security as well as providing the information worker with accurate and up to date information on which to base decisions. The ability of the selector to obtain information rapidly within the electronic environment and make the relationship between the user and the information librarian and between the information librarian and library management will help the users largely in finding the information they require. In the present day the information librarian plays an intermediary role, not only between the user and information, but also between the library management structure and end user.

6 ROLE IN WEB PUBLISHING

Librarian can help in bringing scholarly information to the web in a number of different ways. Firstly, librarian can be very assertive in prompting web publishing. This can take the form of encouraging others to publish their material on the issue of web publishing to the forefront of the campus administrative agenda. Secondly, we may be actually publishing full text articles on the web. These articles can be placed on home page or placed in prominence on the library web server as an advertising message. Thirdly, librarian may be indexing these web publications. Full-text indexing has often proved to be less than helpful in term of precision and recall issue. These published articles deserve at least the base intellectual access point of author, title, and subject. Fourthly, we may keep adding value to web publication through internal and external hyper links. These links make the web just another intellectual platform. The value added aspect of the web, especially its almost universal accessibility, its immediacy, and its hypertext nature make a powerful and compelling argument for the concept of scholarly web publishing.

7 ROLE IN INFORMATION MANAGEMENT

In the area of information management, the librarian-

- is responsible for the overall design, graphics, functionalities, and technologies of the site,
- mounts, maintains, and updates significant portions of the site,
- maintains a master list of all subscription databases on the site, with appropriate links, "about" files, etc.,

- maintains aspects of the Citrix database project,
- in close coordination with the Head of Library Systems, oversees and coordinates the technical needs of the site with Academic Computing,
- oversees the expansion of the directory tree,
- coordinates the inclusion of all new Web builders into the site,
- solves technical problems for Web builders contributing to the site,
- link checks the site, mounts reports on the staff Intranet,
- maintains the staff Intranet, assists in planning for a "true" Intranet Maps SAMBA to staff PCs as requested to create a user-friendly Web building environment,
- maintains subject resource pages,
- maintains the Webmaster e-mail account, and
- works with Library Systems and others to plan for Web technologies that might be maintained within the Libraries.

8 TRAINS, INSTRUCTS, SUPPORTS STAFF AND USERS IN INTERNET-RELATED TOPICS AND TECHNOLOGIES

The librarian of today-

1. teaches HTML to library staff; serves as the primary HTML support for the University Libraries,
2. provides bibliographic instruction to staff and users on using the Internet for research, Internet-related software, non-Web Internet technologies, etc.,
3. solves Internet-related problems that occur on public and staff workstations, and that with remote users,
4. creates/maintains informational handouts for the reference of Internet workstations,

5. creates/maintains a large number of Web-based Internet tutorials,
6. coordinates the reference of Internet workstation area, maintains signage, posting of use policies, etc.
7. contributes to choosing the layout, furniture, equipment, and workability of this area with the Head of Reference and Library Systems.

9 COORDINATES THE INTRODUCTION AND UPGRADING OF INTERNET-RELATED SOFTWARE

The librarian is-

1. responsible for testing, recommending, and training for each Web browser upgrade,
2. responsible for the same with Web browser plug-ins and viewers,
3. recommends other Internet-related software as needed, and
4. meets regularly with other librarians, faculty and staff to ensure effective communication on issues and new developments; plans and revises services in response to needs.

10 CONCLUSION

The library professionals and those, working and managing modern information system are required to possess the knowledge and skill to handle challenge of 21st century. They are required to constantly update their knowledge and skill base so as to work in today's information and knowledge system. Librarian can show the users that they still have the human and organisational skill to fulfil their true purpose in society.

BIBLIOGRAPHY

Pantry, Sheila. (1997). Whither the information professional? Challenges and opportunities. The cultivation of information professionals for the new millennium. *Aslib Proceedings*. Vol. 49, No. 6, June, pp. 170 - 172.

Creth, Sheila D. (1996). The Electronic Library: Slouching Toward the Future or Creating a New Information Environment. *Follett Lecture Series*. Available from-http://www.ukoln.ac.uk/services/ papers/follett/creth/paper.html

Lancaster, F. Wilfrid. (1997). Artificial Intelligence and Expert System Technologies: Prospects. In: *Libraries for the New Millennium: Implications for Managers*. London: Library Association Publishing, pp. 19 - 37.

Hastings, Kirk and Tennant, Roy. (1996). How to Build a Digital Librarian. *Follett Lecture Series*. November. Available from-http://mirrored.ukoln.ac.uk/lis/november96/ucb/11hastings.html

Medhurst, Jamie. (1995). Do or Die: The Librarian in the 21st Century. *Managing Information*. Vol. 2, No. 9, September, pp.30 - 31.

Crawford, W. and Gorman, M. (1995). Future libraries: dreams, madness and reality, American library Association, Chicago.

Lancaster, R. W. (1995). Networked scholarly publishing, Theme issue of library trends, 43(4) spring.

Duckitt, P. The intermediary today and tomorrow, Aslib proceeding. Vol. 36, No. 2, Feb. pp. 79-86.

Devenport, Thomas H (eds). Mastering information management. London: Prentice Hall, 2000.

Saiful, Amin (2002). Role of librarian in content management, available at http://drtc.isibang.ac.in/saiful/

Crowley, B. (2001). Tacit knowledge tacit ignorance and the future of academic librarianship. College and Research Libraries, 62(6), pp 565-584.

Integrated Services Digital Network (ISDN)

Kulesh Kumar

Librarian, Govt. College, Chharra, Aligarh (UP).

1. INTRODUCTION

Integrated Services Digital Network i.e. in short ISDN is one of the important development held in the field of telecommunication. ISDN is a wide area network becoming widely available to the users. Due to rapid advances in computer and communication technologies, these two fields, have virtually merged into each other. ISDN is the product of such a merger of these technologies. The most fascinating fact about ISDN is that, it is related to information and the integrated services digital network.

Integrated Services Digital Network was first launched in 1990 in Singapore, which is a most powerful tool for various services such as voice, images, audio-video and multimedia data communication of the telephone network. It may be viewed as a logical extension to the digitalization of telephone network and has become very common. The most important and main characteristic of ISDN is that, any subscriber can simultaneously send and receive voice, data, image or a combination there of from his premises in digital form on a telephone line from this network. Thus ISDN provides direct digital access to the digital switching technology used in the telephone exchange. The digital access can be used for voice and data signals. In this way, we see that ISDN is capable of transmitting video and high speed data as well as voice. Due to its so many beneficial features, so many industrial countries of the world like Japan, Germany, UK, USA etc. have digitalised their own telecommunication systems and converted them into integrated Services Digital Networks. In our country, the various mail network services as well as DOT, VSNL and MTNL have been providing this service to the users. At present ISDN services are available to and from India for other foreign countries such as Australia, Austria, Belgium, Canada, Denmark, France, Germany, Ireland, Italy, Israel, Japan, Malaysia, Netherland, Norway, Phillipines, Singapore, Switzerland, Thailand, UAE, UK, USA etc.

2. ISDN : TYPES OF ACCESS

There are two types of access (connections) for ISDN.

(a) Basic Rate Access (BRA)

(b) Primary Rate Access (PRA)

The users can opt for a BRA connection from the local ISP or they can opt for PRA connection. In BRA connection 2 B+D channels are available to the users, where 2 channels of 64 kbps for speech and data and 1 channel of 16 Kbps for signalling is provided. (2 x 64 = 128 + 16 = 144 kbps). The other PRA connection is used for ISDN compatible EPABX etc. It is connection of 30 B + D channels, where 30 Channels of 64 kbps for speech and data and 1 channel of 64 kbps for signalling (30 x 64 = 1920 + 64 = 1984 kbps = 2 Mbps).

3. PRINCIPLE OF ISDN

A number of standard organizations are involved in different aspects of ISDN, but its controlling body was International Telegraph and Telephone Consultive Committee (CCITT), which is presently said as TTU-T. The principle of ISDN according to present committee (TTU-T) is state here. The ISDN is supported by a wide range of voice and non-voice applications of the same network. It provides a range of services using a limited set of connections and multi-purpose use network interface arrangements. ISDN supports a variety of applications that include both switched and non-switched and packet switched connections. As far as possible, new services introduced into an ISDN should be arranged to be compatible with the 64 kbps switched digital connections. An ISDN will contain the intelligence for providing service features, maintenance and network management functions. A layered protocol structure should be used for the specification of access to an ISDN. This is same as the Open System Interconnection (OSI) reference model.

4. FEATURES OF ISDN

Following are the main features of ISDN :

(a) In ISDN, a digital link of 144 kbps is available between the telephone exchange and subscribers premises. This link is further divided to form three channels.

(b) The users of ISDN can transmit or receive data at a very high speed of 128 kbps by using ISDN controller cards is their PCs.

(c) These services are also provided by Bharat Sanchar Nigam Limited (BSNL) to the users, hence BSNL is providing these services on the basis of fee to be the member of this network.

5. ARCHITECTURE OF ISDN

The architecture of ISDN is shown in the figure given at below. A new physical connector called digital subscriber loop is being supported by ISDN. The digital subscriber loop is basically a link for end user to the central or end office. A common physical interface has been provided. The same interface can be used for telephone, computer terminals and video text terminals as well. The control of information between the user device and the network is exchanged using protocols. It is necessary to make provision for the high speed interface, for example, a digital PBX or a LAN. The subscriber loop belonging to the telephone network users a twisted pair link to connect the subscribers and the office and the link carries 4 kHz analog signals. But, under ISDN, they use one or two twisted pairs to provide a basic full duplex digital communication link.

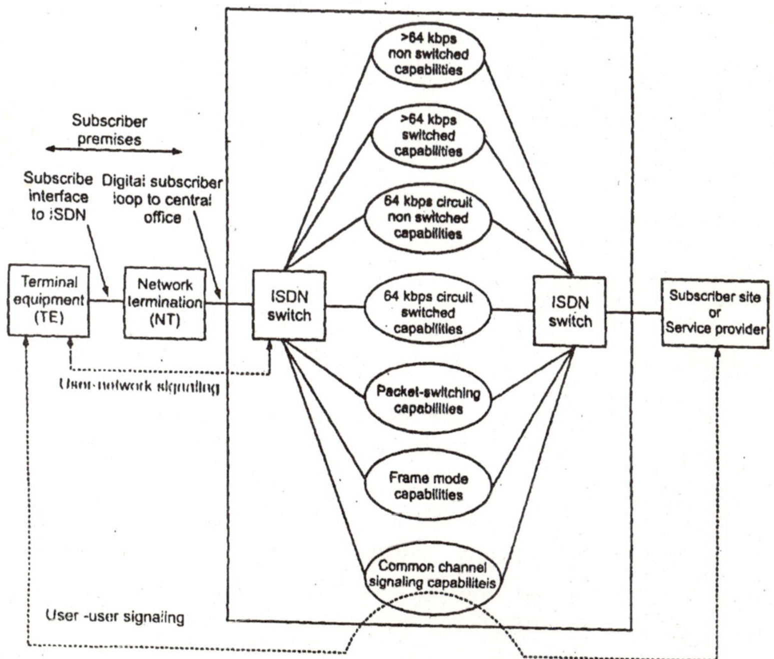

Fig. 1. Architecture of ISDN

The digital central office connects a large number of ISDN subscribers loop signals to the digital network. The central office performs the following operations:

(a) Provides access to the circuit switched network.

(b) Provides subscriber access to the dedicated lines.

(c) Provides subscriber access to the packet switched network and time share transaction oriented computer services.

(d) To accomodate multiplexed access via digital PBX and LAN.

6. TYPES OF ISDN

There are two types of ISDN namely narrowband ISDN and broadband ISDN. The narrowband ISDN is the first generation of ISDN. It has a smaller bandwidth and it can support the data rates of upto 64 kbps only. Due to low bit rates, the quality of service provided by the narrowband ISDN is poor. This means that the quality of video signals in the narrowband ISDN is very poor. So the quality of service is improved by using the broadband ISDN, which can support higher data rates due to the use of optical fibre cables. The bandwidth of an optical fibre cable is very high, So, the broadband ISDN can allow transmission of very high quality video images through it.

7. ISDN NARROWBAND CONNECTION

The figure shows how the connections are made using the ISDN. As shown in the figure, a subscriber can have access to the ISDN by means of a local interface to a digital pipe of certain bit rate. Such digital pipes of various sizes are available to satisfy different needs. For example, a residential user will require a less capacity digital pipe than the capacity required for an office and naturally would require a much higher capacity pipe. The data rate on the pipe will vary depending on the need of application. The user will be charged according to the capacity of ISDN interface and not according to the connection time. As shown in the figure, the ISDN interface supports the telephone service, data terminals, private telephone exchanges, local area networks etc. This is the meaning of integrated services. The customer ISDN interface is than connected to ISDN central office via digital pipe. The digital pipes are also called ISDN lines. The ISDN central office is connected to the Integrated Digital Network (IDN) as shown in the figure. The IDN consists of packet switched network, circuit switched network, databases etc.

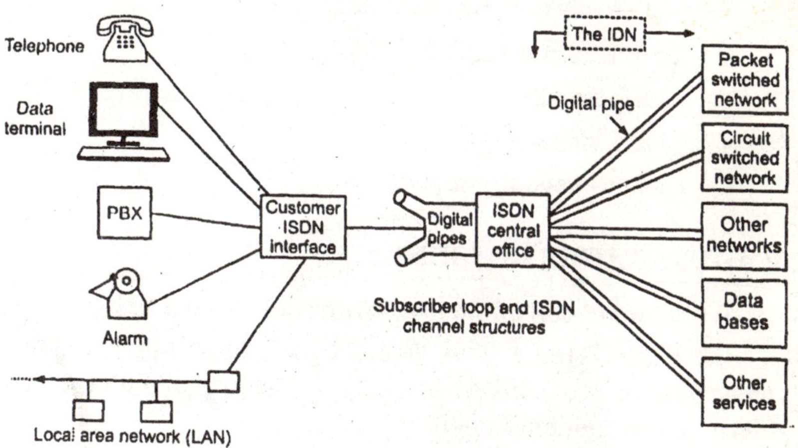

Fig. 2. How to make connections using ISDN

8. SERVICES PROVIDED BY ISDN

The following services are offered by ISDN on dial up basis between any two subscribers.

(a) Existing voice applications

(b) Data applications

(c) Fascinate (Fax)

(d) Teletext and videotext services.

In providing teletext and videotext services, the video conferencing service is the main service. The advantage of video conferencing is that the user may talk to each other at distant places thus saving time and money. This is done by transmission of voice and video images of both users as well as by transmitting images, drawings, text or still products of documents at a high speed. Data files on the PCs may also be transmitted at a very high speed of 64 kbps.

Alongwith above main services, it provides following additional supplementary services also.

- Calling line identification Presentation (CLIP)
- Calling line identification Registration (CLIR)
- Multiuser institution (MUI)
- Terminal mortability (TM)
- Call hold (CH)
- Call waiting (CW)
- User to user signaling.

9. ADVANTAGES OF ISDN

We may get the following advantages from ISDN :

(a) Efficiency : It is useful to transmit quickly data, voice, images etc. continuously applying in place of various voices, faxes, modem lines.

(b) Connection: Through it, we can communicate information to any distant place of the world and it can also be connected with protocols, hardwares, standards & softwares.

(c) Suitability : This technique is useful for multiuser applications.

(d) Speed and Quality - It can communicate data at the rate of 8 times more of the rate by which a modem transmit, and in contraction, this rate may increase upto 64 to 230 kbps. In it, the digital signals are free from pollution. The voice and images are transmitted as their original form.

(e) Cost effective - In developed form, it provides access of many telephone lines on a single line in comparison to different dial up lines.

10. IMPORTANCE OF ISDN

Following are the advantages of ISDN in comparison to simple telephone network.

(a) In the normal telephone network, the user can make a voice call and the voice data are transmitted in analog form, which is normally vulnerable to distortions. In ISDN, the multimedia data (i.e, data image, graphics) is transmitted over the telephone lines in digital form. Thereby noiseless telephone service and very high quality of data service are provided.

(b) The signal level at subscriber premises is independent of line length and line noise, which further enhances the quality of reception.

(c) An ISDN subscriber can establish two simultaneous independent calls which could be voice, data, image or combination of any two whereas only one call possible on ordinary telephone line at one time.

(d) The call set up time between two subscribers of ISDN is extremely short.

(e) ISDN subscribers have full connectivity to all other ordinary subscribers both at national and international levels and vice-versa.

11. APPLICATIONS OF ISDN

This network technology is being used for the following purposes :

- To get Internet access.
- To link local area network (LAN).
- To Video-conferencing.
- To corporate communication.
- To high speed data communication.
- To develop voice services.
- To desktop publishing.

- To marketing work.

12. CONCLUSION

Now we have come to know that ISDN network has been emerged as a wide area network for providing different services like voice, data and image over the local telephone wires, which some years back was impossible. Through ISDN, any one now can connect directly his computer to the telephone network without connectivity first their signals to an analog audio signals, as modem does in ordinary telephone network. With this facility any ISDN subscriber can establish two simultaneous independent calls on existing telephone lines, whereas only one call was possible on the telephone network.

13. REFERENCES

(i) Ali, Amjad : Information technology and libraries. New Delhi : Ess Ess Publications; 2004, p. 43-44 and 359-65.

(ii) Kumar, K. : Integrated Services Digital Network - ISDN. Granthalay Vigyan (Hindi) : Vol. 37 (No. 1 and 2); 2006, p. 15-19.

(iii) Singh, Shanker : Information technology and libraries (Hindi). New Delhi : Ess Ess Publications; 2003, p. 30-31 and 296-98.

(iv) Sharma, Sanjay : Computer Networks, New Delhi : Kataria, S.K.; 2007, p. 284-85.

(v) Tripathi, S.M. and Lal, C. : Descriptive questions in library and information science. New Delhi : Ess Ess Publications; 2002, p. 264.

Internet: It's Impact on Future of Libraries and Books

B. Seenaiah

Library Assistant, NALSAR, University of Law, Shameerpet,
Hyderabad -500 078
E-mail: seenaiah9@yahoo.co.in; seenaiah9@gmail.com

ABSTRACT

The article presents scenario in which Internet is an important source of Information. We need Internet for some how or the other. The Internet makes the world simpler, shrinks time, and enables more effective information resource. Libraries still hold significance role, but libraries alone cannot provide access to the latest knowledge.

Discusses how in today's context of Information Technology driven education, it is important for us to realize that the books of the 21st century will have to be written differently than the books of the 20th century, and this difference will be mainly because of Internet.

It explains the need to club Internet with Library book stores as the Internet is booming. At present there are about 400 World Wide Web bookstores. So in a way Internet is going to be very beneficial to us. Libraries and education system in 21st century should take advantage of the development in the Information Technology.

Suggests caution that libraries are to provide the Internet service in a responsible manner and has to be diligent in developing, training and the context in which recognizes the particular importance of helping users in accessing, important information resource appropriately. Also submits that library staff should be more competent technically to manage networks, avoid dependency on others, and impart information literary programs.

INTRODUCTION

The new millennium has brought us face to face with the new realities of 21st century. These new realities are visible in all sphere of human activity whether it is the world of learning, world of scientific and technology innovations and R&D, the world of business, the world of industry, the system of governance, and in the world of national and international co-operation. Everywhere the new global environment has compelled us to think afresh about the way we work, the way we transact our business and lastly the way we manage and govern an activity. In fact, the new global environment has given rise to the fast emergence of a new information environment, which is exerting a powerful influe-nce on the global economic order, the new social order as the new education order. We have to examine the compelling influence which the new information order is exerting on the world of learning, the world of education and the world of higher education. We have also to understand as to how best to exploit the advances in information technology for the best benefits of modernizing our library information systems.

21st Century is a period of change and quality and the impact could be far reaching as has never been seen before. The current digital revolution especially internet technology integrated with treasure of information has emerged in the past few years, as an indispensable tool for people in pursuit of knowledge and information. It is packed with both primary and secondary sources of information, to track, which one has to develop the ability to shift through millions of search engines hits. The internet makes the world simpler, shrinks time, distance and enables more effective information resource and communication tool to individual knowledge workers to use their time more efficiently and focus on more productive tasks.

The benefits and opportunities, the Internet is offering today, have been widely recognized and appreciated by the citizens. On the contrary, the same Internet is not without any problems, particularly in the context of use in academic and research libraries. Libraries have to strike a balance between assisting the public in accessing relevant, quality resources available on the Internet and preventing access to illegal or objectionable materials, without straying into the realms of censorship.

2. IMPACT OF INTERNET ON BOOKS

We all are aware that the libraries in our country and for that reason abroad were originally conceived as "Pustakalaya" a "Granthalaya" i.e., a storehouse of books and literature meant for dissemination of knowledge to its users. The libraries were therefore expected to store in a systematic manner the literature, records, books and encyclopedias so as to facilitate their users to have an access to the knowledge contained in these publications. A Librarian was supposed to maintain the records of the library through a well-defined accession and issue and return system. He was also required to preserve the records, books and literature so that it could be utilized over a long period of time. New books and periodicals were procured and kept in library to provide in those days what was referred to as up-to-date knowledge. The librarian, therefore, was the custodian of the rich intellectual wealth kept in the library.

In today's context when we look at the role of the libraries, we are confronted with the new challenges, a new reality which has arisen because of the advent of the rapid changes in the knowledge. The changes taking place in the scientific and technical arena are such that the half-life of knowledge, i.e., at least half of the knowledge base in the modern disciplines of Science and Engineering is changing at such a fast pace that the published books being made available in the library are no longer a guarantee of the availability of the up-to-date knowledge. It has happened primarily because of the compelling being exerted in all domains of human activities. It is, therefore, quite clear that printed books and publications in the library cannot provide access to the latest knowledge and know-how, vital for working in today's IT driven environment. The libraries of today and undoubtedly of tomorrow have to tackle this challenge of rapidly reducing half-life of knowledge.

In today's context of Information Technology driven education, it is important for us to realize that the books of the 21st century will have to be written differently than-the books of the 20th century and this difference will be in the style of writing the books. Today's books have to be written from the point of view of facilitating interactive learning i.e., they should be user friendly enabling the cultivation of knowledge thorough, by and large, self learning. Therefore, there is a paradigm shift that has taken place in the modern education systems. The teacher-centered education system has changed to a learner-centered system. The teacher is performing the role of a facilitator rather than that of a preacher. It is this shift, which is to be supported and facilitated by the books and libraries of the 21st century. We are already on the verge of witnessing an IT led revolution in the education sector. Online learning, virtual classrooms, virtual institutions and virtual universities are fast becoming a reality and as the integration of technology inputs is accelerated in the education system in India, we shall witness a sea change in the teaching-learning environment. The challenge, however, is how to retain using of electronic media and reduce the enormous stresses, which the electronic media creates in the human mind.

The books of 21st century will have to be written in such a manner that they facilitate interactive learning and are written using the modern digital communication systems so that they are made available in the libraries of the 21st century on the CDs and databases. Let them not deprive the reader the joy of reading.

3. IMPACT OF INTERNET ON PROCURMENT OF BOOKS

Bookstores on the INTERNET are booming. In USA, cyberspace book vendors have been well-established for year now on the information superhighway, and users are quickly growing accustomed to having an almost limitless selection of books of choose from metropolitan areas of the United States, the only traditional booksellers that can survive are those megastores offering millions of titles under one roof. Cyberspace booksellers like Amazon. Com (www.amazon. com) take millions of orders per day from people all over the world and carry more books than many well-stocked University libraries. The company's stock price has skyrocketed over the past few months, as investors are betting that selling books over and internet is the wave of the future. But so far, selling books over the Net is largely an American phenomenon. In Europe, on-line bookstores are still in their infancy by comparison. Success stories like that of Amazon.com are luring book sellers from around the world to hop on the Internet book-selling bandwagon. It took Amazon.com founder Jeff Bezos only three years to create the world's largest Internet-based book store. Amazon's estimated yearly sales now total over $100 million. Presently, it delivers any book in English in less than four days to any place on the globe. There are 610,000 clients in 160 countries, and they can choose from among 2.5 million titles.

In USA, it is not uncommon for books to be marked down 20 to 30 per cent their listed retail price. Among Internet bookstores, such discounts are typically the starting point when it comes to price. Often, Internet-based book sellers pass on even greater savings to customers because online sales eliminate the need to hire retail personnel. Cyberspace book sellers based in other countries, however, sometimes are not able to offer customers such generous discounts, despite their savings on personnel, since retail prices are fixed by law in some countries. That helps to explain why many international book vendors have not experienced nearly the same degree to success as companies like Amazon. But there are other factors at play as well on the international front. The slower acceptance of the Internet among the general public, continuing anxiety about the security of online transactions, and the ready availability of acceptable local booksellers are frequently cited as reasons why, internationally, Cyberspace book selling has not been as profitable outside of the USA. ABC Bookworld in Regensburg, Germany, for instance, has been on the Internet for well over two years now, and expects its on-line book selling efforts to generate some $5.8 million every year. Still, that is a long way off from the success of US-based Internet bookstores and founder Ulrike Standler expects a tought fight ahead.

At present, there are about 400 bookstores around the world who have opened up shop on World Wide Web. But that does not mean they are all doing well. Germany's Eugen Emmerling the Association of German Booksellers says, "Selling books through the Internet is still in infancy. So far, few companies are out of the red with their on-line operations. Emmerling and others feel that virtual bookstores will thrive in the next few years, as more people around the world log on the Net and come to see Cyberspace shopping as a real alternative to traditional shopping. Few expect on-line bookstores to put real-world booksellers out of business any time soon, especially not outside of the USA. Emmerling says, "We do not have American conditions in Europe. There, the next bookstore is sometimes hundreds of kilometers away, making buying books over the internet that much more attractive".

To get an overview of the range and types of bookstores currently on the Internet, it helps us to check out the Internet site that does nothing more than to provide links to Cyberspace booksellers. The books, magazines, and other media section of the internet mall is a good place to start. Browser may point to http: /internet mail.com/lbkstrs. Html, and then choose from among then many links presented. There, one can move directly to dozens of the best established booksellers on the Internet and browse at his/her leisure.

4. ADVANTAGES OF INTERNET

The libraries of the 21st century have to be conceived not merely as the store-house of knowledge, but an effective mechanism to facilitate dissemination of knowledge, promoting information and knowledge sharing, while, at the same time, supporting the growth of intellectual property. In essence the libraries of 21st century have to be an effective support mechanism for both the dissemination as well as cultivation of knowledge. The libraries of 21st century should facilitate the transition of today's literate society to a knowledge-based society of tomorrow. This undoubtedly requires that the libraries and education systems in 21st century should take advantage of the development in the information Technology. One has to go beyond automation of libraries. One has to create local and national networks to the global network of libraries and information systems so as to facilitate global access of knowledge and promote information and knowledge sharing. Networking, therefore, is one of thc frontal areas of focus for the libraries of 21s1 century. The digitization of records and rich intellectual wealth currently available in the form of print media, books, periodicals and other forms of literature is an emergent task to be addressed to in this country. This would require a committed and sustained effort so that we are in a position to download the available in our libraries and integrate our information and knowledge base with the global databases.

The penetration of IT in the libraries and information system is already exerting a compelling influence in this regard and I would invite the library professionals and IT experts present here to spare no efforts to take the best advantage of the developments in IT for significantly impr-oving our information systems and for modernizing our libraries.

Finding information on the Web is like finding needle in the haystack. Searching may be the most confusing of all the topics of Internet. Not only this but also the quality of information is quite variable. Usually professional assist-ance lacks when user gets confused and lost in the ocean of information. Internet, in fact, is the place to find an answer in three days for a query that would take three hours in a library. Irrespective of the search or metasearch engines (Lycos, AltaVista, Google, etc.) one finds as if Internet is a vast uncatalogued library. Quite a few sites, in spite of their advertisements, do not get updated frequently. The basic problem in finding information on Internet is that even if one knows the exact URL and has it book marked or written down, there is no guarantee it will work next year, or even next week. If MSNBC decides to move that information to a different directory, web browser shows an error when it is tried out.

It is estimated that over one billion web pages are available on the Internet. But out of these many pages very few are free of cost. If some one wants to access Medical Journal or **chemical Abstract**, he needs to pay thousands of dollars for getting access to these journals.

One of the problems with Internet is that when one wants to have access to articles, one finds sites or foot notes or any other things of the site often missing. Not only this but tables, graphs and forumulae do not often show up in a reasonable way.

Journal titles in digitized package change regularly without warning or prior notification. Sometimes one may find that page is not accessible as it has been moved from one place to another without giving new site location. While TCP/IP is a great way to get computers talking to each other, it is a lousy way to manage the information that is on these computers.

Very little is known about what type of information is available as well as the collection of documents that constitute the web. Web is a collection of documents contributed from any authors and publishers who buy a web server. There is no quality control over the Web and there is not likely to be any. Anyone can put up anything on the Web. Most of the information available on the Internet is trash. So problem does not consist in too much irrelevant materials, but in finding what one wants to know in a sea of potentially interesting data, then turning it into useful information, perhaps even wisdom. Users who are discovering the quality of information retrieved from large heterogeneous databases may be lost in a flood of irrelevant results. The major reason for having too much irrelevant material on the Web is that Web does not have a selection policy such as libraries where conscious efforts are made about what works will be acquired and maintained in the collection. In contrast to libraries clearly defined development policies, the web looks more like the result of a fantastically successful gifts programme; it includes the good, the bad, and the ugly.

The problem with the Internet is with copyright and other protections of intellectual property. Users on the Net can easily and freely trade files regardless of any such protection. Thus Internet information must provide for confidential, automated rights and royalty exchange ensuring users and owners that information is protected from unauthorized, accidental, or intentional misattribution, alteration, or misuse. Also ensuring rapid, seamless, efficient linking of requests to authorizations for information use and encompassing effective billing and accounting mechanisms.

Electronic information is still accessible only to a privileged few. Access required equipment, there are connection costs, and also some training is required for accessing digital information. It is very difficult to ensure free inexpensive access to information in a digital environment. Even if the information can be provided at little or no cost, in a developing country like India how will poorer people gain access to the telecommunications and computing infrastructures so that they can find what's there? The cost of access is going to remain high and for the vast majority of the world's population in developing countries having widespread Internet access, may be the equivalent of walking on the moon. Furthermore, the connections that do exist for more people are slow. In contrast, public libraries, even today are the information reference points serving the least privileged in society.

Librarians organize knowledge through the processes of subject analysis and cataloguing-creating information about information, or what is known as 'metadata'. On Internet there needs to develop methods of consistently and uniquely identifying and retrieving networked information, no matter what format they are or where they reside. Metadata standards are still in their infancy. Initiative and research such as the Dublin core/Warwick Framework for metadata, Government Information Locator Services (GILS), and Uniform Resource Characteristics (URC) are promising ways forward. But still a solution to the global resource discovery problem remains distant.

Librarians provide another role in supporting resource discovery, one in which digital technologies or Internet play only a small role. This is in providing a 'trusted' service. This trust and authority is based upon librarians' making choices, evaluating information as a part of collection development and with a thorough understanding of what users need. Librarians do not only created pathfinders and guides for their users, but they, in fact, are the pathfinders and guides.

The volume of information available on Internet is becoming a problem. Many of us feel we may become less informed rather than better informed because we find the screen version of a valued publication much less, user-friendly than its print equivalent or we cannot afford search time spent at a terminal to reach the page that used to arrive automatically in an in-tray. And then there is so much information available online it is often difficult to rate it in terms of relevance and quality.

From the contents prospective, the Web remains somewhat of a mystery. We know very little about the sources of its materials, the type of documents available, the authoritativeness of the documents, the languages in which information is available, the age or longevity of the documents, the scope of subjects available, and other descriptive characteristics of an information collection. There is even wide disagreement on the size of the Web.

Electronic text is subtly different from print. An electronic mail message differs from a letter or office memorandum. There is no concept of leisure reading in digital environment as we can have in print media. We can borrow a book from a library and can read it at our leisure time over a cup of coffee which is not otherwise possible.

5 CONCLUSION

The ultimate aim of the Library in extending Internet service is to provide public access to the Internet to fulfill its mission to preserve and promote universal access to a broad range of human knowledge, experience, information and ideas to support their academic and research endeavors. Thereby the Internet connects electronically to ideas, information and knowledge around the world creating the concept of Global village under one umbrella. The Internet is not free from adverse comments also, as it contained unregulated, unreliable and indecent materials. Developing an Internet use policy approved by the Board and posting the policy online and in Library; developing consistent booking guidelines for Internet computers to facilitate equity of access for customers; providing training to staff on managing Internet services; restricting the use of e-mail and chat to specific workstations.

The Library is to provide the Internet service in a responsible and balanced manner, and has to be diligent in developing training and content which recognizes the particular importance of helping users in accessing important information resource appropriately. In order to ensure that this approach is continued, the library staff should be more competent technically to manage the network and avoid dependency on others; and also to impart user education for optimum utilization of Internet by means of users training including library staff training and also to develop Internet Use Policy. More importantly, the library has to create an atmosphere and impression that, Internet is an integral part of library service and none else in the university environment, with their commitment, dedication, technical skill and personalized service.

REFERENCES

Design and Usability of Digital Libraries: Case Studies in the Asia-Pacifi. Yin-Leng Theng and Schubert Foo, Editors; Hershey: Information Science Publishing, 2004.

McMenemy, David,"Delivering Digital Services: A Handbook for Public Libraries and Learning Centres.". London: Facet, 2005

Prodhani, M.A and Gaufam, J.N. "*Impact of INTERNET on Worldwide Research activities in 21 Century.* Indian Journal of Information Library & Society, 14(12), 2001, 55-64.

Taylor, Arlene G. *'The Organization of Information.* "*2d ed.* London: Libraries Unlimited, 2005.

The Role and Impact of the Internet on Library and Information *Services.* Edited by Lewis-Guodo Liu; United Kingdom: Greenwood, 2001.

Role of Information and Communication Technology in Agricultural Production and Marketing

Kundan Mal Gawaria and B.L. Gajja

Central Arid Zone Research Institute, Jodhpur 342 003

INTRODUCTION

The agricultural research institute programmes help to produce new and improved crop varieties and better crop management practices to enhance human capacity for research and development. These programmes have direct, indirect and intermediate impacts in -production of the countries. Direct impact refers to the impact on the welfare of people and the environment as a result of adopting a technology. It is reflected mainly as an increase in productivity, a reduction in per unit cost of production, increase employment opportunity and/or reduced pressure on expansion into fragile ecosystems because of improved yields in existing systems. Indirect impact includes flow-on impacts to other crops and activities. For example, increase in crops productivity can benefit not only for other crops but also other sectors of the economy. Intermediate impact refers to increase in the knowledge that could subsequently have a direct impact. Information on the evaluation of the gene pool, prototype technologies, new skills and knowledge of researchers are intermediate benefits. From the initial stages of research output to the final impact on a society, these different forms of impact are interrelated.

TECHNOLOGY AND ECONOMIC DEVELOPMENT

The opportunities for the use of new technologies in economic development are vast. There are some speculation among policy-makers and donors with the relevance of these technologies to the lives of the poor. Investing in ICTs (Information and Communication Technology) may mean investing less in other development priorities such as water, sanitation, health, education etc. There is a clear need to demonstrate the usefulness of ICTs for development and to show that these technologies play important role in alleviating poverty and developing sustainable communities.

Information and Communications Technologies, such as the World Wide Web, e-mail, telephones and satellites are revolutionizing the way in perofrming their businesses, competition in international markets and set their economic and human development agendas. These technologies can enable societies to produce, access, adapt and apply greater amount of information, more rapidly at reduced costs, and offer enormous opportunities for enhancing business productivity and economic activity. They can also contribute towards strengthening democracy, increasing social participation and removing barriers to modernization, making poor populations fuller agents in the sustainable developmental process. The information gathered from impact of new technology in terms of economic performance can be put on web site which can play vital source of communication for far-reach farmers. The information and communication techno-logies are spread all over country. Presently medium towns in Tehsils have also I.T. centers. Besides this they are getting wide publicity through television, radio, internet, etc and have become the most strong source to provide information at distant and interior part of country.

Impact assessment exercises are visible in other enterprise development sectors, but documented cases exist in ICTs are scanty. In developing countries there is little serious, impartial and representative research on the impact of ICTs. The introduction of new technology in mainstream societies is revolutionizing the way in which societies interact, conduct their businesses, compete with the international market, set their economic and human development agendas, access and participate in promotion of a popular democratic culture.

ICTs may become the driving force for a new business and economic paradigm with far reaching efforts for all types of industries to make the competitive position of developing countries. The rate of adoption of ICTs differs from country to country, as well as from firm to firm. Due to their potential impacts on the productivity and competitiveness of firms, ICTs are important to all types of enterprises, including micro, small and medium scale enterprises. ICTs offer enormous opportunities to transfer and acquisition of skills, technical knowledge and business-related information.

Enterprises function on the basis of four tangible resources, namely Money, People, Materials and Technology. Enterprises require information and knowledge about four main aspects of their operation i.e. supply, demand, operating environment and internal processes. Information is the most crucial part for effective management of any enterprise, without quality information, unwanted decisions may be made and learning may not take place. Information poverty in small enterprises results in wrong decisions and entrepreneurs' inability to learn from their wrong decisions. This in turn results in the loss of valuable resources such as money, time, income and business relationships. ICTs can change this scenario by enabling small entrepreneurs to gain/access timely and quality information, and thus empower them to take decisions.

ICTs have the potential to empower and provide greater opportunity for individuals, groups and communities, regardless of their age, sex, skill colour, race, creed, class, or position in society, and thus aid in the development of human rights. Poverty elimination is about providing greater empowerment, opportunity and security, and ICT's directly provide information, knowledge, and political and cultural participation.

A case study of Impact Assessment of Information Communication Technology on Marketing of Agricultural Inputs and Production

The agricultural marketing system in the country is ongoing revamping, the need for establishing a sound Agricultural Marketing Information System in the country has been strongly felt. Such a system will ensure proper utilization of the emerging trade opportunities by the farming community. Market information is needed by farmers for planning, production and marketing. Other market participants also need it for taking appropriate trade decisions. For example, the non-availability of latest information on price trend and status of arrivals/stock in different markets of the country and abroad is a major handicap for producers/traders/ processors and exporters. There are several other areas of agricultural marketing with which the users need to be fully familiarized for adopting best marketing practices for improving price realization. Knowledge has to be imparted in areas such as market driven production programmes, post-harvest management, market finance, facilities for quality assurance and standards, packaging and labeling, etc. In order to ensure fair returns to the farmers, it is essential that the agricultural marketing policies should also be based on reliable and comprehensive database on market information. Access to such an up to-date information base would also enable the farmers to plan their strategies for sale of their products at remunerative prices. Besides producers, the traders and consumers would also be benefited from such a countrywide database.

ICT TOOLS

Almost all the States and Union Territories have their own system of providing market information to the users. However, mostly the prevailing systems of dissemination of marketing information is based on conventional methods due to which the communication of information to the target groups usually gets delayed thereby loosing its relevance. Keeping in view the time sensitiveness of market information, it is important that gap between generation and dissemination of information is minimized. Information and Communication Technology (ICT) can play a vital role in bridging this gap. Appropriate use of ICT will strengthen the interface between Government and the farming community, by providing a channel for reaping the benefits accruing from the reforms.

Information and Communication Technologies (ICT) refers to the forms of technology that are used to transmit, store, create, share or exchange information. This broad definition of ICT includes radio, television, DVD, telephone (both fixed line and mobile phones), satellite systems, computer and network hardware and software, as well as the equipment and services associated with these technologies, such as video conferencing and electronic mail.

Many countries, alarmed by the digital divide, have started to address the problem and are making progress in narrowing some of the gaps. In November 2002, India added more mobile phone customers than ever before, bringing the total number of mobile users to almost 10 million resulting one in 100 Indians uses a mobile phone. ICT plays a more important role in enhancing the activities of the poor by increasing their access to market information or lowering the transaction costs of poor farmers and traders.

ICT and Agricultural Extension

ICTs and agricultural extension together can play a vitle role in improving rural livelihoods. It is always a matter of challenge faced by extension planners and policy-makers that how to grapple with unfamiliar issues that are not strictly in the domain of agriculture. In order to enable agricultural extension to harness ICTs are enabling tools that can help rural poor women and men to capitalize on emerging opportunities, especially in education and income generation and disasters, such as disease and hunger. This focus on rural livelihoods over agriculture-specific extension services was also a key theme of the pre-consultation email dialogue (Ballantyne and Bokre, 2003) which defined extension as aiming to:

- Improve the well being of individuals and communities.
- Change production systems so that they improve rural livelihoods and sustain the life.
- Resource base.
- Improve agriculture, social, economic and political status of rural communities.
- Improve the well being of farm families.
- Improve productivity and livelihoods for farmers.
- Increase and improve farmers' incomes and productivity on a sustainable basis.
- Enhance farmers' production.

ICTs – Transforming Agricultural Extension!

- Attain higher levels of efficiency in the farm enterprise; and
- Attain food security and improve rural livelihoods.

In the past, agricultural extension has been seen as an approach for transferring technologies and practices to farmers, often in the context of commercial agriculture.

Several major trends shaping the delivery of extension services, moving extension far beyond technology transfer were identified as summarized as follows:

- Dwindling government budgets for extension, leading to the privatisation of formerly public services.
- Emergence of new service providers in the context of privatisation.
- Increase differentiation among client groups and issue areas (private demand-driven extension for commercial farmers; public livelihoods-focused extension for poor and subsistence farmers; community management support for environmental and natural resource management challenges).
- User demand for effective and appropriate extension – related to higher expectations of rural communities and farm families, and their growing capacity to voice demands.
- Globalisation and liberalisation of agricultural markets.
- Increased presence of agri-business and commercialised farming.
- Environmental imperatives.
- Climate change.
- Increased use of biotechnologies.

The impact of new ICTs, including telephone and Internet access in rural areas were common now a days. However, at the time of collection of data the telephone both land line and mobile were the important source of information communication technology. The use of ICTs in relation to marketing of most important inputs and output were collected and their impact, were assessed.

ACCESS to ICT

Telephones lines as well as mobiles have reached in the study area through introduction of public call office and small exchange and mobile towers. The mode of use of telephones were assessed and the results are presented in the Table 1. It is revealed that majority of farmers used the ICT in shared basis. The other source of ICT were not much popular due to its non-accessibility. The information collected from the owner of telephones were shared with other farmers who do not have this facility. The shared information was on the basis of 50-50% in case of two farmers. If the same information were shared, the expenditure were neared on equal proportion basis.

Table 1. Access to source of Information Communication Technology

Source	Personnel Ownership (%)	Shared basis (%)	Not-Available (%)
Radio	22.6	13.9	53.5
Television	16.9	26.7	56.4
Telephone (land line)	39.5	58.7	7.8
Telephone (mobile)	33.9	66.1	-
Others (including Internet)	-	-	-

Types of Information

Generally farmers were mostly interested to know about on the following aspects which they considered more important for getting more revenue.

- New technology
- Availability of important inputs
- Price of inputs
- Market arrivals of important crop produce
- Market price disease control technology

Use of ICT in input marketing

Traditionally, for any information related to agricultural purpose includes crop production, suggestion from private dealers for important inputs, carrying farm produce nearby local agricultural market (Mandy) and stay till he receive attractive price and/or some time come back without selling produce. Generally private dealer do not spend enough time to provide any information due to his market interest but now the entire scenario has been changed. Most of the farmers now gathere the information on availability of inputs and its price well in advance i.e. at least 3 to 4 weeks before on set of sowing. The inputs are seeds, fertilizers and their quality and price. At the time of harvesting, they started to gather information about markets situation specially price of products. Farmers were interested to sell their produce if they receive reasonable price at the time of harvesting or they would wait till such price prevail in the market. However, small farmers could not wait for such price, so they have to sell a fraction of their produce just after the crop is harvested. Some progressive farmers close to research organizations (i.e. Agricultural Research Station, Rajasthan Agricultural University, Bikaner campus at Mandore, Central Arid Zone Research Institute, Jodhpur and extension wing of Agricultural Department, Govt. of Rajasthan) visited frequently to know about latest technology as well as insect and pest management techniques. The frequent visit to such organisation were costly in comparison to contact on telephone. The extension Officers are also prefers to contact on telephone to provide necessary information and chalk out some programme to demonstrate the latest technology and policies of government for betterment of farmers community. In other words, agricultural officer has now started to use ICTs to inform about technical knowledge and suggestions time to time especially during incurrence of disease/pest attack on crop and provide necessary instruction so that farmers could use cost effective medicine.

The scenario has changed due to use of ICT on behaviour of farmers and cost incurred in transaction and cost for purchasing of inputs etc. The most of farmers (89%) used these information in purchasing inputs. The transaction cost include 'distance traveled" means cost of equivalent of labour hours and cost of travel per visit. The details of information on such cost in purchasing inputs were estimated and same are presented in Table 2.

Table 2. Component – wise cost per visit (Rs)

Component	Expenditure
1. Labour – hours foregone	120.00
2. Traveling (t and fro)	65.00
Miscellaneous	22.00
Total	207.00

It is revealed from the Table 2, that farmers spent whole one day to acquire inputs if available. However, the farmers' experiences revealed the required inputs were made available after three to four visits. The local dealers do not have technical knowledge as well interest to sell available inputs which may not be effective, were the major reasons. Such expenditures either increase the cost of cultivation or reduce the farm income. The cost involved in procuring inputs was estimated under traditional way was Rs. 621/- (Rupee six hundred twenty one only) which was beard by farmers themselves. With the introduction of ICT, farmers first choice was to contact above mentioned research organization and seek the appropriate technical know how for controlling disease and then visit the nearby local market. Such information was gathered by some advance/ innovative farmers and shared to the affected farmers. One group of the farmers (a group of 5 to 7 farmers) visited the local market and shared the expenditure. This indicated the reduction in transaction cost. The average cost in procuring appropriate well effective medicine was Rs. 36.83 which indicated reduction in transaction cost nearly by 94%.

Use of ICT in marketing

Traditionally, farmers were spending more time to sell out his crop produce in the market. To receive reaso-nable price farmers had to stay two to five days and spent unnecessary more money. If they do not get the reasonable or expected price, they have only two option, either they put their produce in nearby godown or in mandi itself or return back with out selling the produce. For both the reasons they have to bear extra burden. Due to ICT, farmer were getting frequently information about the market situation and prevailing price of the particular farm produce. As mentioned above, during the study period, it was noticed that telephone facility was more appropriate technology to collect the required information. The cost incurred in disposal of farm produce in the market at reasonable price at nearby local regulated market from traditional way and with the help of ICT were estimated and the results are presented in the Table 3.

Table 3. Cost structure in marketing of farm produce.

Cost structure	Expenditure Incurred under (Rs.)	
	Traditional Way	ICT Way
Transportation cost (from village to local market)	1260.00	1565.00
Transportation cost (from local market to village)	1260.00	-
Transportation cost (from village to local market)	1260.00	-
Stay (5 days total including second time)	750.00	135.00
Telephone charges	-	36.00
Total	4530.00	1736.00

From the Table 3, it is seen that average transportation cost was 83.4% and remaining cost was on stay at local market or *Mandy*. The cost incurred on weighing, labour charges etc. were not account for as it has to be paid under both methods. The total cost incurred by farmers using ICT was only 38% to total cost under traditional method. It showed that farmers can save, an average, 62% in the transaction cost due to ICT which helped in decision – making and efficient marketing of farm produce (wheat and mustard crop). However, in case of cumin crop, farmers choice was *Ujha Mandy* famous for cumin marketing where the farmers expected an attractive prevailing price. ICT played a vital role in decision-making and efficient marketing of cumin crop. Farmers were in close contact with local dealers and watch the market movement. As and when market favours the farmers expectation then they proceed for selling of their products. Some time they fixed the price on telephone and then deliver the cumin crop in *Ujha* market. The cost saving remains the same as cost of transportation and others remains of similar nature.

From the above discussion, it is evident that ICT has played a vital and positive impact on reducing the transaction cost in acquiring inputs and selling of agricultural produce efficiently.

REFERENCES

Ballantyne, P. and Bokre, D. (2003) `Report from Prepcom for CTA's Sixth Consultative expert meeting of its observator on ICT's, Wageningen, The Netherlands: CTA.

Greenridge, C. (2003). Well come address: ICTs transforming extension? Presentation to CTA's Sixth consultative expert meeting of its observator on ICT's. Wageningen, The Netherlands: CTA.

O'Farrell, C. (2003). Gender and agriculture in the information Society. Presentation to CTA's Sixth Consultative expert meeting of its observator on ICT's, Wageningen, The Netherlands: CTA.

OSI Reference Model

Kulesh Kumar

Librarian, Govt. College, Chharra, Aligarh (UP).

1. INTRODUCTION

A few years back no one was aware with the term network architecture. At that time companies implemented rather rude, crude and socially unacceptable software and hardware for communication purposes in the computers without thinking about the implementation of an architecture for network. The idea of network architecture really took with the introduction of an international standard called Open System Interconnection (OSI) model, which was developed by International Standards Organis-ation (ISO) in 1982. The ISO covers all aspects of networks communication in the OSI model. The OSI model defines seven layers of functions that take place at each end of communication. It is a model for communication between two end users in a network and is used in developing products and understanding networks.

2. GENESIS OF OSI REFERENCE MODEL

The users of a computer network are located over a wide physical range, i.e, all over the world. Therefore, to ensure that nationwide and worldwide data communication systems can be developed and can compatible to each other, an international group of standards has been developed. These standards have been fit into a framework, which was developed by the International Standards Organisation (ISO). This framework is called as Open System Interconnection (OSI). OSI originally was intended to be detailed specification of interfaces. It was officially adopted as an international standard by the ISO. After that ISO started to think for developing on architecture and reference model, which may serve as the foundation for future standard activities. So ISO formed a Technical Sub-Committee (TC97/SC16) in 1978 to develop an architecture and reference model, that can serve as the foundation for future standards activities. From 1978 onwards the above committee worked very hard at providing a flexible reasonable communication architecture that can be implemented on a variety of systems and can provide inter and intra system communication capabilities in a variety of environments. Oddly enough, the committee could not done most of the work on defining there protocols for each layer of architecture of OSI model. An other ISO committee have done this using the model specified by the previous committee. In 1982, the ISO proposed a broad model for mainframe WAN communication, which was titled OSI Reference Model.

3. WHAT IS OSI REFERENCE MODEL

OSI Reference model is a layered framework for the structure of network systems that allows communication across all types of computer systems. As a matter of fact, to reduce the design complexity, most networks are organised as a series of layers or levels, on above the other. The number of layers, the name, the contents and the functions of each layer differ from network to network. The purpose of each layer is to offer certain services to the higher layers. In OSI reference model seven layers have been used to organise a network into well defined functional modules. In the model, the lowest layer is physical layer and the highest one is called the application layer. It is not essential to use all the seven layers in all the applications. The lower 3 layers are enough for most of the applications. Each layer is built from electronic circuits and/or softwares, and has a separate existence from the remaining layers. Each layer is supposed to handle message or data from the layers which are immediately above or below it. This is done by following the protocol rules. Thus each layer takes data from the adjacent layer, and handles it according to these rules and then passes the process data to the next layer on the other side.

Thus we see that the purpose of OSI reference model is to guide product implementors, so that their products will consistently work with other products. In this way in the last we can say that OSI reference model refers to the exchange of information among terminal devices, computers and networks.

OSI Reference model is not, by itself, a standard, nor a lateral description of computer communication, while it defines where to perform tasks, it does not detail how to perform them. The OSI reference model is intended to provide a common basis for coordinating the development of standards aimed at systems interconnection, while allowing existing standards to be placed in perspective within a common framework. OSI reference model refers to the exchange of information among terminal devices, computers, persons, processes and networks. In it, individual services and protocols are not specified. Communication functions are addressed from the perspective of computer to communication on network interconnection. Thus OSI reference model defines a set of procedures and standards grouped into seven layers or levels, for the exchange of information between terminals and computers.

4. USE OF LAYERS IN OSI REFERENCE MODEL

OSI Reference model uses seven layers. Network designers use the model's description of these seven layers to build real network. The seven layers of the model are : Physical layer, Data Link layer, Network layer, Transport layer, Session layer, Presentation layer and the list is Application layer. All these seven layers are shown in the following figure :

Layer 7	Application layer
Layer 6	Presentation layer
Layer 5	Session layer
Layer 4	Transport layer
Layer 3	Network layer
Layer 2	Data link layer
Layer 1	Physical layer
Layer 0	Transmission media

In this model each layer performs a well defined functions and uses one or more protocols to platform its functions. The purpose of each layer in the model, is to offer certain services to the higher layers. Layer n on one machine (source) carries on a conversation with layer n on the machine (destination). The rules and connections used in the conversation are collectively known as the layer n protocol. Basically, a protocol is an agreement between the two computers as how communication link should be established, maintained can released. As a matter of fact, a set of layers or protocols is called network architecture.

Following five major principles are used to develops the layers in OSI reference model.

(i) Create a new network whenever the network software needs a different level of abstraction.

(ii) Each layer should perform a well defined function.

(iii) Choose function of each layer with an eye toward defining internationally standardized protocols.

(iv) Choose layer boundaries to minimize the information flow across the interfaces.

(v) The number of layers should be large enough so that the network designers do not need to place dissimilar functions in the same layer. However, the number of layers should not be so large that they become unwieldy.

5. FUNCTIONS OF LAYERS

Functions of each layer in OSI reference model are as follows :

5.1 Physical Layers

The physical layer is responsible for sending bits from one computer to another. The physical layer is not concerned with the meaning of the bits, but it deals with physical connection to the network and with transmission and reception of signals. The physical layer is used to define physical and electrical details such as what will represent a 1 or a 0, how many pins a network will have, how data will be synchronized and when the network adapter may or may not transmit the data.

Functions of the physical layer are as follows :

- It activities, maintains and deactivates the physical connection.
- It defines voltages and data rates needed for transmission.
- It converts the digital bits into electrical signal.
- It decides whether the transmission is simplex, half duplex or full duplex. A physical layer does not perform the following operations :
- It does not detect or correct errors.
- It does not decide the medium or modulation.

5.2 Data Link layer

This layer is responsible for reliable node to node delivery of the data. It accepts packets from the network layer and forms frames and gives it to the physical layer.

Functions of Data link layer are as follows :

- It enables the error ditection, it adds error detection bits to the data which are to be transmitted.
- The encoded data are then passed to the physical layer.
- These error detection bits are used by the Data link layer on the other side to detect and correct the errors.
- At this level, the outgoing messages are assembled into frames, and the system waits for the acknowledgements to be received after every frame transmitted.
- Correct operation of the data link layer ensures reliable transmission of each message.

5.3 Network layer

The main function of this layer is to deliver packets from source to destination across multiple networks (Links). If two systems are connected on the same link, these is no need for a network layer. The other functions of this layer are as follows :

- It routes the signals through various channels to the other end.
- It acts as the network controller by deciding which route data should take.
- It devides the outgoing messages into packets and to assemble incoming packets into message for the higher levels.

5.4 Transport Layer

This layer is responsible for source to destination delivery of the entire message. It ensures that the whole message arrives intact and in order, ensuring both error control and flow control at the source to destination level. The functions of this layer are as follows :

- It devides each message into packets at the source and re-assembles then at the destination.
- It does not functions such as multiplexing, spliting or segmenting on the data.
- It guarantees transmission of data from one end to the other.
- It breaks the data groups into smaller units so that they are handled more efficiently by the network layer.
- It makes sure that the entire message arrives at the receiving transport layer without error.

5.5 Session Layer

The main job of the Session layer is to establish, maintain and synchronize the interaction between the communicating systems. The other functions of this layer are the following :

- It allows two systems to start a dialogue with each other. The communication initiated between two processes can be either in half duplex or full duplex.
- It manages and synchoronizes conversations between two different applications. This is the level at which the user will establish system to system connection.
- It controls logging on and off, user identification, billing and session management.
- It allows addition of check points i.e, synchronization points into a stream of data. In case of crash doing the transmission of the data can be re-transmitted from the check point inspite of re-transmitting it from the start.

5.6 Presentation Layer

This layer takes care of the syntax and semantics of the information exchanged between two communicating systems. The main functions of this layer are as follows :

- It translates data between the formats the network requires and the format the computer expects.
- It does the protocol conversion.
- For security and primary purposes, it carries out convection at the transmitter and description at the recover.
- It carries out data compression to reduce the bandwidth of the data to be transmitted.

5.7 Application Layer

It is the job most layer of OSI model. The functions of this layer are as follows :

- It provides different services such as manipulation of information in various ways, retransferring the files of information, distributing the results etc. to the user who is setting above this layer.
- It allows application to communicate with applications on other computers as through they were on the same computer.
- It provides a basis for e-mail forwarding and string.
- It provides distributed database sources and access to the worldwide information about various objects and services.
- The functions such as Login, or password check wing are also performed by the application layer.

6. INFORMATION EXCHANGE IN OSI REFERENCE MODEL

We have come to know that OSI reference model uses seven layers in communication of information. In communication of information at the physical layer of the model, the communication is held directly, i.e., the computer A sends a stream of bits to computer B. At higher layers each layer in the sending computer A adds its own information to the message it receives from the layer just above it and passes the whole package to the layer just below it as shown in the following figure. The information added by each layer is in the form of headers or trailers. Headers are added to the messages at layers 6, 5, 4, 3, and 2. A trailer is added at layer 2. At layer 1, the entire package is converted to a form that can be transferred to the receiving machine, where the message is unwrapped layer by layer with each process receiving and removing the data meant for it.

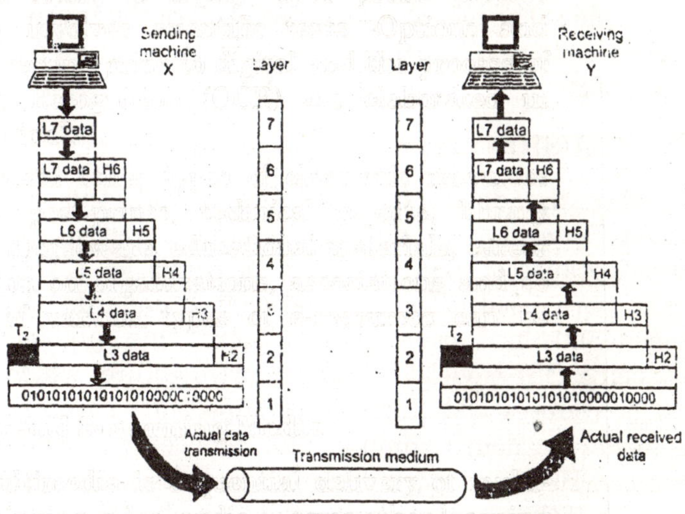

Fig. 1. An exchange using the OSI model

The upper layers (4, 5, 6 and 7) are always implemented in software and lower layers (2 and 3) are combination of hardware and software except for the physical layer which is mostly hardware. Layer 1, 2, 3 i.e. physical layer, data link layer and network layer are the network support layers. They deal with the physical aspects of moving data from one device to another such as electrical specifications, physical connections, physical addressing and transport timing and reliability. Layer 4, the transport layer ensures end to end reliable data transmission. Layer 5, 6 and 7 (i.e., session, presentation and application) they allow interpretability among unrelated software systems.

7. MERITS AND DEMERITS

OSI reference model very clearly distinguishes between the services, interfaces and protocols. The protocols in this model are better hidden. So, they can be easily replaced by new protocols as the technology changes. OSI model is truly a general model. This model supports connection oriented as well as connectionless services. The session and presentation layers of OSI model are not of much use, hence they both are unusable. The model was devised before the invention of protocols, so in real life, there is a problem of felting protocol into a model.

8. CONCLUSION

Before the development of OSI model, the communication between two different systems was a difficult process because of many different protocols for LANS and WANS were used. The international Standards Organisation (ISO) has attempted to solve this problem by introducing OSI model for network architecture, which is a set of procedures and standards grouped into seven layers. This model has done communication between two computers very easy. Hence network designers use the architecture of the layers of this model to built real networks.

9. REFERENCES

(i) Ali, Amjad : Information technology and libraries. New Delhi : Ess Ess Publication, 2004, p. 43.

(ii) Lal, C. and Kumar, K. : Descriptive questions in library and impernation science. New Delhi : Ess Ess Publication, 2004, p. 376-378.

(iii) Sharma, Sanjay: Computer networks. New Delhi: S.K. Katariya; 2007, p. 38-42.

Management of Digital Collection in Modern Libraries

D.V. Kothari & Parvinder Kaur

HOD, L & IS, Jodhpur National University, Jodhpur

ABSTRACT

The paper highlights the management of digital collection. Different steps in management of digital documents have been elaborated in detail. Basic functions in digital document management have been discussed.

INTRODUCTION

By thinking about library, the picture of traditional library i.e., stack room with full of books on all the shelves, issue/return counters, comes in front of our eyes. Computer and communication media have changed and revolutionized the whole world. Library is not a exception to this change. Earlier, in the past, the aim of the librarian was to keep and conserve the documents in the library organization. The library which became rich in collection was called a good library. Now the concept of library has been changed. The library which provides services to the users satisfac-torily is now called a good library.

The library has now become paperless and the services of a library which is special in nature have gone beyond the boundaries of the concerned library. This is due to emergence of electronic media such as computer, internet, E-mail etc. Information desired by a reader of a particular library can be obtained from outside sources of other libraries. The modern library is equipped with website, e-mail, internet, TQM etc. In other words, these modern equipments and methods are more challenging, helping and modernizing to extend the facilities of the boundary less institutions to the information seekers.

Digital era is concerned with creating, sharing and using information in digital form. Libraries are an important and indispensable source of information and knowledge which can be applied in various applications such as trade, commerce, economics, scientific research and development and many other areas. The rapid pace and with which computer and information technology have entered into our lives with new opportunities and libraries have not been left behind. Right information at the right time to right person is the demand of today.

The task of librarians and information professionals has increased manifold as they now have to perform dual responsibility of collecting, organizing information in both physical as well as in digital form to help the information users in accessing the same.

In this information age, we require digital libraries. Emergence of digital technology and computer networks have provided a means whereby the information can be stored, retrieved and disseminated in faster and efficient manner.

1. DOCUMENT MANAGEMENT IN DIGITAL ERA

A general discussion on document management in digital form has been attempted here. Some of the purposes of digital library that are of the direct concern to document management as :

(i) Collect, store and organize information and knowledge in digital form; and

(ii) Promote economic & efficient delivery of information.

1.1 Options in a Library

Some of the activities in the library concerned with managing digital documents may include;

(i) CD-ROM Networking: Networking CD-ROMs with juke box/CD tower or high capacity hard disk mirroring to serve bibliographic or full text databases, electronic supplements with printed books. CDs cut in-house out of publications/reports of internal activity.

(ii) Web access of journals : Current journals could be made accessible from the publisher's websites either through login and passwords or by specific IP address of the institution, without paying extra fee on subscriptions. There are also options to join consortia based electronic access of primary resources through MHRD's INDEST consortium, UGC Infonet project, etc. Seeing the rapidity by which librry automation and CD-ROM technology precolated in the country, there may be many more consortia or at least more and more members to participate in the existing consortia.

(iii) e-books : Free/fee books in electronic form.

1.2 Type of Documents

In the library perspective, the term content encompasses all types of information sources or documents which will be of interest to clientele, though the term is getting wider usage now to denote electronic information resources and the subject matter covered in them. ``Content may be anything, including oral language and natural phenomena, that upon observation appears to have a pattern that can be analyzed for descriptive or inferential purposes" (Penland). If we rephrase the paradigm of Yovits *et al.* ``information to be data of value", then we get `content to be information of value, as the flood of information forces us to be more and more selective and calls for strict measures to identify, collect, organize, and disseminate vital contents. Document management or content management is nothing but the systematic application of various tools and techn-iques for the efficient management of information sources in diverse forms (monograph, journal, reports, conference papers, website resources, email/listserv messages, etc.) and media (print, optical, magnetic, electronic, etc.). Here we should also consider the shift undergoing from traditional library management practices and the attempts towards achieving futuristic knowledge management systems. Since the contents comprise, to a large extent from formal printed monographs and serials in paper or microforms, the collection development concerns were thrust upon providing ``right resource to the right user at the right time" to satisfy the fundamental laws of library science. Whereas in the aftermath of electronic information products and Internet/ Web, the barriers between formal and informal sources are becoming greatly reduced and collection development is leading to access arrangement mechanism.

In the electronic scenario, it is not the document (often regarded as the carrier or physical form of content), but the content is pervasive and more important. This needs new management principles and alertness as well as trained information support staff to trace, track and control electronic resources procured and available free on the web. The availability of local information that institutions would like to share with others and the computer/communication infrastructure emerging also enabled institutions to publish local contents. Well processed and properly connected information that an institution should use significantly to enhance its utility in its sphere of activity becomes knowledge. Thus information-intensive industries are putting considerable amount of money, machines and manpower to conserve and do value-addition to this knowledge. Information Managers identified the various strategies to be adopted while implementing knowledge management, such as, document management, improved access to information, use and reuse of information, access to people, learning by participation, networking/synergies, process orientation, human capital and management culture.

Contents Fall in two Groups, Internal and External

Internal (Local) : Research or annual reports and other publications issued by the parent institution affiliating the library. In addition, there are also p/reprints of research publications and proceedings of conferences hosted by the institution.

External : Contents procured from publishers or vendors such as full-text databases, online access of subscribed primary journals. There are also offline electronic media like CDs, floppies etc. Contents in this category are sourced from a wide range of options such as web access rights, open access materials like web information resources, contents licensed through consortia, etc.

1.3 Steps in Document Management

The basic functions in digital document management are :

- Identification and collection of contents to be digitized;
- Classification and digitization of these contents;
- Editing, formatting and storage of the contents;
- Designing search engines to selectively search and access the contents;
- Publishing contents digitally for end-user access.

(i) Subtasks

Each of these functions involves certain subtasks like :

- Transforming printed information into digital form

- Storage, retrieval and handling of ``easy-to-use" electronic information.
- Converting data from diverse media or formats into digitl format.
- Classification techniques for improving retrieval efficiency.
- Managing devices for large massive storage, with multilevel hierarchical storage structures, supporting different speed storage devices and varied capacity processors.
- Editing and formating of contents in different formats such as, HTML, VRML, XML, PDF, JPEG, MPEG, etc.
- Browsing and querying facilities for content based retrieval.
- Options to promptly distribute and safety access information via standard communication and computing infrastructure.
- Security of delivered contents by different cryptographic/encrycption methods and appropriate firewell mechanisms and access methods through password/IP authentication of clients.

Capturing may involve data capturing equipments such as high-resolution scanners, VCP and compatible capture cards to handle audio, video, images and text. Storage needs servers with multiple CPUs, with RAM in GB range and HDD of few 100 GB to TB and workstations of decent configuration with enhanced processor speed and storage. Search engines/retrieval software deals with software for database management, Webservers, content authoring/editing, application software, etc. Dissemination requires good network infrastructure with ATM/155 mbps card and high-speed routers, large display terminals for servers and workstations, optical disc reproduction/CD-Writers, LCD displays for projections and high/low resolution printers.

(ii) Capturing

Let us identify only textual sources in the beginning, and focus on internal contents first. Retrospective data could be digitized either by keying or by scanning. So some data entry terminals (PCs) and scanners are essential and these may be procured from the market for as low as Rs. 30000. Sophisticated contents like images, video and sound (not so important in an academic library where majority of the collection is textual) may be converted later when the digital library development acquires enhanced monetary support by procuring equipments such as high resolution scanners, VCP, multimedia machines (workstations as well as servers) and compatible capture cards to handle audio, video, images.

(iii) Formatting, encoding and Compression

How data is formatted (written to magnetic media), compressed, and encoded (how internal semantic or syntactic features are represented) will determine its portability across hardware and software platforms and how it may be stored, manipulated and subsequently enriched according to Beegrie and Greenstein. Crucial decisions on these counts are not only required for proper implementation but for efficient use too. Computing formats change continually. Arms warns that file formats of ten years ago may be hard to read. To store digitized files, there are many formats to choose from such as MS Word, LaTeX, Troff, GIF (Graphic Interchange Formate), RTF (Rich Text Format), or MIF (Maker Interchange Format), SGML in compliance with their DTDs (Document Type Definitions). Archive images are saved as TIFF (Tag Image File Format) which is the standard for high quality uncompressed raster images captured by scanners where as full-sized and thumbnail Web Images are saved as JPEG (Joint Photographic Expert Group), the dominant standard in imaging applications. TIFF is the most prevalent for conversion of paper back-files, HTML/SGML (Standard General-sized Mark-up Language) is used by many large publishers after conversion from proprietary formats, and PDF is the most prevalent format for purely electronic documents. The easiest option for web access is to convert the electronic full text availble in the pre-production stage into html format. Added materials like figures/tables may be converted into formats like gif/jpg whichever is convenient in the individual institution. According to Weisser and Walker PDF documents retain all formatting and graphics, permits easy indexing and search by keywords and also allow including links to ther sites on the Web or annotations within the articles. PDF offers a number of benefits as stated by Beebe and Meyers such as read on differnt platforms; editing can be made at any stage; files much smaller than PostScript files, use less space and transmit more quickly; offers a one-file solution for both print and online; and can view using a free reader. The software to read PDF files Acrobat reader is freely downloadable from many sites (for examples, http://www. adobe.com) thus requiring no investment at the client side. Over 95% of the 600 international journals out of the 800 subscribed at a premier library in the country provide the table of contents with abstracts as html files and the full text in PDF. The remaining uses different formats of HTML, PS; etc. Arms stresses the importance to create the information in formats that are widely adopted today as this increases the chance that conversion programmes to new formats will be available as in the case of HTML and PDF so widely used that viewers will surely be available many years from now.

Lossless compression removes redundant information in a manner that is completely reversible and the original data can be reconstructed exactly as it was. Lossy compression can not be reversed as approximations are made during the compression that losses some of the information. Thibdean and Benoit illustrates the cage of Antique Books conversion, the original page image of over twenty megabytes, but the processed image, both print and background is around 50 kilobytes (400 to 1 compression is achieved by this technique). Compression techniques may be used not only for saving space at the server side but also to effect fast transfer and retrieval over limited bandwidth.

(iv) Content Indexing and Metadata

Decisions are to be taken regarding what to be indexed (author, subject, keywords, phrases, etc.), usage of stop words, vocabulary control, proximity searches, language and period limiting etc. Indexing strategy comprises not only of what types of fields are to be indexed, but how they are to be treated (exhaustive or sparse). Implementation of indexes and metadata on the database management systems is also of concern. The popular metadata framework, Dublin Core, contains the following elements : Subject and key words, Title, Author or Creator, Publisher, Description (textural description of content); Other agent (the person(s), such as editors and transcribers); Date (of publication); Object type (the genre of the object, such as novel); Form (the data representation of the object, such as postscript file); Identifier (string or number used to uniquely identify the object); Relation (the relationship to other objects); Source (Objects, either print or electronic from which this object is defined); Language, Coverage (Special locations and temporal duration characteristic); and Right management. Using the Dublin Core framework as the basis, Bishoff states that the CDP identified eight optional elements and seven mandatory elements of creator, title, subject, description, identifier, date, and format. According to Hodge many project managers acknowledge that the best practice would be to create the metadata at the object-creation stage, or to create the metadata in stages, with the metadata provided at creation augmented by additional elements during the cataloguing stage.

The information about a data resource's structure, contents, context, provenance, and history as suggested by (Hedstrom and Montgomery) influences how a resource is located, managed and used, and frequently reflects data acquisition decisions and the documentation standards and practices. A database system to keep stock of digitized collection is important, as the task is to provide selective access to the data. Necessary front end to accept search queries and flash matched results would also be developed. Technical processing done for other documents will be attempted for digital elements here. On digitizing an item marked in the OPAC, it can also link digital images of contents with associated information in the database.

(v) Organization

Indexing required for the digitized contents to search and access them in a selective way like OPAC for printed contents. How the contents and index files are linked and what sort of access points provided is another area of concern? May be the library is going for a modular fashion; they can follow a hypertext link and access to the digitized contents. Once the contents acquire sufficient volume, they can look for a database management system to link the index and contents. A document has different physical parts, links at the file level; they are either stored as independent files or as stored as records in a database at the record level and in most cases identified by a URL/DOI.

(vi) Storage

PCs are marketed now with 20/40GD HDDs and 128 or 256 MB RAMs for Rs. 25000 and entry level servers for less than a lakh. So with limited investment, the library may be able to order a 100 GB HDD system with 512/1024 MB RAM. If money is a problem to get Unix Operating system, they can do with Linux. During the initial stage, it is also appropriate to work with Windows servers. Configure at least one machine with good configuration as a server to hold and service the digital contents. Text in general, is stored at one byte per character and assumed two bytes per character for multi-lingual, with 100% indexing overhead. According to Wolf and Holland, the storage required for a small collection of 100,000 articles averaging five pages (2000 characters per page), all in English stored in full text, and indexed for proximity and structural searching is three GB.

(vii) Search Engines/Retrieval

The library needs software for database management, Web servers, content authoring/editing, etc., and developmental software (Visual studio, C++, Java and Internet tools etc.). As most of these tools are in the public domain, the library does not find it difficult to use at least a few of these in its in-house digitization and document management routines.

(viii) Dissemination

If the campus is well networked, then without much investment from the library side, the contents may be made accessible on the Intranet. It is easier to host the borrowed external contents also in this mode. However, access restrictions are to be put on these contents either with login/ password or and IP filtering when access is provided over Internet. The library is always free to host its internal contents on the Internet. The Internet infrastructure required for hosting the digital library depends upon different parameters such as the quantum of contents to be hosted, number of simultaneous users expected, over and above the bandwidth constraints at the national level. 1 Mbps bandwidth will play videos in real time and internal LAN technology has already crossed the 1 Gbit barrier. Thus institutions with a functional Intranet and leased line connection from VSNL or other Internet Service Providers (ISPs) will not face much hindrances for content delivery.

CONCLUSION

Libraries in India are slowly waking up to the needs of managing digital documents to a large extent for rendering current services. Digital document management unlike print document managment has its own advantages and challenges and it is upto the library adminstration and professionals to frame proper programmes and effective action plans to transform these new media of information resources to the benefit of library and its readers. The INFLIBNET in India has been making efforts to digitize libraries of all universities and research organizations.

REFERENCES

ARMS (William, Y.). 2000. Digital Libraries. Cambridge, Mass : MIT Press, 287 pp.

JEEVAN (V.K.J.). 2005. Digital archives and document management and others. In Advances In Library and Information Science. Vol. 5, Digital Library. By D.C. Ojha & D.V. Kothari, Scientific Publishers (India), Jodhpur, 85-91 pp.

SHARMA (R.S.) 2005. Perspective in Digital Library. In Advances In Library and Information Science. Vol. 5, Digital Library. By D.C. Ojha & D.V. Kothari. Scientific Publishers (India), Jodhpur.

Academic Libraries in 21st Century — Changes experienced

S.D. Vyas

Librarian, NALSAR University of Law, Hyderabad 500 078 (AP)

1. INTRODUCTION

The change goes on endlessly. Change occurs everyday when we look at the clock, river or at the sun rise and sun set. This is part of change. Rivers changes its course every year and seasons change every third month in this part of the world. Since change is constant and reality then the very effort to resist change is like trying to stop a gushing river. Seed becomes a sapling and then tree. This metamorphism is also well explained by S.R. Ranganathan in his fifth law of Library Science i.e. "a **Library is a Growing Organism**". Thus change is very essence of life. Likewise in terms of time and continuous development in technology and knowledge our objectives and needs change. While 20th century paid more attention on production, present century is a century of self renewal. It means we have to put a new life and vigor into our library profession as well as in bringing quality in doing everything in the library work. Now a days we do not come across anything as evolutionary process, but revolutionary, as dramatic changes are occurring. We are doing the earlier things in new ways. Earlier we have transformed book records in catalogue cards, now same records are being fed in machine readable format. Today's libraries have undergone changes from clay tables to papyrus scrolls to sheets of paper to bound books to electronic books. Stephan Juran says that twenty first century is devoted to quality.

2. EDUCATION

We have to remember that in our library science education no one has been taught as to how to deal with 'constant change'. Hence to cope with new learning we have to be prepared to become life long learners. We have to continue to learn about resources and users need outside our area of specialization. Hence Departments of Library and Information Science should touch upon this aspect of constant change. Let it be included in Library Science teaching.

3. SHARING OF KNOWLEDGE

Librarian should share the knowledge with other professionals because lot of research is being done in Library and Information Science. The professionals need to share their knowledge and experience with others. If one is hiding knowledge he is doing it at his own peril. Even developed nations have realized that they cannot take liberty of hiding the information and knowledge from developing nations. Usually we do not discuss with each other because of fear that perhaps others may be benefitted.

4. SCHOLARSHIP AND LEARNING

Continuous learning will develop our own individual strengths. It will assist us in responding to the changing needs of the customers. Library and Informational Science professionals are supposed to develop values of intellectual discourse and scholarship to participate fully in the collegial undertakings of the university. Whether or not we understand the new technology, we have to read about it regularly. This will help us to change ourselves according to change in circumstances. There is changing nature of learning. Being librarian one should study and love his own subject in whom he possesses Masters Degree as well as other subjects also. In addition to reading, librarians are supposed to involve in research methodology, knowing secondary sources in print as well as in electronic format.

5. INFORMATION TECHNOLOGY

To expand our searches, technology has to be understood. Technology is likely to change over coming years and influence every walk of life. We have to have sufficient knowledge of technology not only knowledge, but how to teach to users. Users are at receiving end. If library professionals do not keep on up- dating knowledge, they will fail in educating the users in telling them about library resources and services. This is very much visible as we do not involve ourselves in information literacy programmes.

Internet being a tool of technology is helping users to get information, but its use is like getting fast food. Only libraries can provide nutritious food to the users in order to make them knowledgeable. There is no wisdom involved in information that we get from the Internet. Information landscape in changing and we think will Internet replace libraries. If we look at the present scenario, perhaps it will not because users still do not have full faith in Internet to give the desired information or knowledge. Ever changing nature of electronic information gathering forces us to be on our toe in order to incorporate new services.

6. INTERNET

Use of Internet began in 1970's in USA, but in India it was in 1996, when we witnessed Internet revolution. Perhaps no other recent innovation impacted the library profession so much as the Internet and other networked resources. Not only is our world becoming an interconnected global community, but this early use of the Internet has changed the fundamental roles, paradigms, and organizational cultures of libraries and librarians as well.

It is reported that in 1991 there were 2900 computer networks connected to the Internet, and over 200 online library systems. There will not be any place for librarians who are not willing to interact with technology. Unprecedented changes have occurred in late 1980's and 1990's not only in library profession, but in society as a whole. Internet is an information storage and retrieval tool which provides useful information whenever and wherever we want. Internet helps in getting the knowledge at your fingertips twenty four hours. We need not feel the pinch of missing the library. All these years we have been hankering for need of public libraries. Now it is available on Internet - a tool at your disposal. Thus Internet is trying to prove its utility like learning resource centre. On Internet one finds journal articles, books, reports, open source material and much useful reference information. The criticism leveled against Internet is that retrieval of information is not easy as it is very chaotic. Sometimes one gets information within no time and sometimes one may not get it for hours together. Hopefully in near future Internet will prove to be better user friendly tool of information and knowledge. It is roughly estimated that 3 to 4 per cent of India's population now uses internet which will increase to ten per cent in next one decade. Thus it will make a lot of difference to country's economic development if more people use it.

7. INFORMATION LITERACY

Information literacy is the ability to make significant connections to form interpretations to evaluate situations, and to provide context. Who will give information literacy skills to users of the library? It is the reference librarian's duty to guide users to develop Information Literacy skills so that they become skillful and critical consumers. Thus we have to develop teaching skills to provide education to users in the area of Information Literacy.

8. PROFESSION

Library profession is in dramatic change and this situation will be there in foreseeable future. 'Constant change' is the hall mark of the profession. Thus 'constant change' will have significant impact on this skill of the professionals to whom we recruit and hire. We have to be honest with ourselves as how much comfortable we are with changes. Thus life long learning is essential for librarians. It is not only with Library Science professionals, it has affected the professionals of all subjects.

Jose Ortega y Gasset says that "librarians must function as a filter between the users and the torrents of books." The above statement has got deeper meaning and implications. This is a matter of discussion what we can do and offer as library professionals. Someone says that the price of arrogance is the constant struggle to stay abreast of your expertise in the subject.

9. LIBRARIAN'S QUALITIES

It should be essential qualification for a librarian that he should be good at communication skills, and he should know more than a little of computer equipments and electronic devices. As a matter of fact librarian should have the following qualities:

- Flexible
- Articulate
- Kind, and
- Tenacious

However, the general picture of librarian is that he lacks the above qualities. Librarians should know that users' need rapidly change. They have to up to date their skills. They have to be master learners, communicators, educators and change masters. We have to know more about our subject. We must conduct survey chronologically as to what we have attained till today if Library Science has to grow further for the purpose of research.

We have to use jargon i.e. professional language. We have to be touchy. No one can trample all over if we maintain our expertise in the subject. For this we have to be on our feet i.e. ready to learn anything useful in fulfilling duties as librarian. We need not be extinct reptiles like dinosaurs which mean we have to constantly change according to needs of the time. Senior librarians should engage in discussion about library profession. Such librarians should be entrusted with the job of teaching library profession to younger generation so that they get to know what is expected of them in their professional career as a professional.

10. REFERENCE SERVICE

An ideal reference service librarian is one who is not afraid of 'constant change'. This professional work could not be sustained longer and it is not known whether libraries are involving themselves in giving reference service to the users. Reference librarians have to have a broad knowledge of paper and electronic resources. Moreover we have the responsibility to reduce the fear psychosis of users as most of them remain fearful about asking for help in the library.

11. MARKETING

We have to market ourselves which means our introduction to faculty, staff and students. We should prepare homepage placed prominently on department web page. We have to make teacher aware i.e. what we can offer to them, download a copy of faculty members' syllabus and send them alerts of articles. We should be ready to extend help in teaching and research.

12. CO-ORDINATION WITH THE FACULTY

Another important aspect of changes experienced is co-ordination with the faculty. It is predicted that future of libraries lies in the ability of its librarian to collaborate with faculty. After all our users are basically faculty and students. So they should have confidence in our abilities that what we can offer to them.

13. CONCLUSION

We have discussed about the 'constant changes' occurring in technology every after few years. We have to plan ourselves to cope with 'constant change' as we all feel the impact of technology. Hence we have to keep in mind Darwin's biological principle i.e. 'survival of the fittest' or else we will become dinosaurs. So we have to prepare programmes for Continuous Professional Development. Let us be prepared to do everything in a new way for betterment of our library services and resources. It is recommended that our departments of library and information science in the universities prepare our students to grapple with the problem of 'constant change', encourage lifelong learning, start sharing of knowledge, learn basics of marketing, and improve exceptional communication skills.

REFERENCES

Brophy, Peter. The Academic Library. 2nd ed. London, Facet, 2005.

Brophy, Peter. The Library in the Twenty First Century: New Services for the Information Age. London, Facet, 2001.

Butler, Pierce. *An Introduction to Library Science.* Chicago, University of Chicago Press, 1933

Change Management (people) Wikipedia. 5p.

Clyde, Laurel A. Continuous Professional Education for the Information Society. *IFLA Journal.*

Expectations of Librarians in the 21st Century. Edited by Karl Bridges. Westport, Green Press, 2003.

International Encyclopedia of Information and Library Science. Edited by John Feathers and Paul Sturges. London, Routledge, 2003, 2nd edtion

Mishra, Bal Krishna. Change is Constant, Go with the Flow. *Times of India.*21st May 2009.

Myburgh, Sue. Education Directions for NIPS(New Informational Professionals)10 p.

Narayani, Ganesh. Change is Constant. *Times of India.* 28th December 2008

National Knowledge Commission. *Recommendations for LIS Sector.* 16 p.

Vyas, S.D. *Constant Changes Experienced in Academic Libraries in 21st Century.* Paper Presented in National Seminar on Library and Information Services in Changing Era 22nd.-23rd June 2009 on the Occasion of Golden Jubilee of the Department of Library and Information Science, University of Pune, Pune. p.1-6.

Vyas, S.D. Role of Library and Information Professionals in the Emerging Knowledge Society: A Discussion. Paper Presented in CALIBER Conference held in Pune. February 2000.

Growth and Development of Open Source Software for Libraries

Satynarayan Sharma

Librarian, R.N. Modi Engineering College, Kota

1. INTRODUCTION

Information is now considered as an essential resource for all round development of the society. It provides tremendous opportunities to accelerate the pace of development both at national and international level. Information is a key factor in day-to-day life. It can be considered as the lifeblood of communication and interaction. In a way, research is also a kind of collection of information from various sources and analyzing it to solve the problems or to satisfy the quest for knowledge. The process of research is entirely dependent on information, from the selection of a research problem, till the printing of the report.

Now in information era, in order to avoid obsolescence of information a library professional should apply the advanced technologies to make his user community satisfied. One such application is library automation. Developments in electronic and communication technologies have affected every profession and libraries are no exception. All types of libraries are challenged to provide greater information access and improved levels of service, while coping with the pace of technological change and ever-increasing budget pressure, use of software applications in libraries has become essential. The most visible reasons are :

Growth of Electronic Resources

Large databases from periodicals, magazines, and journals, are available in digital format- at first on CD-ROM, later via online services. Library services are transitioning from local traditional collections to global resources provided on demand via the most advanced networking technologies. Today, library collections are used by people on campus as well as by individuals who could not even locate the information in physical environment.

Anytime Anywhere Access

Access to online digital information from anywhere is the need of the hour. This is forcing the library to shift its role from a repository to a gatewy. Advanced users are expecting online libraries that can provide round the clock service.

Library users have become accustomed to use the Internet as a research tool and do not always appreciate the difference in quality of information available through a library's specialized collections, especially when compared to what can be located through an Internet search engine. Thus, libraries with substantial collections of information often find that collection under utilized if the user interface is not designed to make it easy to locate the required information.

Resource Sharing

Libraries of all types also need to utilize new application systems to automate resource sharing. Union Catalogues and Inter-Librry Loan modules are needed to allow cooperating institutions to combine their catalogues and allow patrons of one library to request and borrow materials from linked libraries. These technologies will foster the growth of library consortia and the extension of offering beyond the organizational boundaries of individual libraries. However, implementing new technologies and tools into library environments may be a highly challenging task. Despite significant benefits, many libraries do not have the definite resources and infrastructure to maintain and upgrade availble technologies. In addition, there is a significant demand for standard-based, open systems to promote interoperability. Open Source Software (OSS), as will be discussed in the present study, comes to the rescue of less privileged libraries to deal with the increasing demands for use of technology. OSS enables democrtization of technology. OSS has definite advantages over proprietary systems in the Total Cost of Ownership (TCO), since it is available free to download on the internet. Thus OSS bears great importance to the libraries in developing countries like India. OSS also gives freedom to the users of the software to customize it to his/her needs since one has access to the source code of the software.

Open Source Software is provided with a license that gives the end user the right to use it freely for private or commercial use. User also has the right to inspect and even modify the underlying source code. One can give away or sell the original version you received or one with your modification. In turn, you may be required to pass on the modified source code so that others may be benefitted from the changes you have made. This last clause protects the developer's work from unfair explitation by others, while allowing the source code to be released to the community. User is not required to pay royalties to previous developers, but he is still permitted to charge money for the sale of OSS. This disc may have been given to you by a friend; or sold to you for a small fee, in both cases it is permited. Keep in mind that there are many different licenses, each of which has its own particular set of conditions. If you plan to distribute or modify one of the programme on this disc, please double check the license before you begin. It will make you clear on both your rights and obligations.

If you have no interest in source code, you may aks for the availability of this matter. One answer is that the release of source allows external observers to inspect the internal functions of the programme, which means you can be confident that the programme treats your private data with respect. One problem with proprietary software is that it tends to use closed file formats to store your data. Once the parent company stops supporting older versions of a proprietary programme you may have to upgrade to newer versions of that prograamme at significant expense in order to retain access to your data. This does not happen with OSS, because when the source code for opening and saving files is available, a third party can easily write an import filter for the next generation of software, ensuring that your data will always be available. Finally, the release of source code has in some cases spawned large communities of volunteer developers who have in turn provided the world with highly useful and entirely free software such as Linux. This software is available free of charge to schools or anyone else who may not have a huge budget available for buying software. So, you can see that the freedom of software is important for everyone not just software developers.

1. MOVEMENT OF OPEN SOURCE SOFTWARE OF LIBRARY

The OSS movement has its roots in this hacker culture of seventies and eighties. OSS is both a philosophy and a process. As a philosophy it describes the intended use of software and method for its distribution. Depending on your persepective the concept of OSS is relatively new idea being only four or five years old. OSS is also having process for the creation and maintenance of software. This is not a formalized process, but rather a process of convention with common characteristics between software projects (Morgan, 2002).

The History of Open Source Software began with the early stages of computer and developers used to share their software freely. Advent of companies in software development with the aim of profit making restricted the culture of sharing source code of software. Milestones in the history of OSS are :-

1983 - Richard Stall Formed GNU project;

1985 - Creation of free software foundation;

1991 - Development of Linux kernel by linus morale's;

1998 - Open source Initiative (OSI) formed by Eric Raymond

1999 - ``October GNOME'' The most stable release of the GNOME system is released

The two terms ``Free'' and ``Open Source'' are used as synonymous for free distribution of software. Popular licenses used for this purpose are the GNU general public license (GPL) BSD license, GNU Lesser general public license, MIT license, mozilla public license and apache license. All these licenses have some differences in their terms and conditions; they ensure users freedom to use copying, distribution and improvement of software fundamentals of these licenses are similar to the philosophy of free software foundation. ``Free sotware is a matter of the users'' Freedom to run, copy, distribute, study, change and improve the software''

According to free software foundation users can enjoy the following freedom with free software :

- The freedom to run the programme for any purpose;
- The freedom to study and modify the programme;
- The freedom to copy the programme; and
- The freedom to improve the programme.

1.1 Open Source

Open source as the many says allows the creation process and its information to be open modifiable to anyone.

A clear definition of the term can be found in a wikipedia entry a relevnt OS project (Sanger, 2006, P. 307).

Open Source describes practices in production and development that promote access to the production sources, the term open source gained popularity with the rise of the Internet and its enabling of diverse production models. Communication paths and interactive communities. {wikipedi 2006 [online]}

1.2 Open Source Software

The Open Source Research Community describes this software as a software for which the human readable source code is made available to the user of the software, who can then modify the code in order to fit the software to the user's needs. The source code is the set of written instructions that define a programe in its original form and when it is made fully accessible, programmers can read it, modify it and redistribute it, thereby improving and adopting the softwre.

The term ``Open Source Software" was coined in 1998 in order to market the ``free software".

The fundamental difference between the two movements is in their values and their ways of looking at the world. [. . . .] open source is a development methodology; free software is a social movement.

Open Source means several things (Chudnov, 1999);

- Open source software is typically created and maintained by developers crossing institutional and national boundaries collaborating by using internet based communications and development toos.
- Products are typically a certain kind of `free often through a license that specifies that applications and source code (The programming instructions written to create the applications) are free to use. Modify and redistribute as long as all uses,

modification and redistributions are similarly licensed;

- Successful applications tend to be developed more quickly and with better responsiveness to the needs of users who can readily use and evaluate open source applications because they are free;
- Quality not profit drives open source developers who take personal pride in seeing their working solutions adopted;
- International property right to open source software belong to everyone who help in building it or simply uses it. Not just the vendor or institution who created or sold the software.

Need for OSS

- Cost of commercial software's is very high.
- Commercial developers do not reveal the source code of their programmes.

OSS Tools

Here are the few general purpose open source software tools:

- Apache - a Web server
- MySQL - a rational databaase application
- Linux - an operating system
- Perl - a scripting/programming languge
- Python - another scripting/programming language
- Swish-e - an indexer/search engine
- Lucene and Plucene - another indexer / search engine

Websites which provide detailed listing of Open Source Software are

1. Free software foundation software directory (www.fsf.org/)

2. UNESCO free & OSS portal (www.unesco.org/)
3. Sourceforge (http://sourceforge.net/)
4. Freshmeat (http://Freshmeat.net/)

Library Open Source Projects

1. Koha : The First Open Source Integrated Library System

Description : Koha is the first open source fully featured Integrated Librry System (ILS) used by a considerable number of libraries in USA, New Zealand, and Europe. The Koha ILS includes catalogue, OPAC, circulation, member management and acquisitions package. Koh is used by public libraries, private collectors, non-profit organizations, churches, schools aand corporates.

Special Features : Some of the key features are

- Simple clear interface for librarians and members (patrons) to serch right from the front page.
- Customizable search - you choose which fields you want on your search forms when you set it up.
- Reading lists for members - now one can find the name of that great book you read last year.
- Full acquisition including budgets and pricing information (including supplier and currency conversion), being kept so that you can see what you've ordered and received - so handy at end of the year and at the time of audit.
- Simple acquisition for the smaller library.
- Able to catalogue websites as items, or have them as links to existing records.

History : Koha was developed in 1999 and the first library went live in January of 2000. Koha's code has been in production since then and is continuing to move towards higher levels of functionality and standards compliance, including embracing the international records and cataloguing standards MARC and Z39.50.

Project Sponsors/Administrators : Katipo Communications, and funding by Horowhenua Library Trust and other libraries. Current project leader is Patrick Eyler.

Dependency : Apache, Perl, MySQL (or any RDBMS)

Supported Platforms : Windows (without Z39.50 support), Linux and UNIX

License : GNU General Public License

Availability : http://sourceforge.net/projects/koha,

http://www.koha.org/download/

Further Information

1. Project Homepage : http://www.koha.org/
2. Koha Wiki Page :
3. http://www.saas.nsw.edu.au/wiki/index.php?page=KohaProject
4. Koha Labs : http://www.kohalabs.com/

2. Greenstone

Description : Greenstone is a suite of software for building and distributing digital library collections. It provides a new way of organizing information and publishing it on the Internet or on CD-ROM.

Special Features : Some of the important features are:

- Support for image, video, and text collection;
- Support for multilingual collection building;
- Z39.50 client available on Linux system; and
- Highly portable collection, can easily be distributed even on a CD-ROM.

History - Greenstone is produced by the New Zealand Digital Library Project at the University of Wikato, and developed and distributed in cooperation with UNESCO and the Human Info NGO.

Project Sponsors/Administrators: University of Waikato, New Zealand.

Dependency : Apache, Perl, GDBM

Supported Platform: UNIX, Windows, Linux, MacOSX

License : GNU GPL

Availability:

http://www.greenstone.org/english/download.html

Further Information: Project Home Page : http://www.greenstone.org/

3. MyLibrary

Description : MyLibrary is a user-driven, customizable interface for collection of Internet resources - a portal. Primarily designed for libraries, the system's purpose is to reduce information overload by allowing patrons to select as little or as much information as they so desire for their personal pages.

Special Features :- Some of the important are :

- Web based administration to add, delete, modify user access;
- Web-based report generation;
- Current awareness service based on cron job; and
- Search engine support based on Swish-E.

History : Unknown

Project Sponsors/Administrators : Eric Lease Morgan

Dependency : Apache, Perl, MySQL/PostgreSQL

Supported Platforms : UNIX, Linux

License : GNU General Public License

Availability:

http://dewey.library.nd.edu/mylibrary/download/

Further Information : Project Home Page : http://dewey.library.nd.edu/mylibrary/

4. DSpace

Description : DSpace is a specialized type of digital asset management or content management system. It manages and distributes digital items, made up of digital files and allows for the creation, indexing, and searching of associated metadata to locate and retrieve the items. It is designed to support the long-term preservation of the digital material stored in the repository.

Special Features : The important features of DSpace are :

- **Institutional Repository :** DSpace is organized to accommodate the multidisciplinary and organizational needs of a large institution.

- **Document Formats :** Support for a Variety of Digital Formats and Content types including text, images, audio and video.

- **Access Control :** DSpace allows contributors to limit access to items in DSpace - at the collection and the individual item level.

- **Digital Preservation :** DSpace provides long-term physical storage and management of digital items in a secured, profressionally managed repository, including standard operating procedures such as backup, mirroring, refreshing media, and disaster recovery.

- **Search and Retrieval :** The DSpace submission process allows for the description of each item using a qualified version of the Dublin Core metadata scheme. (Go to http://dspace.org/technology/features.html for more detailed description on features).

History : DSpace was developed out of collaboration between MIT Libraries and Hewlett-Packard Company.

Project Sponsors/Administrators : MIT Libraries & Hewlett-Packard Company

Dependency : Apache, Tomcat, PostgreSQL, Java

Supported Platforms : Claimed to be Platform Independent, but installation manual suggests only UNIX-like platform.

License : BSD License

Availability :

http://dspace.org/technology/download.html,

http://sourceforge.net/project/showfiles.php?group_id=19984

Further Information : Project Home Page : http://www.dspace.org/

5. E-prints

Description : The primary purpose of the E-Prints software is to help and create open access to the peer-reviewed research output of all scholarly and scientific research institutions. The default configuration creates a research papers archive, but could be used for other purposes.

Special Features : Unknown.

History: E-Prints was part of the Open Citation Project, a DL12 International Digital Libraries Project funded by the Joint Information Systems Committee (JISC) of the Higher Education Funding Councils, in collaboration with the National Science Foundation. E-Prints was previously supported by CogPrints, funded by JISC as part of its Electronic Libraries (eLib) Programme.

Project Sponsors/Administrators : University of Southamptom, UK

Dependency : Apache, Perl, mod_perl, MySQL

Supported Platforms : Linux, UNIX

License : GNU GPL

Availability : http://software.eprints.org/

Further Information : Project Home Page : http://www.eprints.org/

OSS is useful for the libraries

According to Chudnov (1999) there are three factors pushing the use of OSS in libraries :

1. OSS licenses allow libraries to cut budget on software and use it to other issues needing more funds.
2. OSS product is not locked in to a single vendor, thus even if a library buys an open source system from one vendor, it might choose to buy technical support from another company or get it from in-house experts.
3. The entire library community might share the responsibility of solving information systems accessibility issues.

According to the draft report (2001) of digital library federation (USA) to consider OSS for libraries there virtues of OSS in libraries are :

- OSS is an economical alternative to libraries reliance upon commercially supplied software. That is depute the real costs involved in the development maintenance and use of OSS software but these are lower than those associated with library reliance upon commerical software.
- OSS is essential if libraries are to develop software and systems that meet their patrons needs. with OSS the IT infrastructure that is essential to library operations and services can be:
    - Open (that is built according to open standards and as such potentially inter operable with other essential software and systems);
    - Ubiquitously available to libraries;

  - Capable of being loved to suit the needs and circumstances of individual libraries;
  - Documented (documentation must be available); and
  - Errors can more effectively be divetrified and corrected (``Many eyeballs make bugs shallow")

- OSS ensures that library systems and online services will be more functional for libraries and their patrons and as much be good for library patrons. This hypothesis is posited because, through OSS developments, libraries are reinserted in to the research and development process that results in systems and software.
  - Share a stake in software development and as such have greater influence over (and as a result take a greater interest in specification) the functional and performance requirements associated with particular software tools and systems.
  - Motivate and empower librarians and related technical staff by encouraging creativity and positioning them to make a difference and are able more easily to collaborate with other information science communities involved in common research and development.

OSS democratizes the use of software applications in libraries irrespective of the size and scope of the library.

Barriers in Using OSS

There are number of barriers in using of OSS in libraries. Library adminstrators are often reluctant to adopt OSS due to number of factors. According to the Draft Report (2001) of Digital Library Federation (USA) :

- OSS may lack formal support making it difficult for libraries without significant capacity in their systems department to participte in OSS development or to use OSS.
- OSS needs to develop a participatory organizational model that allows many to contribute perhaps in different ways to OSS development.
- OSS is not always easy to use. It is therefore largely inaccessible to the many libraries and library system departments that require plug-and-play software that is well documented and supported and can be easily installed and uninstalled.
- OSS initiatives do not always do enough to get non-systems librarians and library patrons involved in designing and testing of OSS. As such, they are seen as being something that exclusively offers benefits to and holds interest for library systems staff and not for the wider library community.

Another factor that often comes up is the usability of open source software. The basic problem is that most open source systems are written by programmers who do not understand the end user needs and whose software is often complex and difficult to use. Thus, people argue that open source software projects need to adapt in order to produce systems that can be used by a typical and non-technical user.

Another issue related to its usability is the documentation of open source software. A particular piece of software cannot be used easily without proper documentation. While proprietary software vendors can afford to employ documentation people to do the job for open source but world largely lacks the resources to do it. Programmers work in open source projects because they love programming and they do it as a hobby. But documenting the product may not be as challenging to them as writing the software. This factor sometimes reduces the usefulness of a software product to great extent.

Advantages of open source software

A paradigm of software development that allows customization and is based on distribution notion of property can potentially appeal to libraries, which could utilize open source values and principles to better meet their institutional and user needs. The collaborative aspect of open source softwre development mirrors the information and resources sharing ethics of libraries.

Clarke (2000), in an unpublished Master's thesis entitled *Open Source Software and the Library Community* discusses how the library and open source community's principles and values are similar, arguing that open source software is the best way to accomplish the library's goals and to ensure that the library remains a relevant institution in the future. Clarke's (2000) research provides an important framework for understanding the open source movement in libraries. For instance, open source software created by librarians would have the advantage of incorporating the experience of librarians, something that most commercial vendors do not do. This benefit of open source software goes back to the issues of customizability and user input. Softwre developed by and for librarians and library users conceivably will produce softwaare more attuned to the specific needs of libraries. A practical consideration of open source software is the fact that since libraries share many of the same problems, releasing home grown software to the library community allows for a collaboration that fosters the development of solutions to shared problems (Clarke, 2000). In addition, the sharing of open source solutions can quickly lead to enhanced communication with peer institutions, providing another collaborative opportunity for libraries with a long tradition of resource sharing in other forms (Chudnov, 2006).

Another advantage of open source for libraries is that the response time for changes to a library's system can be faster than proprietary software (Clarke, 2000). Library vendors often have multiple library clients and attending to the technical needs of one particular library understandably can take time. Cost advantages have also been seen with library open source products, as libraries do not have to pay often expensive vendor fees (Clarke, 2000). However, this point is debatable and is rooted in some of the challenges of open source software in libraries.

Some of the major successes thus so far in library Open Source Software are found in standards and protocol implementations such as OAI-PMH (Chudnov, 2006). Various library-based applications exist with differing levels of success and promise; however, the potential for more open source development in libraries appears encouraging. This growth in open source development within libraries is driven largely by the modularity and "layering" of open source components (Chudnov, 2006). Different open source components can be built upon each other - for instance, open source servers can be built on open source network infrastructure, and open source applications can be built upon open source servers (Chudnov, 2006). In addition, Dan Chudnov, advocates for one of the leading library-based open source software, sees potential in libraries partnering with non-library institutions in the development of software. For instance, a librarian needs to think of his software needs less as library-specific issues, as many non-library search interfaces and web application frameworks can be relevant for libraries (Chudnov, 2006). By not restricting library open source development to just librarians, more collaborative solutions might be possible.

Motivations for using and developing open source software ranges from philosophical and ethical reasons to pure practical issues. The first perceived advantage of open source models is the fact that open source software is made available as gratis or at a low cost. But this characteristic is not exclusive to open source model as several proprietary software products are made available in similar ways (ex. Microsoft Explorer).

1- The availability of the source code and the right to modify. It enables the unlimited tuning and improvement of a software product. It also makes it possible to port the code to new hardware, to adapt it to changing conditions, and to reach a detailed understanding of how the system works. Source code availability also makes it much easier to isolate bugs, and to fix them.

2- The right to redistribute modifications and improvements to the code and to reuse other open source code permits all the advantages due to the modifiability of the software to be shared by large communities. The right to redistribute which is universal and cannot be revoked is what attracts a substantial crowd of developers to work around the open source software projects.

3- The right to use the software in any way. This ensures a large population of users, which helps in turn to build up a market for support and customization of software, which can only attract more and more developers to work in the project. This in turn helps to improve the quality of the product and improve its functionality.

4- There is no one with the power to restrict in a unilateral way how the software is used, even in a retroactive way. For instance, a proprietary software vendor may decide not to upgrade some software product for some old platform and the customers can only stick to the old version of the software or switch to another product. But with OSS the customers can find some vendors to provide the upgrades.

5- There is no single entity on which the future of the software depends. If a proprietary software vendor closes doors or decides to discontinue development of the product, no one has the right to take the program and continue development on it, thus effectively killing its usability in the market. But

OSS effectively protects against this, because if the group or company that originated the code decides to stop development, it is always possible to find another software group to continue the maintenance and improvement with legal or practical limitations.

Disadvantages of the Open Source Software

There are some potential problems that one should be aware of when evaluating the feasibility of using open source software :

1. Compatibility

It's not always easy to get open source software to work with other applications. More and more institutions are requiring nonprofits to use databases to track information, and those databases must operate with the standard set by the institution. Often, that standard is the office suite most often used. Microsoft Office, which isn't compatible with most open source programs.

2. Lack of control and responsibility

The decentralized distribution of OSS process is a disadvantage in some contexts, particularly for fixing bugs and problems, which become the responsibility of user if the OSS community doesn't mobilize to address the programs. The lack of central controlling hand in OSS development also means that programs can be chaotic and undirected. Organizations should have a very conservative approach in selecting the code and implement that which is used by large numbers of people.

3. Technical support

Support may be sometimes difficult to understand because it is frequently aimed at developers and not end users. Lack of proper guiadance on many open source software, there is lack of user documentation because development of the code enthuse many as compared to documentation. Libraries and librarians have for many years been using, creating and sharing software, scripts and batch files. Recently, with the growing popularity of the open source movement, some libraries have started extending patronage to open source software.

REFERENCES

Afuah, Allan, *Internet Business Models and Strategies.* McGraw Hill, 2003. ISBN 0-07-251166-4

Available from http://www.firstmonday.dk/issues/issue3_3/torvalds/index.html (Accessed July 20, 2003)

Cervone, Frank (2003). The Open Source Option [online] Available from: http://libraryjournal.reviewsnews.com/index.asp?layout=articlePrint&articleI

Chawner, Brenda (2003). Open Source Software and Libraries Bibliographies (Version 0.5) [online] Available from : http://www.vuw.ac.nz/staff/brenda_chawner/biblio.html (accessed on July 23, 2003)

Chudnov, Daniel (1999). Open Source Library Systems : Getting Started [online] Available from : http://www.oss4lib.org/readings/oss4lib- gettingstarted. php (accessed on July 23, 2003)

D=CA304084&publication=libraryjournal (Accessed on August 27, 2003)

Fink, Martin, *The Business and Economics of Linux and Open Source.* Prentice Hall PTR, 2002. ISBN 0-13-04-7677-3

Ghosh, R.A. (1998). FM Interview with Linus Torvalds : What motivates free software developers? First Monday [online] (2 March 1998) Vol. 3 (3)

Greenstein, D. (2001). DLF Architectures : Evaluation of Open Source Software for Libraries [online] Available from : http://www.diglib.org/architectures/ossrep.htm (Accessed on August 26, 2003)

Hahn, Robert William (Editor), *Government Policy Toward Open Source Software.* The Brookings Institution, 2003. ISBN 0-8157-3393-3

MacFarlane, Andrew (2003). On Open Source IR. In Aslib Proceedings, 55 (4), pp. 217-222.

Moody, Glymm (2001). Rebel Code : Linux and the Open Source Revolution. Allen Lane, London.

Morgan, Eric Lease (2002). Open Source Software in Libraries [online] Available from : http://dewey.library.nd.edu/morgan/musings/ossnlibraries/(accessed on July 20, 2003)

Morgan, Eric Lease (2003). Building Your Library's Portal [online] Available from : http://dewey.library.nd.edu/morgan/ musings/portals/(Accessed on August 27, 2003)

Nielsen, Jakob *Usability Engineering*. Boston, MA : Academic Press (1993), ISBN : 0125184069.

OSS4Lib. Oss4lib - Projects [online] Available from : http://www.oss4lib.org/projects/(accessed on July 23, 2003).

OSS-Open Source Software [online] Available from : http://www.eifl.net/opensoft/soft/html (accessed on July 23, 2003)

Pasquinelli, Art (2003). Information Technology Advances in Libraries [online] Available from : http://www.sun.com/products-nsolutions/edu/whitepapers/pdf/it_advances.pdf (Accessed on August 16, 2003)

Rasch, Chris (2000). A Brief History of Free/Open Source Software Movement [online] Available from : http://www.openknowledge.org/writing/open-source/scb/breif-open source history.html (accessed on July 20, 2003)

Raymond, Eric S. (2001). The Cathedral and the Bazaar : Musings on Linux and Open Source by an Accidental Revolutionary. Revised edition. Sebastopol, CA; O'Reilly and Associates.

Raymond, Eric S., *The Cathedral and the Bazaar,* O'Reilly, Sebastopol, C.A., 1999, ISBN : 0596001088

Rosenberg, Donald K., *Open Source : The Unauthorized White Papers*. John Wiley & Sons, 2000. ISBN 0-7645-4660-0

Sandred, Jan, *Managing Open Source Projects : A Wiley Tech Brief.* John Wiley & Sons, 2001, ISBN 0-471-40396-2

Digital Technology in School Libraries: A Futuristic Vision

Dayal Singh Bhati

Librarian, Army Public School, Jodhpur - 342 001

INTRODUCTION

As we all know that today is the era of technology and we can't survive in this global world without technology. We can say that today's man without technology is like a fish without water. In higher education, U.G.C., C.S.I.R., N.I.S.C.A.I.R, INFLIBNET, and many more national institutes and organisations are there to support their libraries and innovative services but surprisingly no such organisation has been thought of for school libraries which basically finds a foundation for the future generation who is going to use this technology. It is unfortunate that school libraries which form the foundation for academic hierarchy, yet they have largely remained neglected when compared with universities and colleges. Essential provisions for organizing library and resource centers are often not provided. Even physical facilities are not there to show existence of a Library Resource Centre in the scheme of thoughts. In fact nothing wroth mentioning has been done at all India level to improve the lot of school Library Resource Centers. The situation of school library differs from state to state. With exception of a few states the situation in almost all states is below the mark. For want of copies of Classification Schedule, Catalogue Codes, Catalogue card Cabinets the entire collection of books remains unclassified, uncatalogued and unorganized. It speaks about the ill health of a School Library.

In this situation only way is to improve the position of school library by using modern digital technology at nationwide.

Why Digital Technology in Schools: Many more Indian schools have traditional libraries with insufficient books and magazines and journals and if few schools have sufficient books and magazines then the relevant data and information are very old. Thus those books can't help the readers for specific information and with the result reader goes away from the library.

Mostly schools donot have any separate building for library and also not sufficient place for reading room. The fifth law of library "Library is a growing organism" and as we know that day by day the information and literature is coming in very large amount and the school library building is unable to handle and arrange it on stacks to this material as a result the librarian can't provide the better service to its readers quickly.

The next one is so many school libraries are poor in library budget because the administration does not take proper interest and they think it is avoidable for school. Inspite of CBSE guidelines for school library the private and govt. schools both don't take any step. Some big and expensive convent and public schools have budget for library but it is very scanty to meet demands of resources because the cost of books has increased very high so a library can't purchase sufficient books and magazines.

Today's era is information era. Readers want to seek very quick information from the library and at that moment the librarian is unable to provide the relevant information due to lack of modern digital technology.

How Digital Technology is Useful: As we know that in information explosion era we cannot survive without technology because the literature comes very fast and a librarian can't collect all literature and information which is helpful for students e.g. career information, new innovative research and ready reference within a certain time. So if a school library wants to march forward then new technology will be a great asset for any school library. With this a library can do its routine work in very less time and a librarian can save his/her time to provide better services to its readers. Budget is the major problem for any school. Secondly, recent innovative donot reach into the hands of students and thirdly there is no sufficient space in the school library to store information, books and journals. As a result the new digital technology will be a great help for school library.

It has more space to store data and information within a very little space in comparison to a traditional library. It takes very less cost to set up and provide world wide knowledge, text books, magazines and journals with nominal cost or free. It has expendable storage capacity for future in the form of microfilms, DVD's, CD's and Pen drives etc. It can be handled by a very less staff. One can carry the whole library in his beg any where he wants.

WHAT IS DIGITAL LIBRAY?

A digital library is a collection of documents in organized electronic form, available on the Internet or on CD-ROM (compact-disk read-only memory) disks. Depending on the specific library, a user may be able to access magazine articles, books, papers, images, sound films, and videos. A digital library is a library in which collections are stored in digital formats (as against to print, microform, or other media) and accessible by computers. The digital content may be stored locally, or accessed remotely via computer networks. A digital library is a type of information retrieval system. Controlled collections of information bearing objects that are in digital form and that may be organized, accessed, evaluated and used by means of heterogeneous and extensible set of distributed services that are supported by digital technology.

HOW DIGITAL LIBRARY WORKS ?

In digital library the analogue information includes printed books, periodical articles, photographs, microforms, video and audiotapes. It is broken down into 0's and 1s. It is the process through which all literature is converted into digital format. This process has some steps for proper work and these are as follows-

1. Selection of material for digitization.
2. Selection of Audio: Sound quality has to be checked and required corrections are made together by the librarian and computer sound editor.
3. Video: The video clippings are edited on Beta max tapes.
4. Photographs: It requires high resolution for photographic image and slides.
5. Documents: Those documents which are much in demand may be reviewed and selected for the process of digitization.

Steps in the Process of Digitization

1 Scanning : Electronic scanners are used for scanning. It may be photographs, text, image etc.

Steps in the process of scanning

1. Placing picture on the scanner's glass.
2. Start software.
3. Select the area to be scanned.
4. Choose the image type.

5. Sharpen the image.
6. Set the image size.
7. Save the scanned image using a desirable format (TIFF, GIF or JPEG).

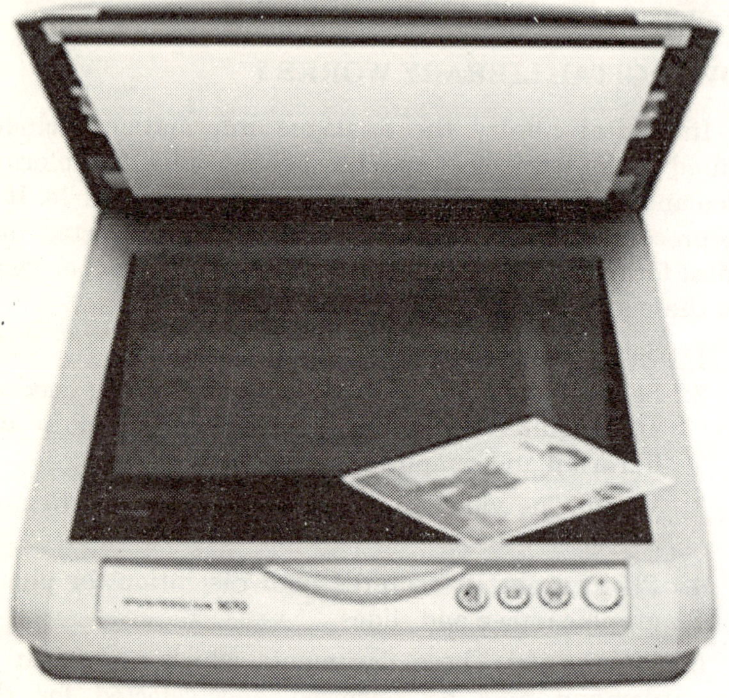

Scanner

Organizing and Indexing: If one wants a document to convert into an image or text file then following steps will be followed:

1. Develop metadata scheme.
2. Assign metadata to each digital object.
3. Link digital objects with associated metadata to facilitate browsing and searching.
4. Organize digital objects and associated metadata into a database.
5. Build browse, search and navigational facilities.

3 SPACE

At this moment all school libraries are facing this problem because they have a very little space to store text books, magazines and newspapers, old issues and rare books but digitization of literature in the form of CDs, DVDs has emerged as a great solution of the space and storing problem.

1 CD's

2 DVD' s

3 NAS.

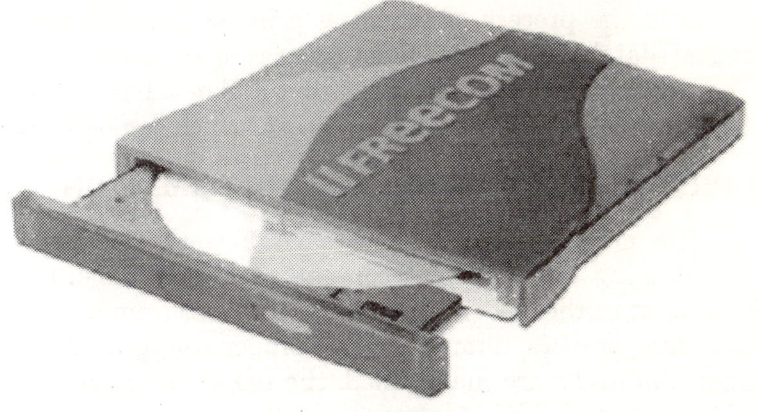

CD ROM

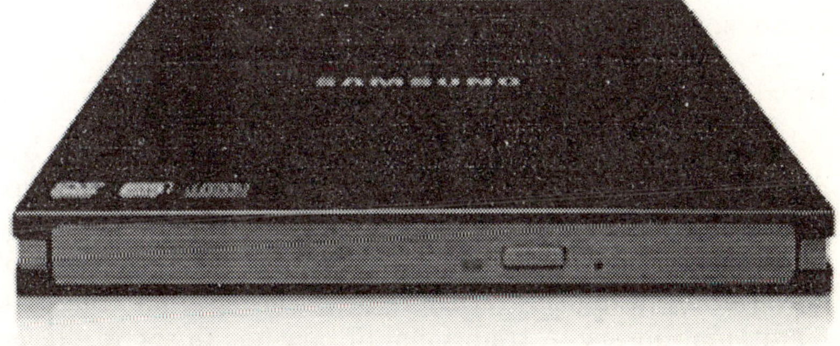

DVD ROM

4 PROVIDING ACCESS: SEARCH AND RETRIEVAL

Scanned images and text are saved as a file, thus we can prepare a database for retrieval. Digital library software use database management system as backend, sophisticated search engines and user friendly search D space is the software which uses Postgres database and Lucene search engine. All digital softwares provides for elaborate search options like that Boolean, proximity operators and wild cards.

5 OPTICAL CHARACTER RECOGNITION

It is the process of scanning printed pages to build a digital database of text. This process uses OCR (Optical Character Recognition) software that makes a picture of the page and then turns it into digital text, which can be edited.

6 PRESERVATION OF DIGITAL INFORMATION

The normal way of doing such a work involves the microfilming the physical content of the document and keeping it in the controlled environment free from moisture, dust, temperature, humidity etc. If proper storage and controlled conditions are maintained, the life of the microfilmed documents would be in centuries. Although digital information preservation is a complex process but the stored digital information may deteriorate sharply owing to known reasons, and prone to corruption of data.

DIGITAL LIBRARY - ADVANTAGES

The traditional libraries have limited storage space but digital libraries have the potential to store much more information, simply because digital information require very little physical space to contain them. As such, the cost of maintaining a digital library is much lower than that of a traditional library. A traditional library has to spent a large sums of money as salary for staff, book maintenance, rent etc. Digital libraries do away with all these taxes.

Digital libraries can immediately adopt innovations in technology providing users with improvements in electronic and audio book technology as well as presenting new forms of communication such as wikis and blogs.

- **No physical boundary**. The user of a digital library need not to go to the library physically. People from all over the world can access to the same information, as long as an Internet connection is available.
- **Round the clock availability**. A major advantage of digital library is that people from all over the world can access to the information at any time and any where, as long as an Internet connection is available.
- **Multiple accesses**. The same resources can be used at the same time by a number of users.
- **Structured approach**. Digital library provides access to much richer content in a more structured manner, i.e. we can easily move from the catalog to the particular book then to a particular chapter and so on.
- **Information retrieval**. The user is able to use any search term and can search the entire collection. Digital library can provide very user friendly interfaces, giving click able access to its resources.
- **Preservation and conservation**. An exact copy of the original can be made any number of times without any degradation in quality.
- **Space.** Whereas traditional libraries are limited by storage space, digital libraries have the potential to store much more information, simply because digital information requires very little physical space to contain them. When the library had no space for extension digitization is the only solution.
- **Networking.** A particular digital library can provide the link to any other resources of other

digital library very easily thus a integrated resource sharing can be achieved.

Cost. In theory, the cost of maintaining a digital library is lower than that of a traditional library. A traditional library has to spent large sums of amount for staff, book maintains, rent, and journals. Although digital libraries do away with these fees, it has since been found that digital libraries can be no less expensive in their own way to operate. Digital libraries can and do incur large costs for the conversion of print materials into digital format, for the technical skills of staff to maintain them, and for the costs of maintaining online access (i.e servers, bandwidth costs, etc.). Also, the information in a digital library must often be "migrated" for few years to the latest digital media. This process can incur very large costs in hardware, software and skilled personnel.

Digital library - Disadvantages

Some people have criticized that digital libraries are hampered by copyright law.

- Because works cannot be shared over different periods of time in the manner of a traditional library. The content is, in many cases, public domain or self-generated content only. Some digital libraries, such as Project Gutenberg, work to digitize out-of-copyright works and make them freely available to the public. An estimate of the number of distinct books still exist in library catalogues from 2000 B.C. to 1960, has been made.
- Digital libraries cannot reproduce the environment of a traditional library. Many people also find reading printed material to be easier than reading material on a computer screen although this depends heavily on presentation as well as personal preferences [2]. Also, due to technological developments, a digital

library can see some of its content become out-of-date and its data may become inaccessible.

FUTURE OF DIGITAL TECHNOLOGY IN SCHOOL

Integrated virtual libraries of the 21st century will provide integrated access to an increasing number of resources including existing library collections, archives, scientific databases and multimedia presentations. The impact of digital libraries will be great in schools where lack of the infrastructure, lack of budget are the major problems. Access to the world's knowledge will soon be available to anyone with phone line, eliminating the need for expensive and incomplete local collections. It may persevere unlimited information regarding to domestic and international level. In 21st century the era will be digital era and we shall search all type of books, magazines, journals, pictures, audio and video on computer through digital technology.

CONCLUSION

Today everywhere we hear the word digital it means the technology of present to guide future and when we talk about library, especially school library then it will play a great role in every school library where they are facing the problem of infrastructure, lack of budget, better and faster services, lack of staff and to over come these problems digital technology is only the solution. Thus we can say that without digital technology we can't improve our school library system.

REFERENCES

1. www.schoollibraryjournal.com
2. www.librarysupportstaff.com
3. www.schoolcomputing.wiki.com
4. www.meritnation.com
5. www.whatis.techtarget.com

6. www.wikipedia.org.
7. www.images.google.com
8. S.M. Rokade and D. Rajyalakshmi : Integrated Information System in Agricultural University Libraries in Maharashtra in the Context of Digitization: A Case Study, IASLIC Bulletin V.53 No. 2 June, 2008. p. 83-88
9. Organising school Library-Guidelines CBSE 2006
10. www.experiencefestival.com.

Automation in Academic Libraries of India : An Overview

Mihir Ranjan Panda

Library Assistant, NALSAR University of Law, Hyderabad-500 078

ABSTRACT

Paper presents the scenario of library automation in higher education and libraries in India. Academic environment of higher education institutions has gone under drastic changes in the past twenty years. During this period academic libraries have seen numerous waves of technological breakthrough, changing the ways the libraries provide services, and in effect, transforming traditional and print-based libraries into fully automated libraries. It discusses need, importance, slow development and advantages of library automation. Paper highlights the events in library automation that was experienced in India during past 20 years.

1. INTRODUCTION

Though we are in 21st century, we are still moving slowly towards library automation. There are many faactors which have restricted us to go for automation in academic libraries. While British and American higher education libraries have already automated their libraries in early 70s but automation in academic libraries in India began in late 1990s. However, since 2000 it has picked up acceleration, which is again still not enough. As regards to college libraries, library automation is yet to take off owing to various problems.

2. NEED OF LIBRARY AUTOMATION

Earlier (when card catalogues were in operation) a user has to go to search the cards from the catalogue cabinet. He never knows whether that particular material is in the library or issued to someone. If the book is not in the stacks he used to go to the circulation counter where he finds from the record that the book is issued. It used to be a usual practice in the library. It does not fulfill the fourth law of Dr. S.R. Ranganathan i.e., Save the Time of the Reader because a user is actually interested in getting a document and not simply knowing the location. Sometimes a number of users search for the same trays or drawers, and hence other users may have to wait.

The concept of Online Public Access Catalogue (OPAC) came to replace the card catalogue. The bibliographic records stored in the computer memory are printed on the screen in response to a request from a user. Entries may comprise the full bibliographic record, or medium, or only a brief, it is depending on the system and the desires of the users. Online catalogue is the most flexible and current. Additions, deletions, and changes of entries can be made at any time, and the results are immediately available to the users.

In most academic libraries, OPACs have been replaced the card catalog. OPACs offer several advantages over the traditional card catalogue. For example, there are more advanced searching options than the usual author, title, and subject. The biggest advantage to an automated catalogue is the collection becomes 80% more accessible. It can be searched in many more ways and more quickly than with a card catalogue. Almost every part of the bibliographic record is accessible through keyword searching. This capability helps users to find data contained in notes, including content notes. Most OPACs provide author, title, subject heading, call numbers, ISBN, ISSN and keywords, etc., as access points. The primary advantage of the online catalogue is that database can retrieve information in a variety of ways, and it also provides very rapid search. Database in online catalogue is updated online, the moment we enter data.

Circulation section is the gateway between users and documents so it plays a major role to any library and information system. In traditional manual system it takes a few minutes to perform a transaction in circulation section. If there are a number of students in front of the circulation counter for issue/return of books, there is a big queue for it. This again does not follow the fourth law of library science of Dr. S.R. Ranganathan. Some students may have classes/ tutorials. Students may shout for fast transaction at the circulation counter. Such situation may lead to argument between students and the circulation staff. Hence, library automation resulted in better control over materials. Circulation system performs faster and more efficiently. Frequent reminders can be sent out to the patrons for overdue items. Circulation systems instantly can tell what items a patron has checked out.

Other benefits of library automation are to provide Selective Dissemination of Information (SDI) service which is a current awareness system which alerts the users of the latest publications in their specified field(s) of interest. For this a user has to register with keywords representing his or her fields of interest and whenever new publications matches the user's search profile, the system informs the user instantly, periodically or upon request through email. Thus library automation performs tasks less expensively, more accurately and more quickly to handle tasks which can no longer be accommodated by the manual system due to higher volumes, costs and chances for duplication of effort.

Library automation especially becomes familiar because the computers keep getting more powerful and cheaper. Now it is within the reach of any library which provides numerous benefits to the library staff and patrons.

Library automation helps to offer various and improved services to its users. It makes easier for patrons to locate as well as allowing staff to give better services and facilitates a multitude of staff tasks such as acquisitions, cataloguing, circulation, reports and reference services. On the other hand, the financial and staff commitment need to be moved to an automated system. Automation cannot be approached as a solution for systematic problems in a library. Without staff support and training no system can offer its full potential. In India boost in library automation emerged after the establishment of INFLIBNET Centre by UGC in late 80s. Efforts were made for automation in academic libraries attached to IITs, IIMs, Central Universities and some other renowned universities. INFLIBNET provided funds for library automation to specified universities according to their seniority, and today more than 150 universities have automated their library operations. It is all because of financial support received from INFLIBNET.

3. FACTORS INVOLVED IN AUTOMATION

The following factors are involved in library automation in academic libraries.

3.1 Resources

Most important factor is to get funds for library automation. Human resources are also as important as funds. Library staff should be well trained to meet the requirements of the automation of library operations.

3.2 Software

Initially it was CDS/ISIS which was provided to the institutions free of cost by UNESCO. At later stage a number of softwares were made available and most of them failed to fulfill the users requirement. Software which is of high standard to meet users' need is expensive. Roughly it requires Rs. 10.00 lakhs initially to start automation in academic libraries. Since cost involved was huge this confused the librarians to take decision. However librarians should involve some measures to select library software.

3.3 Selection Procedure

Library software or computer based information storage and retrieval systems cover two major functional areas, namely (i) control and management of library resources, and (ii) access to documents and information. These two areas deal with library house-keeping systems and information retrieval systems respectively. Gradually, the distinction between them is vanishing. There are a large number of commercially available library software packages. Studies that enumerate compare and highlight the salient features of these software packages are also in abundance. An effort is made here to review some such selected studies to enable one to fathom the length, breadth and depth of the problem of selecting suitable software for one's use. The following is the selection procedure :

- **Information about the Vendor :** Whether the software developer is a reputed company or local or an individual. As a number of companies have developed their automation software, librarian must call a few vendors for demo and judge which one would fit in library's requirement. He should seek help from computer science department in discussion.
- **Software Modules :** Librarian has to check important modules available in the software like Acquisition (Monographs and Serials), Cataloguing, Circulation, Reports, OPAC (which support all types of search like Browse, Heading Keyword & Keyword and also SDI query) and Inventory etc. available or not. He has to check whether user oriented facilities are there or not, like automatic reminder through

email, online request, renewal, purchase recommendation, chat with librarian for query etc. The above are important functions of the library

- **Functions of Software :** Once the selection part is over the librarian should find out how it is functioning? Whether it has updated or not since inception? There should be provision for annual maintenance and upgradation.
- **Language :** The programming language in which the software is written. We have to see whether compiler or interpreter is available on the given system to run it efficently in terms of machine time and storage requirements. It should support Unicode as the most of the academic libraries have multilingual collection.
- **Ease-in-use** : The quality of the operator-machine interface, menus, commands, screen displays, documentation, etc. will enhance ease in use of the software.
- **ISO Format** : Whether the software has the facility to import and export bibliographic data availale in ISO 2709 format?
- **Maintenance :** Whether there is any maintenance office in same locality ?
- **Trainging Facilities :** Provide training and guidance after installation
- **Compatibility :** Whether compatible with major operating systems and can be accessed through intranet and internet ?

3.4 Users

If the users (either students or faculty) are well acquainted with information technology, there will be a demand from their side to implement library automation.

3.5 Staff Skills

Library professionals must be highly qualified, so that they can perform their duites skillfully towards the progress of the library.

4. REASONS FOR SLOW PROGRESS

The scientific and technical libraries took the early lead in library automation in India. They funded several training programs and software development projects which played an important role in increasing awareness of the potential of the new technologies. Their main emphasis was on database development and information retrieval services. Unfortunately, the academic libraries made little progress in this direction during the same period. The main reasons for slow pace of automation in academic libraries are the following :

- Academic libraries in India function in a relatively less autonomous environment.
- Academic libraries are comparatively smaller unit within a larger setup.
- Libraries have to compete for scarce resources.
- Academic libraries are not under as much pressure to improve their services as are scientific and technical libraries.
- Library automation at all levels needs good co-ordination between librarians and computer services professionals.

5. ADVANTAGES OF LIBRARY AUTOMATION

Advantages of library automation to users and the library staff are as follows :

5.1 Advantages to Users

- Online Public Access Catalogue (OPAC) allows users to :

- Use search engine like `browse search', `keyword search', `heading keyword search' and `quick search' from which a user can use Boolean operators like ``AND'', ``OR'', ``NOT'' and ``NEAR'' to truncate and expand the search.
- Know about their account regarding the books due with her/him, satisfied request and the status of a particular book.
- Reserve book or books and make renewal online.
- Make recommendation for purchase.
- Set theri search filter. For example, there are a lot of branches in a library. If a patron wants to serch only in either journal section or thesis or ny other branch, it can be possible.
- Save all search records in cart and can be used in future.

• In case of circulation there should not be long queue. Whereas in traditional manual system it takes time and users have to stay in line. Thus it saves a lot of time of the user.
• Reference Service : The system should be able to answer and querry within no time. It helps users to save thier time from searching here and there.

5.2 Advantages to the Library Staff

The following are the advantages to the library staff :

• Faster response time and accuracy in providing information can improve the quality of library services.
• Availability of statisticaly information from the system which can lead to effective decision making and elimination of wastage.
• Saving of future expenditure in collection development. There is possibility of sharing resources with other libraries by linking through INFLIBNET.

- Provision of new information services like current awareness service, selective dissemination of information, retrospective search, etc. which may help the library staff to give better library services.

Library automation also helps the library staff in performing the following technical jobs.

5.2.1 Acquisition

An automated library acquisition module is designed to handle to ease the paper work involved in buying books. Typically they print purchase orders, maintain book fund accounts and print book fund reports of various types, provide information to orders outstanding, preparing voucher against payment and sometimes on work in progress, i.e. books received but not yet processed.

5.2.2 Serials Management

Automation makes serials management easy. Once MARC tag 853 is set properly it becomes easy to process the current issues. It allows user to prepare bound volume list. If there is a missing issue it generates remider for it.

5.2.3 Circulation

It performs circulation system more efficiently which includes check-in, check-out, renewals, overdue notices, reservations and request. The main advantage is this that it saves both time and labour. It takes a few seconds to generate reports like overdue, daily transactions, patron statement etc.

5.2.4 Cataloguing

Most of the library system fully integrated with the Z39.50 cataloguing client. Z39.50 is an NISO standard defining a protocol for computer to computer information retrieval. It allows users in one system to serch and retrieve information from other systems those have implemented Z39.50. Records can be imported into an automated library within a few hours and without incurring new cost for retrospective conversion. It also allows for cataloguing internet resources and for importing them into a local system. It includes MARC tag 856 to link URLs to MARC21 records by which a user can access data from either internet or from saved location through URL provided in MARC record.

5.2.5 Inventory

It expedites and simplifies the inventory of library materials by using scanner. It may be a barcode scanner or RFID scanner by which a library can generate a report within one or two weeks and with less man power. Where as the same collection may take two months to complete in a non-automated environment.

5.2.6 Reports

Report generating is also an important factor to know the statistics of all the activities in library. If library management software is of better standard then there are a lot of reports which can be generated. For example :

i. In Acquisition: Account Summaries, Items received by month, Nw books list, Order status, Titles in order, Gifts received and Vendor list etc.

ii. In Serials : Serials List, Serials without Holdings. Bindery List etc.

iii. In Cataloguing : Authorities List, Bibliographic Record List, Item Barcode List, Subject Bibliography, Cataloguer Productivity etc.

iv. In Circulation : Daily Circulation Statistics, Reserves, Satisfied/Unsatisfied Requests, Over-due, Active and Expiring Patrons, List of Patrons etc.

Library Automation encourge cooperative collection development and resource sharing. Automated libraries can develop a union catalogue and join bibliographic utilities and consortia. A user can search for a material of interest from the union catalogue if it's not available in the local library. This can be possible through OPAC.

6. CONCLUSION

Library automation plays a pivotal role in modernizing our academic libraries in terms of delivering services to the users and in satisfying their needs. It will changes the way libraries organize themselves in due course. There is a wide range of technology products available by different vendors. It is necessary for librarians to keep a watch on developments in library automation. It may not be possible for vendors to create systems that can accommodate different types of libraries. Hence librarians should develop a checklist of features and requirements that they want in their library system and find out whether it is compatible for its library. New information technology in general and library automation in particular has made users impatient for quick access to library materials. Thus libraries must carefully plan the introduction and management of new technology. As we are in 21st century, librarians and library managements must be prepared to take risks and try new ideas to modernizing their operations by using the best posible library management software. It is hoped that in near future almost academic libraries will go for library automation to give best library services to clients. Now important aspect of the library automation is how quickly our remaining academic libraries go for it.

REFERENCES

Aswal, Rajinder Singh, *Library Automation for 21st Century*. New Delhi, Ess Ess Publication, 2006.

Carande, Robert, Automation in Library Reference Services : A Handbook. Westport, Greenwood Press, 1992.

Head, John, W. and Gerard B. McCabe, Ed. *Introducing and Managing Academic Library Automation Projects*. Westport, Greenwood Press, 1996.

Kochar, R.S. and K.N. Sudarshan, *Library Automation.* New Delhi, APH Publishing Corp., 1997.

Malwad, N.M. Selection Criteria for Library Automation Software. *DESIDOC Bulletin of Information Technology.* 15, 2, March 1995, pp. 17-26.

Manjunath, G.K., *Library Automation : Why and How?,* Paper Presented at a `Workshop on Information Technology and Library Automation held at Thane, Maharashtra on August 16, 1998.

Prabha, Neelam, *Automation in Academic Libraries.* Agra, YK Publishers, 2004.

Pruet, Nancy Jones. *Scientific and Technical Libraries : Functions and Management.* New York, Academic Press, 1986. pp 267-269.

Ravichandra Rao, I.K. Library Automation : What is Expected of ?. *DESIDOC Bulletin of Information Technology.* 15, 2, March 1995, pp3-10.

Vaishnav, A.A. and N.G. Bapat. *DESIDOC Bulletin of Information Technology.* 15, 2, March 1995, pp 11-16.

Vyas, S.D., Library Automation and Networking in India : Problems and Prospects. *World Libraries.* 8-1 (Fall 1997) pp. 27-35.

www.wikipedia.org.

Staff Relationship Channels in Academic Libraries

K. Krishna

Assistant Librarian, NALSAR university of Law, Shameerpet, Hyderabad -500 078

ABSTRACT

Discusses human relations in library are important for functioning and development. All relations in a corporate body have a mechanism. Few facts which are significant, but remain concealed and once these are identified and acted upon will benefit both the employee and the employer. Explains how exchange of ideas, availability of Communication channels, etc. are important means in developed and sustaining human relationships for long. Suggests that interaction is developed by training and motivation. Library image is boosted by staff who are best in communication skills and interpersonal relations.

INTRODUCTION

There are many channels for communication between the library staff. This can be among supportings, superiors, and colleagues. We may have to consider in this discussion dealings with staff who are smart, normal, abnormal, and of the least the irritating colleagues, and all the characteristics and traits, etc. Staff relationship means relationship which deals with individual to individual, individual to group, and vice versa. All relationships are for mutual co-existence, and all communication is for building a healthy working atmosphere. However it does not overlook the human tendencies to get into stress, strain, boredom, ego, and other physiological, psychological and behavioral issues. It also takes care of the intricacies of relationship between the professionals and supporting staff, or the paraprofessionals. Interpersonal connections are not examined here in isolation. It is also important to note that job satisfaction and library environment are interlinked with the performance of the individual and the productivity of the library. It is concerned with the self and then refers to the other. Hence this exercise is introspection and not at criticizing the world at large, while much of the following is general and common sense, it is applied to the library situation and the profession is brought into discussion as a Central foci.

1. TRANSACTIONS BETWEEN THE COLLEAGUES

The motivation, devotion and commitment of the staff to the fulfillment of the objectives and goals of the institution are the primary purpose of library personnel. In dealing with humans, however, the individual identity gets more prominent and hence creates a problem in fulfilling these goals.

Transactions with the superiors and subordinates: Relationship with the superior can be considered in two different perspectives, like direct dealing and indirect dealing with the subordinates. Direct dealing brings a human touch which mars or promotes the objectives of staff relations. Within the organization everyone agrees that there is a need for good communication, but few only acknowledge the number of obstacles which come in the way. "...Management generally underestimates staff's desire to be informed and staff generally overestimates its own need to be informed" (Euster: 1981: 6}. Not everyone need to know everything. Even if there is non confidential material the management may not like every staff to use office time on it, since this amounts to wasting time and in terms of loss in production and service. Then there is another managerial strategy, that is premature disclosure of uncertain "information" results in unnecessary anxiety and stress.

Relationship builds mainly with communication media, whether it is written, verbal, or electronic. The communication will work well if the communicator and recipient are in the same level and in such a case they can develop good understanding interpersonal relationship.

2. ORGANIZATIONAL HIERARCHY

In the organizational hierarchy the staff relationship is top to down but cooperation and communication is required from either ways. Empathy and sympathy are must for the progress of the individual and the institution. Human relations demand that there is an understanding for the other, irrespective of the fact whether it is homogeneous group or heterogeneous, diversity is a complex issue and requires serious consideration of all its dimensions and perspectives.

A survey conducted by "studies at Florida state-university, Michigan state university and the university of Minnesota demonstrated that the average person remembers only 50% of what he/she heard immediately after hearing it. Two months later only 25% is remembered. The difficulty of effective listening stems from the fact that we think far faster than the we speak. The average rate of speech for most Americans is 125 words per minute. The brain can process the language of our thoughts at much higher speed" (Albritton: 1990: 106). Communication is an art and a skill, which if done in proper fashion will have definite results.

Feelings of an individual are also to be considered for development of interpersonal relationship. Describing one's feeling helps other person's understanding how one feels, so others can respond to it. These feelings may be comfortable, pleasant, and angry. If the feelings are specific and comfortable to receiver the communication helps in improving relationship, otherwise wrong communication may result.

Behavior also effects staff relationship and communication. Describing one's own behavior and observing others behavior leads to improvement of personal relations in any organization. "Rude or brusque behavior to faculty, students, fellow staff, and other members of the community simply cannot be tolerated. Because no administration can afford to permit staff to damage the library's image, the search for a consistently patient and tactful attitude among applicants forms an important part of the search panel's research and line of questioning" (Veaner: 1990: 269). Obviously, the main factor in interpersonal relations is function of the words employed and the actions manifested.

That is, words and actions are the basics within which this exchange of ideas and communication takes place. "Despite the various analysis which have been made, these verbal and nonverbal behavior serve as the currency of group dynamics as well as the operational contexts within which much small group research has been conducted" (Penland: 1973: 228) while it is essential that the individuals have their own psychological and behavioral demands and limitations, it is also true that a group must have a psychological bond strong enough to contain its divergent tendencies. We can find in the literature the variables which constitute this bond, and list includes: size, composition, structure, cohesiveness, tasks, culture and effectiveness.

A large group may have complications like over motivation, different perspectives, and so on. So also variations in the composition of the group like personality, intellectual and demographic factors, effect the performance of the group. Structure of the group is the pattern in which the individuals relate to one another as part of the system, and not the hierarchy of the managerial type. This can be illustrated by the point that an individual, who has a central position in this communication structure, would be sometimes important role player in other structures like power, friendship, etc. Cohesiveness is a factor which relates to congeniality, loyalty and receptivity and this is an important variable in interpersonal relations. Task is a determining factor on the types and amounts of interaction and communication within the group. Interaction helps in establishing the social reality of group culture and norms. The culture of group is composed of its values, beliefs and goals. The group has its own overall behavior which the individuals must relate themselves to and accept the group behavior as a basic survival strategy. This interpersonal relationship will not be constant. It keeps changing from situation to situation. Environment also influences communication process either it improves or worsens.

3. STAFF MEETINGS

Staff meeting can be both formal and informal. Meetings of the staff are definitely a useful exercise for all libraries, and such meetings can be general staff meeting or professional meeting. Meetings provide good opportunities for the communication and interaction, for exchange of ideas and to learn from informal opportunities. Regular meetings give an opportunity to report on problems and achievements, and other issues can be discussed. Lack of meetings reflects on the administration's uncaringness, unwillingness to share information and may build miscommunication all over. Such meetings can be called business sessions. Informal meeting, other than the business and decision meetings are also called grapevine. Such get together are inexpensive, practical, enjoyable and encouraging. The informal meeting must not become a discussion policy decision session, it is sometimes possible that a business meeting can become informal, but it is not always the other way round.

Exchange of ideas between staff take place in study circles, discussion groups, and in programs meant to develop personality of individuals, wherein staff form discussion group and prepare for a workshop or debate on topics of mutual interest. These topics can be professional, social, or academic but will definitely enhance the information base of the participating teams and other staff who share and exchange ideas.

4. ORAL/ WRITTEN COMMUNICATION

Oral/Written communication is also an equally significant factor. The art of writing is a skill which can be developed at any stage. Written communication may vary between staff to staff in terms of quality, ability to express the idea, preciseness, etc. "Writing quality among librarians varies enormously. Despite the fact that the very essence of academic librarianship is communication, startlingly large numbers of persons in the field have difficulty writing coherent, articulate prose. Some of these people are totally unaware of this deficiency. Submissions from staff frequently need considerable reworking before they can be passed on to others or incorporated into proposals and reports. In a large library, one might have an editor, secretary, or other officer to do this; in the smaller institution the chief librarian obviously has to be the editor" (Veaner: 1990: 269).

Written word must be able to convey the message, brief or long, to the audience intended. Obviously, certain matters must be written and documented. This has many advantages and also some disadvantages, Memo is a brief communication and reduces the need of lengthy documentation. Long notes or too many memos produce frustration and waste time and supplies. Written communication some times documentation hinders direct and open discussion. In performance appraisal a lack of written communication does more harm than good to the staff.

5. OFFICE DOCUMENTATION

Staff bulletins, newsletters, circulars, and bulletin boards (in the e-mail) are some important means of written communication. These cover business, social and staff matters. Editing, these in turns, provides a good opportunity for staff-development.

Every library service is ideally oriented towards user friendliness and all library education is to train librarians to be able to find the right things at the right time, which directly relates to the ability to communicate. Communication is an essential skill and requirement for a librarian if he or she has to link the document with the user. It is not that all librarianship is behind the screen, it is a fact that the major part of the professional role is played in the public where maximum time is spent in interacting with the users and the documents. It is essentially a communications skills that the library training must provide to the "would be librarians". If one can not communicate and attend to the information behavior of the user, that person deserves to be called a semi-professional or non-professional library worker. Whereas a Para-professional or as an 'untrained' library worker who is good at communication skills can be upgraded as a library professional.

What is then essential in a professional, irrespective of the position of holds, is a capacity for fluent, tactful oral and written communication. A librarian has to deal with all people and ability to communicate and skillfully handle all situations is a must for successful professional performance.

6. SOCIAL INTERACTION SKILLS

Social interaction skills are "generic term for the exchange of meanings between people..... all the various ways in which people can and do express themselves in face-to-face meetings" (Berelson: 1964: 326). This then is simply the ability which librarians must have to be social and extrovert. If the staff lacks this skill, they can be trained through direct observation and participation in actual events. A simple method of developing a working relationship among the colleagues is by a model (Allen: 1971: 86) which included:

- build interpersonal competencies and social interaction skills in individual staff members

- Strengthen the ability of the staff work effectively as a collaborative team on organizational problems, and
- Initiate the managerial mode of democratic decision-making and provide a basis for its continuation.

Whether this is applied in a laboratory method or on the job training program, it is also noteworthy that it can be a part of the regular education, or continuing education, but it does require some specialists to orient it to the best desired goals. Some institutions support and encourage staff association for the purpose of social, educational, or welfare, this is not to be confused with trade unions. A staff association can arrange for a talk, or debate, or seminar, or visit to other libraries. This may ease some of the departmental rivalries in large libraries. Educational exchanges and visits in such a forum will have positive effect of enhancing opportunities for continuing development. This does not affect the daily routines and still provide the chances for interdepartmental and interpersonal training. Furthermore, shared training and joint involvement can have better results and much more beneficial.

The management of good interpersonal relations also calls for time management, and an understanding of the importance of others time. There are time wasters, gossipers, chatters and all other types of colleagues, who can tell them that they are not paid for all this extra curricular activities. It is their own individual upbringing and conscience which should caution them on these. Time management also requires that staff know when they can have discussions, group meetings, and the like and when they cannot. Similarly telephone interruption and drop-in visitors are also a problem in interpersonal relationship. The callers do not know or do not have the sense of responsibility and create a problem for the colleagues as well as for the management.

Then the skills required for interpersonal relationship are many, and a list can be exhaustive. These include be proactive, good listeners, confident, articulate speakers, keep cool in all situations, active in professional activities, unembarrassed by failure and willing to fail, willing to delegate both authority and responsibility, willing to share ideas, spontaneous in expression, have a good sense of humor, capable of accepting criticism, decisive (not necessarily impulsive or stubborn). Convincing and persuasive, goal and achievement oriented, willing to encourage others, honest and dissembling, technically competent, above the gossip levels, develop ability to communicate, etc.

There is lot of work done by specialists in human relationships, group dynamics, sociometry, and on, Powell's (1949) work is very important in this context, as it has a humanistic orientation to the benefits of group work and to ways in which discussion techniques can work effectively. In the context of group behavior, it is pertinent to note that "the best way to preserve individuality is to give each individual the knowledge and skill necessary to diagnose and withstand the forces toward conformity in modern life and at the same time learn how to express his individuality constructively" (Penland: 1973:210)

Today staff relations are developed and have reached a stage where many studies in qualitative and quantitative aspects are all dealt in. Sociometry is the study of the group structure and social distance in terms of the personal preference of the members of a group. In other words, sociometry is a branch of social psychology which focuses on the quantitative aspects of interpersonal phenomena - with special reference to the measurement of preferences. Then the level of relationship among the staff is measurable by asking the preference of the staff.

One could survey libraries with measures of honesty and kindness and see how far the question of empathy is still valid and how effectively it builds interpersonal and human relations in libraries. One instance reported in literature (Anderson: 1993: 49) is that of staff donating their leave privilege to their colleagues who was seriously ill and had to leaves. Does this mean anything to self-centered and self-conscious humanity?

7. CONCLUSION

To sum up, it is important to note that "As libraries we function within an organizational structure wherein there exists an ongoing social process with our colleagues and clients. To be more effective we need to develop our human skills in order to better understand ourselves, others and our organizations" (Allen: 1971:90) Interpersonal relationship has to be developed with our becoming conscious that without it, it would be detrimental to healthy working atmosphere of academic libraries. There is need to involve in studying the subject in depth. If need be, it should be included in library and information science curriculum. It also reflects to some aspects of best practices followed in the academic libraries. In Indian academic library environment, this aspect should be strengthened to improve working efficiency of our academic library professionals.

APPENDIX

Competencies required for Library Professionals: Current Communications Channels

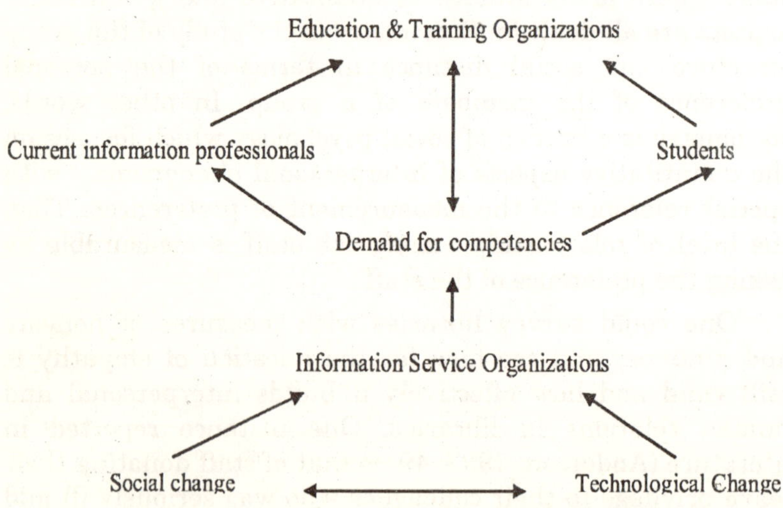

Source: Griffiths, J., 1983.4-5

8. REFERENCES

Albritton, Rosie L and Shaughnessy, Thomas W., Developing Leadership Skills :A Source Book for Librarians", Englewood, Libraries Unlimited , 1990.

Allen, L.A., and Conroy, B., "Social Interaction Skills", Library Trends 20, 1971, 78-90.

Anderson, A. J., "How do you manage: Case Study: Could You Block a Bad Reference", Library Journal, 116 Jan 1991, 71-73.(covers two analyses: six steps to fight fate: and define – then do – the right thing).

Anderson, A. J.: How Do You Manage; Case study : I Refuse to Work with a Right –tolifer", Library Journal, 117 June 1, 1992. 89-92. (covers two analyses:take leadership over turf war: and Hire now , assess objectively).

Anderson, A. J. "How Do You Manage : Case study: The Arrangement", Library Journal, 116 May1, 1991. 56-58. (covers two analyses: Form an esprit de corps: and be more assertive).

Anderson, A. J. "How do you manage: case study : 'I gave at the office' gets new meaning", Library Journal July 1993, 49-50. (deals with a unique way of cooperating with the staff, where the staff donated their leave privilege to a colleague, in need)

"Cartoons Causes Strife', Library Journal, 119 march 1. 1994, 26. (deals with supposedly problematic cartoon which deals with sexual harassment}.

Casteleyn, Mary and W ebb, Sylvia P. Promoting Excellence : Personal Management in Libraries. London, Bowker, 1993.

Cowley, J. Personal Management in Libraries. London , Bingley, 1982.

Deiss, Kathryn J., "Staff -based policy building ", College & Research Library News, 55, 1994, 730, 733.

Euster, Jonne R. Changing Patters in International Communication in Large Academic Libraries. Occasional paper no. 6.Washington, D.C., ARL/OMS, 1981.

Ganguly, S. M. "An ethical code for the library profession in India", 11th National IASLIC Seminar, Hyderabad , 1984, 15-24.

Gossen, E., et al. "Forging new communication links in an academic library: A cross –training experiment" Journal of Academic Librarianship, 16 March, 1990, 18-21 (An experimental cross-training program at SUNY resulted in the development of new lateral lines of communication between the public and technical services divisions of the library. This helped boost morale by decreasing feelings of isolation and reinforced the importance of interdepartmental cooperation in providing the best possible services for patrons).

Griffiths, J., "Competency Requirements for Library and Information Science Professionals," in Linda C Smith, ed., professional competencies – Technology and the librarian. Urbana-Champaign Univ. of Illinois, 1983.

Maher, William J., "improving archives- library relations: User-Centered solutions to a sibling rivalry", Journal of Academic Librarianship 15 Jan 1090, 355-373. (Analysing the relationships between archives and libraries has been a popular topic in the professional literature over the past 10 to 20 years. While this literature has simply explored the fundamental differences and similarities, improvements in library –achieve relations have been limited by a failure to focus on the fact that the tensions between the two need to be resolved at the institutional levels. This paper examines these relations in the college and university setting where tensions are often sharpest but where the reasons and opportunities for improved relations are greatest).

Penland, Patrick R., "Group dynamics," in Encyclopedia of library & Information Science. Edited by Allen kent. New York, Dekker, 19n73. 207-237.

Powell, John W. Education for maturity. New York, Heritage House, 1949.

Scanion, J J., "How to mix oil and water: or , getting Librarians work with programmers", College and Research Libraries news, April 1090,320-322. (deals with building bridge between two workers, whose ultimate purpose is to serve the society).

Shaffer, K.R., Library Personal Administration and Supervision. Shoe string press, 1963, 2nd revised and enlarged edition. (case studies in library administration, series1). (covers issues like absenteeism, forgery and theft, increment, use of library telephones, irritating staff personality, protection of a superior, etc.

Taher, Mohamed and K. Krishna. Interpersonal Relationship: Communications and Miscommunications in Academic and Research Libraries. Paper presented at All India Library Association Annual Conference, held at Vijayawada, January 1996.

"Union Lobbies City to Fire Library Director", American Libraries, Nov.1990, 941-942. (suggest that the concerned officer is considered very uneasy and uncommunicative with the staff, supervisors and subordinates, including women).

Veaner, Allen, B. Academic Librarianship in a Transformal Age Program, Politics and Personnel. Boston, G.K. Hall, 1990.

Cyber Crime and Indian Cyber Law

Vimal Kishore Purohit and Mukesh Gehlot

ARIS Cell, Central Arid Zone Research Institute, Jodhpur - 3

1. INTRODUCTION

The development of any technology is always associated with pros and cons. Development of computer and Information Technology has driven the world in such a way that it is stepping new steps every day. The impact of Internet on the daily life of human being has made the world as global village. The Internet, as we know, has grown rapdily over the last decade. It has given rise to many avenues in every field we can think of be it education, entertainment, business, or sports. However, with every boon there is a cruse too. This cruse is Cyber crime i.e. illegal activities committed over the Internet. The Internet, along with its advantages, has also exposed us to security risks. Computers today are being misused for unlawful activities like e-mail espionage, credit card fraud, Spam, software piracy, spreading or viruses and so on, which invade our privacy and offend our senses. Criminal activities over Internet are on the rise.

2. CYBER CRIME

The first recorded cyber crime took place in the year 1820. Joseph-Marie Jacquard, a textile manufacture in

France, produced the loom. This device allowed the repetition of a series of steps in the weaving of special fabrics. This resulted in a fear amongst Jacquard's employees that their traditional employment and livelihood were being vulnerable. They committed acts of harm to discourage Jacquard from further use of the new technology. At present it is High-tech time when everything from microwave ovens and refrigerators to nuclear power plants are being run on computers, cyber crime has assumed rather distributing implications. Cyber crime can involve criminal activities that are traditional in nature, such as theft, fraud, forgery, defamation and mischief. The abuse of computers has also given birth to a extent of new age crimes such as hacking, web defacement, cyber stalking, web jacking etc.

A simple yet powerful definition of cyber crime would be ``unlawful acts wherein the computer is either a tool or a target or both". The term computer used in this definition does not only mean the conventional desktop or laptop computer. It includes Personal Digital Assistants (PDA), cell phones, sophisticated watches, cars and many more electronic gadgets.

Recent global cyber crime incidents like the targeted rejection of service attacks on Estonia have heightened fears. Intelligence agencies are preparing against coordinated cyber attacks that could disorder rail and air traffic controls, electricity supply, networks, stock markets, banking and insurance systems etc. Calculation of social and financial impact of cyber crime is not possible as most crimes go unreported. Cyber crime is a term used broadly to describe criminal activity in which computers or networks are a tool, a target, or a place of criminal activity. These categories are not exclusive and many activities can be characterized as falling in one or more categories. Although the term cyber crime is usually restricted to describing criminal activity in which the computer or network is an essential part of the crime, this term is also used to include traditional crimes in which computers or networks are used to enable the illicit activity.

Since Computer crime activities are traditional in nature and are subjected to the Indian Penal Code (IPC). Simultaneously it has also given birth to a gamut of new age crimes that are addressed by the Information Technology Act, 2000 and cyber crimes, are punishable by the Information Technology Act.

3. COMMONLY USED CYBER CRIMES

Following are the commonly used cyber crimes:

(i) Cyber pornography

Pornography is the sexually explicit depiction of persons, in words or images, created with the primary, proximate aim, and reasonable hope, of eliciting significant sexual arousal on the part of the consumer of such materials including pornographic websites; pornographic magazines produced using computers (to publish and print the materials) and the Internet (to download and transmit pornographic pictures, photos, writings etc). Recent Indian incidents revolving around cyber pornography include the Air Force School case. A student of the Air Force School, Delhi, was teased by all his classmates for having a covered with spots face. Tired of the cruel jokes, he decided to get back at his tormentors. He scanned photographs of his classmates and teachers, morphed them with nude photographs and put them up on a website that he uploaded on to a free web hosting service. It was only after the father of one of the class girls featured on the website objected and lodged a complaint with the police that any action was taken. In another incident, in Mumbai a Swiss couple gathered slum children and them forced then to appear for obscence photographs. They then upload the photographs to websites specially designed for pedophiles. The Mumbai police arrested the couple for pornography.

(ii) Virus and worm attacks

Viruses are programs that attach themselves to a computer or a file and then circulate to other files and to other computers on a network. They usually affect the data on a computer, either by altering or deleting it. Worms, unlike viruses do not need the host to attach merely make functional copies and do this repeatedly occupy all the available space on the computer's memory. The virus VBS_LOVELETTER (better known as the Love Bug or the I LOVE YOU virus) was reportedly written by a Filipino undergraduate. In May 2000, this deadly virus beat the Melissa virus hollow and became the world's most prevalent virus. It struck one in every five personal computers in the world. When the virus was brought under check the true magnitude of the losses was incomprehensible.

(iii) Financial crimes

Financial crimes often involve fraud and cheating. Financial crimes are carried out via check and credit card fraud, mortgage fraud, medical fraud, corporate fraud, bank account fraud, payment (point of sale) fraud, money laundering and currency fraud. A website offered to sell special quality mangoes at a casual price. Distrusting such a transaction, very few people responded to or supplied the website with their credit card numbers. These people actually sent the special quality mangoes. Thousands of people from all over the country responded and ordered mangoes by providing their credit card numbers. The owner was later proven to be a fake website then fled taking the numerous credit card numbers and proceeded to spend huge amounts of money much to the charging of the card owners decided to get even. On the Valentine Day, he sent Janak a spoofed e-card, which appeared to have come from Sunita's mail account. The e-card actually contained a Trojan. As soon as Janak opened the card, the Trojan was installed on his computer. Trilok now had complete control over Janak's computer and proceeded to harass him thoroughly.

(iv) Information Theft

Information theft means leak of information by any means. Information theft has been referred as computer crime but it is very difficult to lodge case against any person/company for information theft as the employee had access to such data in the course of a normal working day.

(v) Web jacking

This occurs when someone forcefully takes control of a website by cracking the password and later changing it. The actual owner of the website does not have any more control over what appears on that website. It usually comes an unwanted chage of the homepage on browser, and Windows that ``Pop-Up" with unsolicited advertisements and completely invisible Trojans that use computer to attack others.

(vi) Email bombing

Email bombing refers to sending a large number of emails to the victim resulting in the victim's email account or mail crashing. In one case, a foreigner who had been residing in Shimla, India for almost thirty years wanted to avail of a scheme introduced by the Shimla Housing Board to buy land at lower rates and his application was rejected on the grounds that scheme was available only for citizens of India. For taking revenge, he sent thousands of mails to the Shimla Housing Board and repeatedly kept sending e-mails till their mail servers crashed.

(vii) Data diddling

Data diddling is the changing of data before or during entry into the computer system. This kind of an attack involves altering raw data just before a computer processes. Electricity Boards in India have been victims to data diddling programs inserted when private parties were computerizing their systems.

(viii) Denial of service attack

A denial-of-service attack (DoS attack) or distributed denial-of-service attack (DDoS attack) is an attempt to make a computer resource unavailable to its intended users. It generally consists of the planned efforts of a person or people to prevent an Internet site or service from functioning efficiently or at all, temporarily or indefinitely. DoS attacks typically target sites or services hosted on high-profile web servers such as banks, credit card payment gateways, and even root nameservers. This involves flooding a computer resource with more requests than it can handle. This causes the web server to crash thereby denying authorized users the service offered by the resource. The attack is initiated by sending excessive demands to the victim's computer, exceeding the limit that the victim's servers can support and making the server's crash.

(ix) Logic bombs

A logic bomb is a computer program executed at a specific time period or on a specific event implying that these programs are created to do something only when a certain event occurs. A programmer can write a program to instruct the computer to delete all personnel and payroll files. Even some viruses may be termed logic bombs because they lie inactive all through the year and become active only on a particular date.

(x) Trojan attacks

A Trojan horse is the secret placement of instructions inside or a valid program causing the computer to perform unauthorized functions but usually allow the program to perform its intended purpose. This is probably the most common method used in computer-based frauds and sabotage. A Trojan functions from inside seems to be an authorized program, thereby concealing what it is actually doing. Two friends Trilok and Janak (names changed), had a heated argument over one girl, Sunita (name changed) whom they both liked. When the girl, asked to choose, chose Janak over Trilok, Trilok legal regimes in order to promote online commerce. India has enacted the Information Technology Act, 2000 in order to provide the required boost to E-commerce.

NEED OF CYBER LAW

Internet is an irreversible phenomenon, which has set new benchmarks for the entire mankind. Internet has grown in a very rapid, arbitrary and unplanned manner due to unplanned nature. It was felt initially that Internet is a system of disorder. Unplanned activities laid the seeds of origin of Cyber law.

There is no one in-depth definition of the term Cyber law. However, Cyber law is a term, which refers to all the legal and regulatory aspects of Internet and the World Wide Web. In simple language we can say, ``Cyber Law is the law governing cyber space. Cyber space is a very wide term and includes computers, networks, software, data storage devices (such as hard disks, USB disks etc), the Internet, websites, emails and even electronic devices such as cell phones, ATM machines etc".

The growth of electronic commerce has created the need for vibrant and effective regulatory mechanisms, which would strengthen the legal infrastructure that is crucial to the success of electronic commerce. All of these regulatory mechanisms and the legal infrastructure come within the domain of cyber law. Cyber law is important because it touches almost all aspects of transactions and activities concerning the Internet and Cyberspace. As the nature and scope of Internet is changing, it is perceived as the ultimate medium ever-evolved in human history. Every activity in cyberspace needs legal perspective. From the moment a person registers a domain name, sets up and promotes his or her web site, and then conducts electronic commerce and has transactions on the site, various cyber law issues are involved. As the Internet grows, numerous legal issues arise relating to Domain names, Intellectual Property Rights, Electronic commerce, Privacy, Encryption, Cyber crime, Online banking, spamming etc. Today world is moving steadily towards the information society and knowledge economy, it is essential that law must contribute its inputs to promote e-commerce. As cyber law develops around the world, there is a growing realization among different nations that their laws must be harmonized and international best practices and principles must be implemented. Many countries are trying to establish it.

INDIAN CYBER LAW

The primary source of cyber law in India is the Information Technology Act, 2000 (IT Act), which came into, force on 17 October, 2000. The primary purpose of the Act is to provide legal recognition to electronic commerce and to facilitate filing of electronic records with the Government. The IT Act also penalizes various cyber crimes and provides strict punishments including imprisonment terms up to 10 years and compensation up to Rs 1 Crore. The main objectives of IT Act 2000 are :

- Different appraoches for controlling, regulating and facilitating electronic communication and commerce.
- To provide legal recognition for transactions.
- Carried out by means of electronic data interchange.
- Other means of electronic communication commonly referred to as ``electronic commerce'', involving the use of alternatives to paper-based methods of communication and storage of information.
- To facilitate electronic filing of documents with the Government agencies.
- To provide legal infrastructure for E-commerce in India.
- Besides IT act 2000 following cyber laws are also incorporated by Government of India

- The Cyber Regulations Appellate Tribunal (Procedure) Rules, 2000 also came into force on 17th October 2000. These rules prescribe the appointment and working of the Cyber Regulations Appellate Tribunal (CRAT) whose primary role is to hear appeals against orders of the Adjudicating Officers.

On 17th March 2003, The Information Technology (Qualification and Experience of Adjudicating Officers and Manner of Holding Enquiry) Rules 2003 were passed. These rules lay down the qualifications required for Adjudicating Officers. Their chief responsibility under the IT Act is to adjudicating on cases such as unauthorized access, unauthorized copying of data, spread of viruses, denial of service attacks, disruption of computers, computer manipulation etc. These rules also prescribe the manner and mode of inquiry and adjudication by these officers.

Information Technology (Use of Electronic Records and Digital Signatures) Rules, 2004 has provided the necessary legal framework for filing of documents with the Government as well as issue of licenses by the Government. It also provides for payment and receipt of fees in relation to the Government bodies.

The Indian Penal Code (as amended by the IT Act) penalizes several cyber crimes. These include forgery of electronic records, cyber frauds, destroying electronic evidence etc. Digital Evidence is to be collected and proven in court as per the provisions of the Indian Evidence Act (as amended by the IT Act). In case of bank records, the provisions of the Bankers' Book Evidence Act (as amended by the IT Act) are applicable. Investigation and adjudication of cyber crimes is done in accordance with the provisions of the Code of Criminal Procedure and the IT Act. The Reserve Bank of India Act was also amended by the IT Act. Various cyber crimes covered under law are being depicted in Table 1.

Table 1. Computer Related Crimes under IPC and IT Act

S.N.	Cyber Crimes	Laws Under Section
1.	Sending threatening messages by email	Sec 503 IPC
2.	Sending defamatory messages by email	Sec 499, 500 IPC
3.	Forgery of electronic records	Sec 463, 470, 471 IPC
4.	Bogus websites, cyber frauds	Sec 420 IPC
5.	Email spoofing	Sec 416, 417, 463 IPC
6.	Web Jacking	Sec 383 IPC
7.	Cyber Pornography	Sec 67 IT Act
8.	Accessing Protected System	Sec 70 IT Act
9.	Tampering with Computer Source Code	Sec 65 IT Act

IMPLEMENTATION OF CYBER LAW

At present the Adjudicating Officers in India are not aware about how to proceed in to settle or determine an issue or dispute judicially. This is due to the way in which the Central Government by means of notification has only stipulated the Information Technology Secretaries of different states as the Adjudicating Officers. By designating technocrats to perform quasi-judicial functions without giving them appropriate training or orientation, only leads to complications of problems. This has resulted in a scenario where the adjudicating officers are not oriented to perform their quasi-judicial functions. The Government of India also needs to plan and implement special awareness and orientation programmes for police officers. The Information Technology Act 2000 stipulates that cyber crime in India shall only be investigated by a police officer not below the rank of Deputy Superintendent of Police (DSP). Given the practical reality where a DSP in India, as a high-ranking police officer, is already burdened with other critical issues and pressing problems and responsibilities, cyber crime investigation and prosecution becomes an extremely low priority for them. There is no orientation given to the police officers in an organized, systematic basis. Special training programmes are needed for those police officers who are designated to deal with cyber crime.

For the legal profession, there are various areas, which require maximum Capacity-building. Lawyers in India are not much aware of information technology legal provisions and there is a compelling need to educate them. Lawyers need to be trained appropriately about various relevant issues relating to e-commerce law and the technical nuances of the law. Judges also need to be duly trained about the various legal issues pertaining to the Information Technology Act. People in the lower and middle level judiciary are almost completely unaware of the various nuances and other technical details concerning such e-commerce laws. This area needs to be seriously and urgently addressed. Cyber law training also needs to be given to the government departments and the relevant officers engaged in e-commerce and e-governance activities. This is essential, as the preamble of the Information Technology Act specifi-cally states that the objective of this law is to promote e-commerce and electronic filing of documents with government agencies. Nothing much has been done to facilitate access by consumers to the tribunal court alternatives for e-commerce disputes. The Indian e-commerce law has only provided that one statutory authority be established, namely adjudicating officers. At the time of writing, only one case has been filed in India before the adjudicating officer for grant of damages by way of compensation under the Indian Cyber law. This industry and the public at large have been generally starts massive capacity building programmes and initiatives, the situation is likely to continue to remain the same. Various institutes in India conduct courses on cyber law for lawyers, students and other professionals. However, most of these courses are pure commercial ventures and the quality of knowledge and awareness imparted is not up to the standard and often leaves much to be desired. With the media reporting cyber law related issues, as well as various cases conducted under the law, awareness about crimes conducted over the

Internet has been slowly increasing. As time flies fast, e-commerce continues to grow with each passing day. However, a look at the existing laws shows that it will take a large amount of time and effort for South Asian countries to effectively put their legal regimes in agreement with the existing international best practices and procedures.

FUTURE PROSPECTUS

When the law was framed, there were no technologies like MMS or sophisticated devices like mobile phones, Latest News and mobile phones with cameras. The IT Act is struggling to cope up with the changes in modern technology. India is likely to have a tighter data protection and privacy regime in place later, after bowing to pressure from Western users of outsourcing services. The National Association of Software and Service Companies (NASSCOM) in Delhi is confident that new measures will be prepared for Cyber law by Indian parliament. Opponents of offshore outsourcing to India have often cited the absence of a data protection and privacy law in India as a strong reason for stopping the movement of call centre and BPO work to the country. The government is considering an amendment to its Information Technology Act of 2000. NASSCOM is in the process of inserting new clauses in the IT Act 2000, and the government is reviewing these. The Act in its existing form only covers unauthorized access and data theft from computers and networks, with a penalty and does not have specific provisions relating to privacy of data.

CONCLUCSION

The Indian experience has shown that it is easy to enact law on paper. However, it is extremely difficult to enforce laws in actual practice. There are numerous challenges that require appropriate awarenes among citizens about e-commerce laws. This is so because at the end of the day, the e-commerce laws are basically targeted to protect and help those citizens. It is also necessary to ensure that there is adequate training of the relevant department and government officials who would draft and implement policies relating to e-commerce. Cyber law is constantly in evolving process and various legal issues may arise, so we have to keep updating cyber laws constantly. Thus there is a need to adopt a practical approach in dealing with these various legal challenges.

साहित्यिक खोज एवं ग्रंथ सूची
(Literature Search and Bibliography)

Pawan Kumar Gupta* & Usha Pawan**

*Hony. Director, University of Rajasthan, Jaipur – 302055
** Retd. Associate Professor, Department of LIS,
University of Rajasthan, Jaipur 302 055 (Raj.)

ज्ञांन जगत में वर्तमान युग में तीव्र गति से वृद्धि हो रही है तथा सभी विषयों में साहित्य अबाध रूप से प्रकाशित हो रहा है। जितनी वृद्धि शिक्षित व्यक्तियों में हो रही है, जितना धन सरकार शोध एवं विकास कार्यों पर व्यय कर रही है तथा जितने शोध कार्य गैर सरकारी संस्थाओं के द्वारा संचालित किये जा रहे हैं, उतनी ही तीव्रता से प्रकाशित साहित्य में वृद्धि हो रही है। इसीलिये वर्तमान युग को सूचना विस्फोट का युग कहा जाता है। विशेष नया विज्ञान, एवं तकनिकी विषयों में प्राथमिक सूचना स्त्रोत बहुतायत से प्रकाशित हो रहे हैं। एक अनुमान के मुताबिक इन विषयों में दस वर्ष से भी कम अवधि में प्रकाशित साहित्य में वृद्धि दुगनी हो जाती है। इसके साथ ही समाज विज्ञान एवं मानविकी विषयों में भी शोध के फलस्वरूप साहित्य में निरन्तर वृद्धि हो रही है। शोध कार्यक्रम की प्रगति इस पर निर्भर करती हैं कि शोध के विषय से संबंधित सूचना कितनी शीघ्रता से शोध कर्ता को उपलब्ध होती है। इस कार्य का उत्तरदायित्व पुस्तकालय पर डाला गया कि वे प्रकाशित पाठ्य सामग्री में से आवश्यक प्रलेखों की सूचना शोधकर्ता को दे, ताकि शोधकर्ता अपना अधिक से अधिक समय संबंधित

प्रलेखों का अध्ययन करने में लगा सके। इस प्रकार निरन्तर शोध कार्य में प्रगति होती रहे। पुस्तकालय में इस सेवा को साहित्यिक खोज की संज्ञा दी गई है। पुस्तकालय यह सेवा शोधकर्ता द्वारा मांगने पर ही देता है। इस इकाई में साहित्यिक खोज प्रक्रिया एवं उसके फलस्वरूप जिस ग्रंथ का संकलन किया जाता है, उसका विस्तार से वर्णन किया जा रहा है।

साहित्यिक खोज की परिभाषा

आन लाइन डिक्शनरी ऑफ लायब्रेरी एवं इन्फोर्मेशन साइंस (Online dictionary of library and information science) के अनुसार साहित्यिक खोज प्रकाशित पाठ्य सामग्री की एक व्यापक खोज होती है, जिनका उद्देश्य एक सुनियोजित पद्धति के द्वारा एक शोध के विषय पर द्वितीयक सूचना स्त्रोतो की सहायता से अधिकतम पाठ्य सामग्री खोजना होता है। साहित्यिक खोज की तुलना व्यापक संदर्भ सेवा से की जा सकती है क्योंकि व्यापक संदर्भ सेवा में उपभोक्ता द्वारा पूछे गये प्रश्न, जो शोध प्रकृति के होते है, के उत्तर देने के लिये साहित्यिक खोज की जाती है। इस प्रकार की सेवा विशिष्ट पुस्तकालयों में विशेष तौर से दी जाती है। विशिष्ट पुस्तकालयों में ऐसे प्रश्नों का उत्तर देने के लिये प्राथमिक, द्वितीयक, एवं तृतीयक तीनों श्रेणी के सूचना स्त्रोतों का अवलोकन किया जाता है।

साहित्यिक खोज की आवश्यकता

शोध कार्यो में साहित्यिक खोज बहुत महत्वपूर्ण भूमिका अदा करती है। शोध कार्य का यह प्रथम पायदान है। प्रत्येक शोध कार्यक्रम में बहुत धन, श्रम व समय खर्च होता है। अतएव नये शोध कार्यक्रम को आरंभ करने से पहले यह जानना अनिवार्य होता है कि उस पर पूर्व में शोध कार्य हो तो नहीं चुका है। उसी प्रकार शोध कार्य की समाप्ति पर रिपोर्ट बनाते समय विषय पर विगतकालीन व नई प्रकाशित पाठ्य सामग्री की आवश्यकता पड़ती है। शोधकर्ता अपने स्वयं के प्रयासों से विषय पर सम्पूर्ण प्रकाशित सामग्री में से आवश्यक सूचना नहीं खोज सकता है। अतएव उसे पुस्तकालय पर निर्भर रह्ना पड़ता है। वर्तमान समय में प्रकाशित साहित्य में वृद्धि के साथ, वह कई प्रारूपों में भी उपलब्ध होता है। इसके साथ बहुविषयी शोध के कारण एक विषय की सामग्री कई विषय की पत्रिकाओं में बिखरी होती है। यह कार्य प्रायः

सार पत्रिकाओं एवं अनुक्रमणिकरण पत्रिकाओं के माध्यम से किया जाता है। परन्तु फिर भी अन्य सूचना स्त्रोत भी खोजने पड़ते हैं। अतएव एक विषय पर समस्त सामग्री का अवलोकन करने एवं आवश्यक पाठ्य सामग्री पर एक ग्रंथ सूची के निर्माण के लिये एक व्यवस्थित पद्धति काम में लाई जाती है। संक्षेप में यह कह सकते हैं कि साहित्यिक खोज से निम्नलिखित कार्यो में सहायता मिलती है –

1. अध्ययन एवं शोध कार्य में।
2. शोध कार्य की द्विरावृत्ति को रोकने में।
3. शोध समस्याओं को सुलझाने में।
4. शोध के नये क्षेत्र खोजने में।

ग्रंथ सूची का संकलन

विशिष्ट पुस्तकालयों में साहित्यिक खोज एवं ग्रंथ सूची का संकलन, ये दो प्रमुख सेवाएँ उपभोक्ताओं को प्रदान की जाती है। ये सेवाएं अनुरोध पर दी जाती है। पुस्तकालय ग्रंथ सूची का संकलन किसी विभाग के अनुरोध पर भी करते है, जब उस विभाग में सम्मेलन, सेमीनार या कार्यशाला आयोजित की जा रही हो। साहित्यिक खोज एवं ग्रंथ सूची का संकलन कम्प्यूटर या पारम्परिक विधि की सहायता से कर सकते हैं। दोनों विधियों में ही एक व्यवस्थित पद्धति काम में लाई जाती है, जिसका विस्तृत विवरण दिया जा रहा है। साहित्यिक खोज आरंभ करने से पहले यह जानना आवश्यक है कि उपभोक्ताओं द्वारा कैसे प्रश्न पूछे जाते हैं। पाठकों द्वारा जो प्रश्न पूछे जाते हैं हम उन्हें निम्नलिखित श्रेणियों में विभाजित कर सकते हैं –

1 *शब्द एवं कहावतें* – संदर्भ डेस्क पर काफी प्रश्न भाषा के शब्दों मुहावरे, कहावतों आदि से संबंधित पूछे जाते हैं। उपभोक्ता शब्द का अर्थ, पर्याय, विलोम एवं समानार्थक शब्द, मुहावरे का अर्थ, आदि, जानकारी प्राप्त करना चाहता है। यह सूचना शब्दकोष (dictionary)] ग्लौसरी (glossary), थिजोरस (thesaurus)] आदि के माध्यम से दी जाती है।

2 *सामान्य सूचना* – उपभोक्ता किसी विषय पर सामान्य सूचना जैसे – विषय का संक्षिप्त विकास, संबंधित सांख्यिकी, आंकड़े, आदि। इनका उत्तर विश्वकोष की सहायता से देते हैं।

3 अत्यन्त नवीन या प्राचीन विषय – कई बार अत्यन्त नवीन या प्राचीन विषयों के प्रश्न भी सूचना प्राप्ति को जटिल बना देते हैं। अद्यतन सामान्य विषय और तथ्य, नई खोज, आदि की सूचना परम्परागत संदर्भ ग्रंथों में नहीं मिलती है। इनसे संबंधित सूचना प्राप्त करने के लिये नवीन प्रलेखों जैसे पत्रिकाओं में प्रकाशित लेख, शोध विवरण, प्रतिवेदन तथा अस्थाई पाठ्य सामग्री से सूचना एकत्रित की जाती है। इसी प्रकार प्राचीन विषयों से संबंधित प्रश्न भी चाहे वे सामान्य प्रकृति के हो, उत्तर खोजना जटिल बना देते हैं। संदर्भ ग्रन्थों में प्राचीन विषयों की सूचना उपलब्ध नहीं होती है तथा उत्तर खोजने के लिये कई प्रलेख देखने पड़ते हैं।

4 *दृष्टिकोण एवं विविध मत* – अनेक विषयों पर विशेषज्ञों द्वारा भिन्न भिन्न दृष्टिकोण से अध्ययन किया जाता है। उन विषयों के पक्ष व विपक्ष पर विद्वानों के भिन्न भिन्न विचार होते हैं। अतएव एक ही विषय से संबंधित सूचना भिन्न–भिन्न स्त्रोतों में एक जैसी नहीं होती है। अतएव जब सूचना विशेष दृष्टिकोण की व्याख्या से मांगी गई हो तो उस प्रश्न का उत्तर देने के लिये विविध प्रलेखों का उपयोग करना आवश्यक हो जाता है।

5 *सांख्यिकी आँकडे* – शोधकर्ताओं को अक्सर शोध विषय से संबंधित सांख्यिकी आँकड़ो की आवश्यकता पड़ती है। जनगणना रिपोर्ट तथा अन्य सांख्यिकी स्त्रोतों की सहायता से इन प्रश्नों के उत्तर दिये जा सकते हैं।

6 *विषय जिनका प्रचलन नहीं हो* – कई बार ऐसा होता है कि किसी विशेष विषय पर सूचना प्रचलित नहीं रहती है। उदाहरण के लिये विज्ञान एवं प्रौद्योगिकी विधाओं के निरन्तर शोध के कारण नई सूचना का प्रादुर्भाव होता है जिससे विषय को नया रूप मिलता है। इन विषयों के परीक्षित और परिवर्तित रूप की सूचना सामयिक शोध पत्रिकाओं में प्रकाशित लेखों में अंकित रहती है। दूसरे विषय पर नई जानकारी तो संदर्भ ग्रंथों के नये संस्करण में प्राप्त होती है परन्तु कुछ सूचना जो विगतकालीन होती है, इनमें उपलब्ध नहीं होती है। अतएव जब उपभोक्ता आकस्मिक रूप से विगतकालीन सूचना की मांग करता है तो उसे विगतकालीन प्रलेखों में से खोजना पड़ता है।

7 *विशिष्ट खोज से संबंधित प्रश्न* – इस श्रेणी में वे प्रश्न आते हैं जिसमें पाठक किसी विषय पर संक्षिप्त परन्तु व्यापक सूचना चाहता है। उदाहरणार्थः प्रथम महायुद्ध के लिये जर्मनी कहाँ तक उत्तरदायी था? इन प्रश्नों के उत्तर संदर्भ स्त्रोतों की सहायता से नहीं दिये जा सकते बल्कि इनके उत्तर खोजने के लिये विषय से संबंधित प्रलेखों का चयन करके, उपभोक्ता को देना होता है। कई बार प्रलेखों की सूची बनाकर भी दे देते हैं।

8 *शोध प्रकृति के प्रश्न* – इस श्रेणी में वे विषय आते है जो विषय के विशेषज्ञों के द्वारा विशिष्ट विषय पर विस्तृत एवं गहन सूचना के लिये पूछे जाते हैं। इनका उत्तर प्रायः विषय की पत्रिकाओं में प्रकाशित लेखों एवं विषय की पुस्तकों से दिया जाता है। इसके लिये द्वितीयक सूचना स्त्रोतों की सहायता भी ली जाती है।

इसके अतिरिक्त कई प्रश्न संस्थाओं के क्रिया कलापों से, प्रमुख व्यक्तियों की जीवनी, आदि से संबंधित भी पूछे जाते हैं। उपरोक्त वर्णित सभी प्रश्नों को दो श्रेणियों में विभाजित किया जा सकता है –

1. तथ्यात्मक प्रश्न तथा,
2. साहित्यिक खोज के प्रश्न ।

तथ्यात्मक प्रश्नों का उत्तर पारम्परिक संदर्भ स्त्रोतों जैसे विश्वकोष, भाषा कोष, निर्देशिका, आदि की सहायता से दिया जा सकता है, परन्तु जिन प्रश्नों के उत्तर देने के लिये काफी संख्या में प्रलेखों में से सूचना खोजनी पड़ती है, उसके लिये एक विशिष्ट साहित्यिक खोज प्रणाली अपनानी पड़ती है। जिससे उपभोक्ता की आवश्यकता का सही आंकलन करके प्रलेख खोजे जा सकें। आगे साहित्यिक खोज पद्धति का विस्तार से वर्णन किया जा रहा है।

खोज पद्धति – साहित्यिक खोज दो विधियों से की जा सकती है–

1. पारम्परिक विधि तथा,
2. कम्प्यूटर आधारित साहित्यिक खोज पद्धति।

पारम्परिक विधि–इस विधि में पुस्तकालय कर्मचारी स्वयं ही प्रलेखों का अवलोकन करके, विषय से संबंधित पाठ्य सामग्री की सूची का निर्माण करते हैं।

इसमें निम्नलिखित कार्य किये जाते है :

1 विषय को स्पष्टतया समझना।

2 विषय क्षेत्र का निर्धारण करना।

3 खोज प्रक्रिया का निर्धारण करना।

4 सूचना स्त्रोतों का अवलोकन – तृतीयक, द्वितीयक व प्राथमिक सूचना स्त्रोतों का अवलोकन करना।

5 प्रविष्टि निर्माण करना।

6 व्यवस्थापन करना।

7 अनुक्रमणिका का निर्माण करना।

प्रथम पद

विषय को स्पष्टतया समझना – खोज प्रक्रिया आरंभ करने से पहले यह आवश्यक है कि उपभोक्ता द्वारा पूछा गया प्रश्न एवं उसका विषय पुस्तकालय कर्मचारी को पूर्णतया स्पष्ट हो। यह पता होना चाहिये, के वास्तव में इस विषय में कौनसे विषय शीर्षकों एवं सम्बद्ध विषयों की सूचना सम्मिलित की जायेगी। इसके लिये विषय विश्व कोष एवं विषय के कोष की सहायता ली जा सकती है। यदि आवश्यक हो तो विषय को सही परिपेक्ष्य में समझने के लिये विषय के विशेषज्ञों की सहायता भी ली जा सकती है। उपभोक्ता की सही आवश्यकता का पता लगाने के लिये उससे संक्षिप्त वार्तालाप भी किया जा सकता है।

द्वितीय पद

विषय क्षेत्र का निर्धारण (decision on scope): इस पद में ग्रंथ सूची के विषय क्षेत्र का निर्धारण, ग्रंथ सूची चयनात्मक होगी या व्यापक, अवधि का निर्धारण : ग्रंथ सूची सामयिक या पूर्वव्यापी होगी, का निर्धारण किया जाता है।

पाठ्य सामग्री का स्वरूप : ग्रंथ सूची में कौन–कौन सी पाठ्य सामग्री सम्मिलित की जायेगी (पत्रिकाओं में प्रकाशित लेख, सम्मेलन में पढ़े गये लेख, शोध प्रतिवेदन, शोध ग्रंथ, पुस्तक, आदि)।

भाषा : विज्ञान के क्षेत्र में महत्त्वपूर्ण सामग्री का प्रकाशन आंग्ल व अन्य भाषाओं में होता है। अतएव यह भी निश्चित करना पड़ेगा कि

किस किस भाषा में प्रकाशित साहित्य सम्मिलित किया जायेगा या ग्रंथ सूची उपभोक्ता को किस भाषा में दी जायेगी।

उपरोक्त निर्णय लेने के लिये आवश्यक है कि उपभोक्ता से वार्तालाप किया जाये जिसे संदर्भ साक्षात्कार (reference interview) कहा जाता है। इस साक्षात्कार के माध्यम से निम्नलिखित जानकारी प्राप्त हो जाती है :

1 प्रश्न को पूर्ण रूप से समझा जा सकता है।

2 सूचना की आवश्यकता किस उद्देश्य की पूर्ति के लिये है? समझा जा सकता है।

3 उपभोक्ता का शैक्षिक स्तर क्या है?

4 विषय क्षेत्र की जानकारी: क्या विषय पर सामयिक एवं विगतकालीन दोनों प्रकार की सूचना चाहिए? पाठ्य सामग्री का प्रकार—पत्रिकाओं के लेख या अन्य सामग्री, किस प्रकाशन वर्ष तक प्रकाशित प्रलेख चाहियें?

5 उपभोक्ता ने इससे पहले कौन—कौन से सूचना स्त्रोतों का अवलोकन किया है?

6 कितने समय में सूचना चाहिये?

तृतीय पद

खोज प्रक्रिया का निर्धारण (formulation of search strategy): इस पद में खोज करने के लिये एक सुव्यवस्थित योजना बनाई जाती है। इसमें सबसे प्रथम प्रश्न का विश्लेषण करके उसका विषय, उपविषय, विषय शीर्षक, आदि का सोच कर पता लगाना पड़ता है। इस कार्य को करने के लिये वर्गीकरण तथा अनुक्रमणिकरण पद्धतियों की सहायता ली जा सकती है। इसमें मुख विश्लेषण (facet analysis) किया जा सकता है तथा इसमें विभिन्न एकलों (isolates) का पता लगाया जाता है। अनुक्रमणिकरण पद्धति के द्वारा मुख्य विचारों को छांटा जा सकता है, जो एक साथ मिलकर मुख्य विषय को बनाते हैं। इसके पश्चात उन संदर्भ स्त्रोतों की पहचान की जाती है जिनसे खोज आरंभ की जा सकती है। खोज का आरंभ तृतीयक सूचना स्त्रोतों से किया जाता है, उसके पश्चात द्वितीयक सूचना स्त्रोत एवं अन्त में प्राथमिक सूचना स्त्रोतों का अवलोकन किया जाता है। सबसे प्रथम यह

जानकारी प्राप्त की जाती है कि विषय पर कोई ग्रंथ सूची उपलब्ध है या नहीं। यदि प्रकाशित ग्रंथ सूची विषय पर उपलब्ध होगी तो विगतकालीन साहित्य को खोजने में समय कीं बचत होगी। निम्नलिखित स्त्रोतों से यह पता लगाया जा सकता है कि विषय ग्रंथ सूची उपलब्ध हैं या नहीं –

1 Bestermans, T. Physical sciences, bibliography of bibliographies. Totwa, N.J., Rowman and Little field (A reprint of Bestermans bibliography of bibliographies) (4thed 1965-66, 4V and index).

2 Bibliographic index : A cumulative bibliography of bibliographies. N.Y., H.W. Wilson, 1937 to date.

3 Walford's guide to reference material. Ed 8. London, Library Association, 3 Vols.

 Vol. 1 : Science and technology, ed by Muley M. Schlicke. 1999.

 Vol. 2 : Social and historical sciences. philosophy and religion, ed. by Dey, A and Welsh, M. 2000

 Vol. 3 : General language and literature, ed. by Chalcraft, A, Prytherch Raud, Wills, S. 1998

4 Shechy, Eugene P. Guide to reference books. Ed. 10. Chicago, American Library Association, 1986.

बेस्टरमैनस के द्वारा रचित ग्रंथ सूचियों की ग्रंथ सूची से हम विगत कालीन प्रकाशित विषय ग्रंथ सूचियों का पता लगा सकते हैं। बिब्लियोग्राफिक इंडेक्स के द्वारा सामयिक प्रकाशित ग्रंथ सूचियों का पता लगा सकते है। इसके पश्चात विषय शीर्षक पर किसी समीक्षा लेख की खोज करनी चाहिए क्योंकि समीक्षा लेख के अन्त में पाठ्य सामग्री की सूची से हम अपना कार्य आरंभ कर सकते हैं। यदि पाठ्य सामग्री की सूची व्यापक है तो उसमें केवल समकालीन पाठ्यसामग्री की जानकारी सम्मिलित करके काफी हद तक साहित्यिक खोज का कार्य पूरा हो जाता है। ग्रंथ सूची में क्योंकि केवल पुस्तकों की जानकारी होती है अतएव पत्रिकाओं में प्रकाशित लेख व अन्य सामग्री के लिये अनुक्रमणिकरण एवं सार पत्रिकाओं का अवलोकन करना पड़ता है। विषय पर कौनसी सार पत्रिकाएं एवं अनुक्रमणिकरण पत्रिकाएं उपलब्ध है, इसका पता निम्नलिखित स्त्रोतों से चल जाता है :

1 Ulrich's periodicals directory. New Province, N.J. etc. 5 vols. 2004 (Published annually since 1932). (Window Based CD Rom Version since 1986, updated Quarterly) (Web version hllp:/www. ulrichsweb.com updated weekly).

2 Abstracting and indexing directory. Detroit (Michigan), Gale Research Corp. 1982 (3 vols.)

चतुर्थ पद

सूचना स्त्रोतों का अवलोकन (scanning of information sources): इस पद से वास्तविक खोज कार्य आरंभ होता है। सबसे प्रथम द्वितीयक सूचना स्त्रोतों का अवलोकन किया जाता है। इसके माध्यम से प्राथमिक सूचना स्त्रोतों तक आसानी से पहुंचा जा सकता है। ये सूचना स्त्रोत प्राथमिक सूचना स्त्रोतों में उपलब्ध पाठ्य सामग्री की अनुक्रमणिका बनाते हैं तथा उनके साथ मूल लेख का सार भी देते हैं। इनका उद्देश्य एक विषय पर प्रकाशित सूचना की जानकारी देना होता है। अनुक्रमणिकरण एवं सार पत्रिकाएं इस श्रेणी में आते हैं। अनुक्रमणिकरण पत्रिकाओं में विभिन्न विषय पत्रिकाओं में प्रकाशित लेखों के विषय शीर्षकों की व्यवस्थित सूची होती है तथा सार पत्रिका में लेखों के संक्षिप्त सार भी दिये होते हैं।

इसके अतिरिक्त वे सूचना स्त्रोत भी आते हैं जो प्राथमिक साहित्य का सर्वेक्षण करके लिखे जाते हैं तथा जो एक विषय पर विस्तृत सूचनाएं देते हैं, जैसे – समीक्षा पत्रिकाएं। परन्तु इन द्वितीयक सूचना स्त्रोतो के अलावा प्राथमिक सूचना स्त्रोतों का अवलोकन सूचना एकत्रित करने के लिये किया जाता है।

सम्मेलन में पढ़े जाने वाले लेख, शोध प्रतिवेदन शोधग्रंथ, पेटेन्टस, मानक ग्रंथ की पूरी सूचना कई प्रमुख सार एवं अनुक्रमणिकरण पत्रिकाएं नहीं देती है, अतएवं एक विषय पर व्यापक पाठ्य सामग्री की सूचना देने के लिये निम्नलिखित प्रकाशनों का अवलोकन भी किया जाता है ।

1. सम्मेलन कार्यवाही (conference proceedings): वर्तमान समय में सम्मेलन व सेमीनार वैज्ञानिकों एवं शोधकर्ताओं को आपसी विचारों का आदान प्रदान करने के लिये एक मंच की भूमिका निबाहते

हैं। इसमे विशेषज्ञ लेख पढ़ते हैं तथा नई सूचना की जानकारी देते हैं तथा बाकी सदस्य इस पर वाद विवाद करते हैं। अंत में निष्कर्ष निकाले जाते हैं। ये लेख मौलिक सूचना के स्त्रोत होते हैं। ये प्रलेख पूर्ण रूप से प्रमुख सार एवं अनुक्रमणिकरण पत्रिकाओं में सम्मिलित नहीं किये जाते हैं। अतएव इनकी सूचना के लिये निम्नलिखित स्त्रोतों का अवलोकन करना चाहिए।

A. Index to scientific and technical proceeding. Philadelphia, Institute for Scientific Information, 1978 Monthly.

B. Conference paper index. Louisville K.Y. Data Courier 1978, monthly.

2. शोध प्रतिवेदन (research reports) : सरकारी संस्थाओं द्वारा विज्ञान, प्रौद्योगिकी, व्यवसाय, सैन्य विज्ञान, इत्यादि के क्षेत्र में जो शोध प्रतिवेदन प्रस्तुत किये जाते है, शोध कार्य में उनका बहुत महत्व होता है। इनकी जानकारी के लिये निम्न स्त्रोत देखना चाहिये।

A. National Technical Information Service (NTIS), Department of Commerce, 1964। यह USA से प्रकाशित होती है। इसमें अन्तर्राष्ट्रीय संस्थाओं एवं विशेषतया संयुक्त राज्य अमेरिका में संस्थाओं द्वारा जो शोध प्रतिवेदन विभागों को प्रस्तुत किये जाते हैं, उनकी जानकारी होती है।

3. शोध ग्रंथ (thesis): अप्रकाशित शोध ग्रंथो की जानकारी निम्नलिखित स्त्रोतों से प्राप्त की जा सकती है :

A. Dissertation abstracts international. Ann Arbor, Mich., University Microfilms, 1861.

B. 'Thesis of the month' *In* 'University news' (Published weekly), Association of Indian Universities, New Delhi.

4. एकस्व (patents) : एकस्व भी मौलिक सूचना के स्त्रोत होते हैं क्योंकि इसमें नये उत्पाद, आविष्कार, विधि आदि का सम्पूर्ण विवरण उपलब्ध होता है। रसायनशास्त्र, टैक्नोलोजी, औषधि निर्माण विज्ञान, इत्यादि में इसकी काफी उपयोगिता होती है। एकस्व की सूचना निम्न स्त्रोतों से एकत्रित की जाती है।

A. EPIDOS – INPADOC पेटेन्टस का सबसे बड़ा डेटाबेस है, इसमें अनुमानतया 65 राष्ट्रों के पेटेन्टस की सूचना दी हुई होती है।

B. भारत में पेटेन्टस की जाकनारी भारतीय गजट के भाग 3 में दी जाती है। यह साप्ताहिक प्रकाशित होता है।

5. मानक (standards) : मानक अनेक प्रकार के एवं अनेक उद्देश्यों से निर्धारित एवं निर्मित सूचना के मौलिक एवं प्राथमिक स्त्रोत होते हैं। मानक एक ऐसी पुस्तिका होती है जिसमें उत्पादों की परिभाषा, विधि, गुणवत्ता तथा सही माप, इत्यादि के बारे में पूर्ण सूचना दी होती है। विज्ञान, प्रोद्योगिकी, उद्योग, वाणिज्य, स्वास्थ्य एवं शिक्षा के क्षेत्र में मानकों की आवश्यकता पड़ती है। इनकी सूचना इन स्त्रोतों से प्राप्त की जा सकती है।

A. BIS calalogue. Bureau of Indian Standards. (annual)

B. ISO calalogue 2004 – International Organization for Standardization.

ये दोनों ही आन लाइन भी उपयोग किये जा सकते हैं ।

6. उद्धरण अनुक्रमणिकाएं (citation indexes) : कई बार कुछ लेखकों की रचना सामान्य सार एवं अनुक्रमणिकरण पत्रिकाओं में सम्मिलित होने से रह जाती है, उन्हें उद्धरण अनुक्रमाणिकाओं के माध्यम से खोजा जा सकता है। अतएवं विभिन्न विषयों में प्रकाशित उद्धरण अनुक्रमणिकाओं का अवलोकन भी अवश्य करना चाहिये।

A. Science citation index. Philadelphia, Institute for Scientific Information, 1963 – Quarterly (The online version (Science Citation Index Expanded) covers 6,400 of the world's leading journals of science and technology, but mainly those in the English language). This was later acquired by Thomson Scientific.

B. Social science citation index. Philadelphia, Institute for Scientific Information, 1973 (Social Sciences Citation Index covers 1700 journals, beginning with 1956). This was later acquired by Thomson Scientific

C. Arts & Humanities citation index. Philadelphia, Institute for Scientific Information. (Arts and Humanities Citation Index, which covers 1150 journals, beginning with 1975.) This was later acquired by Thomson Scientific.

उपरोक्त सभी स्त्रोतों का अवलोकन करने के पश्चात यदि आवश्यक हो तो पुस्तकालय में विषय से संबंधित जो पत्रिकाएं आती हैं, उनके नये अंकों में प्रकाशित लेखों के साथ संलग्न पाठ्य सामग्री की सूची का अवलोकन करना चाहिए, ताकि सभी प्रकाशित संबंधित पाठ्य सामग्री की सूचना एकत्रित की जा सके।

पांचवां पद

प्रलेखों की खोज के पश्चात यह निर्णय किया जाता है कि किन विषय शीषकों को सूची में सम्मिलित किया जायेगा। इसके पश्चात प्रत्येक विषय शीर्षक (subject heading) के लिये एक प्रविष्टि का निर्माण किया जाता है। प्रत्येक प्रविष्टि में मानक के अनुसार प्रलेख का सम्पूर्ण विवरण दिया जाता है। इसके लिये निम्नलिखित मानकों को ध्यान में रखकर प्रविष्टि बनाई जा सकती है।

A. IS : 2381 : 1978. Bibliographical references, Essential and supplementary items.

B. ISO: 690 : 1975. Documentation – Bibliographical references – Essential and supplementary elements.

प्रत्येक प्रविष्टि को 5" x 6" पर बनाना चाहिये तथा एक व्यवस्थित क्रम में रखना चाहिये।

छठा पद

प्रविष्टियों को वर्णक्रमानुसार या वर्गीकरण पद्धति के अनुसार व्यवस्थित करना चाहिए।

सातवां पद

अंत में उपभोक्ता के विभिन्न अभिगमों की पूर्ति करने के लिये आख्या अनुक्रमणिका, लेखक अनुक्रमणिका या विषय अनुक्रमाणिका का निर्माण करना चाहिये।

संक्षेप में कह सकते हैं कि जब पारम्परिक विधि से साहित्यिक खोज का कार्य किया जाता है तो खोज में प्रकाशित ग्रंथ सूची तथा सार एवं अनुक्रमणिकरण पत्रिकाओं का अवलोकन किया जाता है। परन्तु सूची को व्यापक बनाने के लिये कुछ विशिष्ट प्रलेखों का पता लगाने के लिये कुछ अन्य स्त्रोत भी देखे जाते हैं जैसेः शोध प्रतिवेदनों की सूची। साहित्यिक खोज का एक ही मुख्य उद्देश्य होता है कि विषय पर विस्तृत एवं गहन सूची का निर्माण किया जाये।

कम्प्यूटर आधारित साहित्यिक खोज (Computer assisted literature search): आधुनिक सूचना एवं सम्प्रेषण तकनीक (modern information and communication technology - ICT) के आगमन एवं प्रकाशित साहित्य के ग्रंथपरक संगठन में इसके अनुप्रयोग ने सूचना की खोज एवं पुनः प्राप्ति में अत्याधिक गति एवं दक्षता के नये आयाम जोड़ दिये। आजकल काफी संख्या में प्राथमिक, द्वितीयक एवं तृतीयक श्रेणी के सूचना स्त्रोत मशीन सुवाच्चय स्वरूप (machine readable form) में उपलब्ध हैं। सार एवं अनुक्रमणिकरण पत्रिकाएँ प्रायः निम्नलिखित चार स्वरूपों में उपलब्ध हैं –

1 सीडी–रोम डिस्क संस्करण (CD-ROM disc version)

2 रिमोट एक्सेस आन लाइन संस्करण विक्रेता के माध्यम से (remote access on-line version through vendors) जैसे डायलोग (DIALOG)

3 रिमोट एक्सेस वेब संस्करण (remote access web version)

4 मुद्रित संस्करण (print version)

मुद्रित संस्करण में से सूचना परम्परागत तकनीक से खोजी जा सकती है, जिसका विस्तृत विवरण पहले भाग में किया जा चुका है। परन्तु उपर वर्णित तीनों संस्करणों में से सूचना की खोज कम्प्यूटर के माध्यम से की जाती है। इस भाग में आप कम्प्यूटर के माध्यम से सूचना खोज एवं आन लाइन सूचना की खोज कैसे की जाती है, यह सीखेंगे।

कम्प्यूटर आधारित खोज पद्धति का विकास – कम्प्यूटर के माध्यम से खोज पद्धति का विकास वर्ष 1960 से देख सकते हैं, जब विभिन्न सार एवं अनुक्रमणिकरण पत्रिकाओं ने अपने अंक कम्प्यूटर के माध्यम से मुद्रित करने का कार्य किया तथा सूचना का संग्रह चुम्बकीय टेप पर किया। इन चुम्बकीय टेप को कम्प्यूटर के द्वारा देखा जाने

लगा। सरकारी एवं गैर सरकारी संस्थाओं में कम्प्यूटर सॉफ्टवेयर का निर्माण किया गया, जिसके माध्यम से टेप में संग्रहित सूचना का भिन्न–2 प्रकार से उपयोग किया जाने लगा। आरम्भ में कम्प्यूटर के द्वारा खोज में अधिक समय लगता था, परन्तु जैसे–2 कम्प्यूटर की गति, संग्रहण क्षमता में वृद्धि हुई, उसी के अनुरूप खोज की गति में भी वृद्धि हुई। इसके साथ ही एक स्थान के कम्प्यूटर दूरस्थ स्थान के कम्प्यूटर से टेलीफोन लाइन के द्वारा सम्पक्र स्थापित करने में सफल हो गये। इस प्रकार आन लाइन खोज प्रक्रिया का आरंभ हुआ। आन लाइन खोज के लिये उपलब्ध डेटाबेस में भी वृद्धि हुई। सबसे प्रथम प्रमुख आन लाइन डायल–अप सेवा (dial-up-service) मेडलाइन (MedLine) आरम्भ हुई तथा इसके प्श्चात व्यवसायिक आन लाइन डायल–अप सेवा ड़ायलाग (DIALOG) आरम्भ हुई। इसके पश्चात कई संस्थाओं ने यह सेवा देनी आरंभ कर दी। इसके पश्चात डेटाबेसों की संख्या में निरन्तर वृद्धि होने लगी। 2004 में डेटाबेसों की गेल निर्देशिका (Gale directory of databases) प्रकाशित हुई, जिसके अनुसार 12,000 आन लाइन डेटाबेस बनाये गये।

आरंभ में आन लाइन डेटा बेस में केवल ग्रंथ परक संदर्भ (bibliographical references) ही होते थे, परन्तु समय के साथ साथ ग्रंथपरक संदर्भ के साथ पूर्ण लेख भी प्रस्तुत होने लग गये। इन डेटाबोसो में मूलपाठ (full text) के साथ चित्र, ध्वनी, आंकडे आदि भी उपलब्ध होते हैं। इसके पश्चात इंटरनेट (internet) तथा वर्ल्ड वाइड वेब (World Wide Web) के आगमन से संसार में सभी संस्थाओं में उपलब्ध सूचना स्त्रोतों से खोज की जा सकती है। इन सूचना स्त्रोतों में से सूचना खोजने के लिये उपभोक्ता सीधे ही वेब पेज (web page) पर जा सकता है, जहॉ सूचना उपलब्ध होती है। उसे वेब पेज (web page) का यूनीफार्म रिर्सोस लोकेटर (uniform resource locater - URL) का पता होना चाहिये ।

Rowley (1999) ने आन लाइन खोज की तीन पीढ़ियों का वर्णन किया है जबकि चतुर्थ चौधरी एवं चौधरी ने (2001) में जोड़ी है। वे पीढ़ियां निम्नलिखित हैं :

(1) 1981 तक प्रथम पीढ़ी मानी जाती है जिसमें मूक कम्प्यूटर टर्मिनल (dumb computer terminals) होते थे तथा उसकी सम्प्रेषण की गति धीमी होती थी तथा अधिकतर ग्रंथपरक डेटाबेस ही होते थे ।

(2) द्वितीय पीढ़ी, जो पूरे दशक पर्यन्त चलती रही, के अन्दर मूक कम्प्यूटर टर्मिनल के स्थान पर वर्क स्टेशन (work station) तथा पर्सनल कम्प्यूटर आ गये। इससे सम्प्रेषण की गति मध्यम हो गई तथा ग्रंथ परक डेटाबेस के साथ साथ पूर्ण मूलपाठ डेटाबेस (full text data base) भी उपलब्ध हो गये। इसके साथ डेटाबेस एवं उपयोगकर्ता के बीच में सॉफ्टवेयर मध्यस्थ (interface) के रूप में कार्य करने लगे।

(3) तृतीय पीढ़ी, जिसका आरम्भ 1990 से हुआ, में मल्टी मीडिया कम्प्यूटर (multimedia computer) काम में आने लगे। इससे सम्प्रेषण की गति पहले से अधिक हो गई। इसके साथ ग्रंथ परक डेटाबेस के साथ पूर्ण मूलपाठ डेटाबेस (full text data base) तथा उन्नत मध्यस्थ सॉफ्टवेयर (interface software) भी उपलब्ध हुये। इन मध्यस्थ सॉफ्टवेयर में सहायता (help) टयूटोरियल जैसी सुविधाएं मिलने लगी।

(4) चौथी पीढ़ी, जो बीसवीं सदी तक चलती रही, में वेब एक्सेस (web access) तथा आन लाइन खोज की सुविधा मिलनी आरंभ हो गई। इससे उपभोक्ता सीधे ही आन लाइन सेवा प्रदाता (on line service provider) के वेब पते (web address) पर जाने लगे तथा उनके द्वारा उपलब्ध कराई गई सेवाओं का उपयोग करते हुये वांछित सूचना की पुनः प्राप्ति करने लगे।

आरंभ में आन लाइन खोज महंगी होती थी परन्तु धीरे–धीरे ये सस्ती होने लगी तथा उन्नत उपभोक्ता मध्यस्थ सॉफ्टवेयर (interface software) के कारण तथा मध्यस्थ सॉफ्टवेयर में दिये गये निर्देशों के कारण उपभोक्ता स्वयं ही खोज करने में सक्षम होने लगे। आन लाइन खोज में तीव्र गति से अद्यतन सूचना खोजी जा सकती है। परन्तु सी डी रोम डैटाबेस (CD Rom data base) की तुलना में आन लाइन खोज महंगी होती है। सी डी रोम डैटाबेस को केवल एक बार क्रय करना पड़ता है तथा उससे कितनी ही बार सूचना खोजी जा सकती है।

कम्प्यूटर आधारित साहित्य खोज के लाभ

(1) उन्नत खोज क्षमता (Improved research capacity) – मुद्रित स्त्रोतों में खोज केवल अनुक्रमणिकाओं एवं सार पत्रिकाओं तक ही सीमित रहती है तथा किसी एक पद जैसे लेखक, विषय उपविषय, मुख्य शब्द के अन्तर्गत ही खोज की जाती है। यह उसकी

सीमा होती है। खोज करने के लिये अनुक्रमणिका के सम्मुचित अंक तथा नये अंकों में से भी सूचना एकत्रित करने के लिये खोज की जाती है। इस कार्य में श्रम व समय दोनों ही काफी लगते हैं। परन्तु जबसे अनुक्रमणिकाएं एवं सार पत्रिकाएँ इलैक्ट्रॉनिक रूप में उपलब्ध होने लगे हैं कम्प्यूटर के द्वारा कम समय में ही डेटाबेसों से खोज की जा सकती है। उदाहरणार्थ लीसा पत्रिका (LISA) के 1969 के पश्चात के अंक आन लाइन खोज के लिये वेब पर उपलब्ध है तथा इनकी खोज बहुत शीघ्रता से की जा सकती है। साथ ही खोज के परिणाम कम्प्यूटर स्क्रीन पर देखे जा सकते हैं, तथा जिसमें आवश्यकतानुसार खोज योजना में संशोधन किया जा सकता है। इसके साथ ही संबंधित पाठ्य सामग्री की सूची भी तुरन्त मुद्रित की जा सकती है। इलैक्ट्रोनिक डेटाबेस में कई खोज के विकल्प उपलब्ध है। इलैक्ट्रॉनिक डेटाबेस में से निम्नलिखित विकल्पों में से एक या अधिक सें खोज की जा सकती है –

अ – मुख्य पद या वाक्यांश से खोज (keyword and phrase search)

ब – बूलियन खोज (boolean search)

स –शब्द के एक भाग के द्वारा (search with truncated word)

द – शब्दों की समीपता के अनुसार खोज (proximity search)

य – विशिष्ट अनुच्छेद के अन्तर्गत खोज (field specific search)

र – सीमाओं में खोज (limiting search)

ल – रेंज खोज (Range search)

(अ) मुख्य पद या वाक्यांश से खोज (keyword and phrase search) : एक शब्द या पूरा वाक्य जिसमें दो या तीन पद हो सकते हैं, को कम्प्यूटर में प्रविष्ट करके खोज की जाती है।

(ब) बूलियन खोज (boolean search) : इसमें बूलियन तक्र के आधार पर खोज की जाती है। इसमें दो पदों के मध्य और (AND), अथवा (OR), तथा नहीं (NOT) लगा कर खोज की जाती है। और (AND) लगाकर दो या अधिक पदो को जोड़ कर खोज की जाती है। इस प्रकार उन सभी प्रलेखो में सूचना खोजी जा सकती है जिनमें ये पद उपलब्ध हो। अथवा (OR) दो या अधिक पदों के मध्य में लगाया जाता है, परन्तु खोज एक ही पद में की जाती है। इसमें यह सुविधा

मिलती है कि इस पद में अन्यथा दूसरे पद में खोज की जा सकती है। नहीं (NOT) से खोजकर्ता को यह सुविधा मिलती है कि वह वे पद बताये जिनको छोडकर खोज करनी है।

(स) शब्द के एक भाग के द्वारा (search with truncated word): इस सुविधा के द्वारा उन सभी शब्दों से एक साथ सूचना खोजी जा सकती है जिनका मूल एक हो। विभिन्न खोज पद्धतियों में शब्द को दायें, बायें या मध्य भाग को काट छांट करने की सुविधा होती है और इस कटे हुये भाग से खोज की जा सकती है।

(द) शब्दों की समीपता के अनुसार खोज (proximity search): इसके द्वारा खोजकर्ता को यह सुविधा प्रदान की जाती है कि वह यह बताये कि (1) दो पद साथ आयें, (2) या दो पदों के मध्य अन्य शब्द आयें या, (3) खोज शब्द एक पैरा के मध्य आयें, चाहे उनके मध्य कोई भी शब्द हो।

(य) विशिष्ट अनुच्छेद के अन्तर्गत खोज (field specific search) : यह सुविधा खोजकर्ता को बताती है कि खोज डेटाबेस के किसी भी एक अथवा सभी अनुच्छेदों में एक ही समय में की जा सकती है।

(र) सीमाओं में खोज (limiting search): यहां पर खोज करने से पहले कुछ सीमाएं तय की जाती है। जैसे प्रकाशन का वर्ष, सूचना स्त्रोत की श्रेणी। इन सीमाओं के अनुसार ही इस खोज के द्वारा सूचना प्राप्त की जाती है।

(ल) रेंज खोज (range search): इसमें सूचना का विस्तार तय करना होता है। यह विशेषतया आंकड़ों पर आधारित डेटाबेस की खोज करने में उपयोगी होती है। उदहारणार्थ किसी विशेष अथवा विशिष्ट प्रकाशन वर्षों के प्रलेखों की खोज रेंज खोज कहलाती है।

उपरोक्त वर्णित सभी खोज विकल्प खोज प्रक्रिया को उन्नत बनाते हैं –

(2) अनुक्रमणिका का प्रदर्शन (display of index): इलैक्ट्रोनिक डेटाबेस में पदों को उनके प्रयुक्त संदर्भ में दर्शाया जाता है। यहां पर डेटाबेस की मुख्य अनुक्रमणिका, जिसे विपर्यस्त अनुक्रमणिका (inverted index) कहा जाता है, में सभी पदो को जिनसे खोज की जा सकती है को वर्णक्रमानुसार व्यवस्थित किया जाता है। इस सुविधा के कारण एक पद का उसके पूर्व व पश्चात पद

के साथ संबंध का पता लगाया जा सकता है। इसके अतिरिक्त यह भी पता चल जाता है कि डेटाबेस में कितने प्रलेख हैं जिनमें इस पद की सूचना उपलब्ध है। इस विशेषता के कारण उन सभी पदों का पता लगाया जाता है जो एक विचार को प्रदर्शित करते हैं तथा वे पद जो आपस में समीप है।

(3) उन्नत गति (improved speed) : इलेक्ट्रोनिक डेटाबेस में खोज की गति, मुद्रित स्त्रोतों की तुलना में काफी अधिक होती है। इसमें पाठ्य सामग्री की ग्रंथ परक जानकारी भी हाथ से नहीं लिखनी पड़ती है। यहां प्रलेखों की सूची काफी जल्दी बनाई जा सकती है, या उसे अपने पर्सनल कम्प्यूटर पर डाउन लोड (download) भी किया जा सकता है।

कम्प्यूटर आधारित खोज पद्धति के मुख्य पद : (basic steps for computer – based searching) जैसा पहले वर्णित किया जा चुका है कि आन लाइन खोज के लिये इलेक्ट्रोनिक डेटा बेस विभिन्न प्रारूपों में उपलब्ध है, जैसे सी डी रोम (CD Rom), व्यवसायिक आन लाइन खोज सेवा प्रदाता (जैसे DIALOG) (commerical on line search provider), और वेब पर। मुद्रित प्रलेखों की तुलना में इलेक्ट्रोनिक डेटाबेसों में खोज विकल्प ज्यादा होते हैं, खोज द्रुत गति से की जा सकती है तथा इनमें सूचना बार बार अद्यतन होती है। उदाहरणार्थ अलरिच पीरियोडिकल्स डायरेक्ट्री (Ulrich's periodicals' directory) मुद्रित संस्करण में सूचना एक वर्ष में, सी.डी. रोम (CD Rom version) में सूचना तीन माह में तथा वेब प्रारूप में सूचना सप्ताह में अद्यतन की जाती है। इसके अतिरिक्त इलेक्ट्रोनिक डेटाबेस के वेब (web version) प्रारूप में कुछ अधिक खोज सुविधाएं उपलब्ध होती है। साथ ही इसमें प्रस्तुत सूचना स्त्रोत के अन्य सूचना स्त्रोतों से संबंध स्थापित करने वाले पद होते है जिन्हें लिंक (link) कहते हैं। उदाहरणार्थ अलरिच पीरियोडिकलस डायरेक्ट्री (Ulrich's periodicals' directory) के वेब प्रारूप (web version) में खोज के लिये स्वच्छंद ग्रंथावलोकन अनुक्रमणिकाएँ (browse indexes) जैसे (भाषा तथा प्रकाशन अवधि) होती हैं, परन्तु ये सुविधाएं सी डी रोम या मुद्रित प्रारूप में नहीं होती है। इसके अतिरिक्त वेब प्रारूप उपभोक्ता का वैकल्पिक पत्रिकाओं तथा वैकल्पिक प्रारूपों से संबंध भी स्थापित करते हैं। इसमें वैकल्पिक पत्रिकाओं तथा प्रकाशनों के इलेक्ट्रोनिक मेल का

पता भी दिया होता है तथा उपभोक्ता को पत्रिकाओं की कुछ सूचना देते है जैसे सूची, लेखों का सार, फुल टैक्सट जर्नल (full text journal) आदि। यह उपयोग के आंकड़े भी प्रदान करता है।

इलेक्ट्रोनिक डेटाबेस में जो मुख्य खोज प्रक्रियाएँ की जाती है वे एक माध्यम से दूसरे माध्यम में भिन्न होती है। प्रत्येक माध्यम अथवा सेवा प्रदाता के द्वारा प्रस्तुत खोज प्रक्रिया अपनी विशिष्ट पहचान लिये हुये होती है तथा इसमें अलग अलग खोज सुविधाएँ उपलब्ध होती हैं। अधिकतर आन लाइन सेवा प्रदाता (on line service providers) तथा सीडी रोम उत्पादक निःशुल्क ट्रेनिंग माड्यूल (free training modules) देते हैं जिनके द्वारा नवागुन्तक उपभोक्ता इन डेटाबेसो में से सूचना क्रमबद्ध तरीके से खोज सकता है। कुछ सी डी रोम उत्पादक अपने विभिन्न डेटाबेसों के उपयोग हेतु साझा मध्यस्थ सॉफ्टवेयर (common interface software) उपलब्ध करवाते हैं। यही आन लाइन डेटाबेसेस के संबंध में होता है। इसके अतिरिक्त आन लाइन खोज सेवा में कुछ दूसरे घटक भी होते हैं, जैसे डेटाबेस उत्पादक – जो खोज करने के लिये डेटाबेस उपलब्ध करवाते हैं, खोज सेवा प्रदाता जो सूचना खोजने के लिये सॉफ्टवेयर उपलब्ध करवाते हैं, तथा दूरसंचार की लाइन जो खोजकर्ता, खोज सेवा प्रदाता तथा डेटाबेस के मध्य संबंध स्थापित करती है।

सीडी रोम में भी एक पर्सनल कम्प्यूटर, एक खोज सॉफ्टवेयर आदि की आवश्यकता पड़ती है।

किसी भी विषय पर सूचना खोजने के लिये सबसे प्रथम उपभोक्ता को उस डेटाबेस की सभी विशेषताओं से परिचित होना आवश्यक है। चाहे सी डी रोम डेटाबेस में सूचना खोजनी हो या आन लाइन डेटाबेस में से, एक निश्चित पद्धति काम में लाई जाती है। इस खोज पद्धति के निम्नलिखित पद होते हैं –

1 विषय को समझना (understanding in subject)
2 विषयक्षेत्र, व्यापकता, अवधि का निर्णय (decision on subject area, scope and period)
3 आनलाइन सेवा के लिये इंटरनेट पहुंच का प्रबंध करना (arrange internet access to on line search service)

4 आनलाइन सेवा प्रदाता अथवा उत्पादक के पते पर पहुंच स्थापित करना (log on to the on line search service provider)

5 उपयुक्त डेटाबेस का चयन (select the appropriate data base)

6 विषय शीर्षकों की श्रंखला का निरूपण (formulate the search expression)

7 खोजे गये प्रलेखों की ग्रंथपरक सूचना के प्रदर्शन के लिये उपयुक्त प्रारूप का चयन (select the appropriate format for display of retrieved records)

8 आवश्यक हो तो विषय शीर्षकों की श्रृंखला व प्रश्न का पुनः निरूपण (reformulate the query and search expression if necessary)

9 खोजी गई सूचना की प्राप्ति के लिये उपयुक्त माध्यम का चयन (select the mode of delivery)

प्रथम एवं द्वितीय पद के अन्तर्गत कार्य वैसे ही किये जाते हैं जैसे कि पारम्परिक खोज पद्धिति में किये जाते हैं। पद तीन एवं चार के कार्य सी डी रोम डेटाबेस की खोज करते समय आवश्यक नहीं होते हैं। इनकी आवश्यकता आन लाइन खोज में पड़ती है।

तृतीय पद – इसमें सबसे प्रथम किसी इंटरनेट सेवा प्रदाता से सुविधा प्राप्त करनी पड़ती है। जैसे भारत संचार निगम लिमिटेड या सत्यम से नेट की सुविधा प्राप्त की जाती है। नेट की सुविधा कई स्तर पर उपलब्ध होती है जैसे डायल आप सुविधा (dial-up connection), ब्रॉड बैंड सुविधा (broad band facility), अथवा पट्टे पर ली (leased telephone line) गई टेलिफोन लाइन आदि। इसके पश्चात किसी व्यवसायिक सेवा प्रदाता अथवा डेटाबेस उत्पादक के पास सेवा प्राप्त करने के लिये पंजीकरण करवाना पड़ता है। पंजीकरण प्रक्रिया में वे उपभोक्ता को उपभोक्ता परिचय पद (user ID) तथा संकेत शब्द (password) देते हैं, जिससे डेटाबेस खोजने का अधिकार मिल जाता है। यह कार्य करना, वास्तविक खोज करने से पहले करना आवश्यक है।

चतुर्थ पद - आन लाइन सेवा प्रदाता अथवा उत्पादक के पते पर पहुंच स्थापित करना (log on to the on line service provider) : यह

कार्य आन लाइन सेवा प्रदाता के वेब मध्यस्थ सॉफ्टवेयर के माध्यम से किया जाता है। इस पद में आन लाइन सेवा के लियें उपभोक्ता को प्रदाता अथवा उत्पादक के वेब पते की सूचना होनी चाहिये।

पांचवाँ पद – उपयुक्त डेटाबेस का चयन (**select the appropriate database**) : इस स्तर पर खोज करने के लिये उपयुक्त डेटाबेसों का चयन करना पड़ता है। बहुत सी डेटाबेसों में कुछ सुविधाएं उपलब्ध होती हैं जैसे उपभोक्ता को डेटाबेसों का अवलोकन (**browse**) करने की सुविधा – ताकि उपभोक्ता उपयुक्त डेटाबेसों में से चयन कर सके। जैसे डायलाग (**DIALOG**) में यह सुविधा उपलब्ध है।

छठा पद – विषय शीर्षक की श्रंखला का निरूपण (**formulate search expression**): इस स्तर पर सही पदों या वाक्यांशों का चयन किया जाता है जिनकी सहायता से डेटाबेसों में से प्रलेखो या सूचना का चयन करते है। यदि आवश्यक हो तो सूचना खोजने में पुस्तकालयाध्यक्ष मध्यस्थ की भूमिका अदा करता है। वह उपभोक्ता का एक संक्षिप्त साक्षात्कार भी ले सकता है। इसमें वह सूचना की आवश्यकता, विषय क्षेत्र, भाषा आदि की जानकारी उपभोक्ता से एकत्रित करता है। इसके पश्चात मुख्य विषय शीर्षकों (**key words**) तथा उनके समानार्थक विषय शीर्षकों की सूची बनाई जाती है। कई व्यवसायिक उत्पादक अपनी स्वयं की मानक शब्दावली प्रस्तुत करते हैं तथा उन्हें आन लाइन उपलब्ध भी करवाते हैं। इससे विषय शीर्षकों की श्रृंखला बनाने में सहायता मिलती है। इसके अतिरिक्त यदि खोजकर्ता को डेटाबेस की प्रकृति (**nature**), अर्न्तवस्तु (**contents**), संरचना (**structure**), खोज के लिये उपलब्ध अनुच्छेद (**fields**), खोज सुविधाओं की उपलब्धता तथा उपयुक्त बूलियन तथा अन्य संयोजकों का ज्ञान हो तो विषय शीर्षकों की श्रृंखला बनाने में अत्याधिक सुविधा रहती है। प्रायः आन लाइन डेटाबेसों में दो प्रकार के खोज स्तर होते हैं।

(1) नवागन्तुक खोजकताओं के लिये तथा (2) अभ्यस्त खोजकर्ताओं के लिये। नवागन्तुक खोजकर्ताओं के लिये ग्राफिक यूजर इंटरफेस (graphic user interface) तथा अभ्यस्त खोजकर्ताओं के लिये कमांड ड्रीवन इन्टरफेस (command driven interface) होता है। यहां पर खोजकर्ता को विभिन्न खोज कमांड (commands) का पता होना चाहिये। विषय शीर्षकों की श्रृंखला का निर्माण करने के बाद खोज संतोषप्रद होती है।

सातवां पद – खोजे गये प्रलेखों के प्रदर्शन के लिये उपयुक्त प्रारूप का चयन (select the appropriate format): जब ऑन लाइन खोज प्रणाली में सही निर्देश (commands) उपभोक्ता के द्वारा दे दिये जाते हैं तो खोजे गये प्रलेखों को वर्णक्रमानुसार दर्शाया जाता है। इन प्रलेखों का अवलोकन करने के लिये यह भी बताना आवश्यक होता है कि केवल ग्रंथपरक विवरण चाहिये या पूर्ण मूल पाठ (bibliographical or full text)। सी डी रोम खोज में पूर्ण मूल पाठ को प्रदर्शित करने में अधिक लागत नहीं आती है परन्तु ऑन लाइन खोज सेवा में लागत अधिक आती है।

आठवां पद – आवश्यक हो तो विषय का पुनः निरूपण (formulate search expression if necessary): यदि खोज के परिणाम संतोषप्रद नहीं हों तो विषय शीर्षकों की श्रृंखला को पुनः निरूपित कर सकते हैं। आन लाइन खोज बार–बार करने वाली प्रक्रिया है। इसमें खोजकर्ता कई खोज करता है। परिणामों का तुलनात्मक अध्ययन करता है, खोज वाक्यांशों को संशोधित करता है तथा नये प्रकार से खोज कर सकता है ताकि अच्छे परिणाम प्राप्त हों। इसमें खोज को उन्नत करने के लिये कई खोज विकल्पों को काम में लाया जाता है जैसे बूलियन खोज, शब्द के एक भाग से खोज (truncation), शब्दों की समीपता के अनुसार खोज (proximity search), आदि का चयन।

नवां पद – खोजी गई सूचना के वितरण का माध्यमः (select the mode of delivery): इस पद में उपभोक्ता खोजी गई सूचना दो माध्यम से प्राप्त कर सकता है (1) सूचना की प्रति अपने पर्सनल कम्प्यूटर पर हस्तान्तरित करके, तथा (2) आफ लाइन मुद्रित प्रति का आदेश देकर।

खोज में असफलता – खोज के परिणाम आदि संतोषप्रद नहीं होते हैं तो उसका मुख्य कारण अनुक्रमणिकरण पद्धतियों की शब्दावली का पूर्ण ज्ञान नहीं होना होता है। प्रत्येक डेटाबेस की अपनी शब्दावली होती है जिसका अच्छा ज्ञान खोजकर्ता को होना चाहिये। जो अनुक्रमणिकाएं डेटाबेस के साथ बनाई जाती हैं, उसमें समानार्थक पदों को सम्मिलित किया जाता है। अतएव मानक शब्दावली को अद्यतन बनाये रखना चाहिये। इन परिस्थितियों में खोजकर्ता को अनुभवी पुस्तकालयाध्यक्ष का सहयोग लेना चहिये।

पारम्परिक खोज या आन लाइन खोज

पारम्परिक खोज निम्नलिखित परिस्थितियों में करनी चाहिए –

1 – विषय पर एक या दो प्रलेखो की आवश्यकता हो।

2 – किसी वृहत् विषय पर खोज करनी हो।

3 – किसी विषय की सम्पूर्ण परन्तु सरसरी जानकारी चाहिए हो।

4 – एक ही अनुक्रमाणिका से खोज करनी हो।

ऑनलाइन खोज प्रणाली निम्नलिखित परिस्थितियों में करनी चाहिये –

1. किसी विषय पर पिछले कई वर्षों में प्रकाशित सूचना स्त्रोत में से व्यापक खोज करनी हो।
2. सूचना खोजने के लिये कई डेटाबेस काम में लाने हों।
3. जब सूचना की खोज किसी विषय पर बहुत विशिष्ट प्रकृति की हो।

सारांश

संक्षेप में कह सकते हैं कि हमने शोध एवं विकास कार्यो में साहित्यिक खोज की महत्ता एव आवश्यकता का वर्णन किया है। यह भी बताया है कि साहित्यिक खोज एवं ग्रंथ सूची के संकलन में क्या होता है। पारम्परिक खोज एवं कम्पूटर आधारित साहित्यिक खोज के मुख्य पद क्या हैं। कम्प्यूटर आधारित खोज प्रक्रिया का विवरण भी दिया है। ग्रंथ सूची का संकलन करने में कौन–कौन से तृतीयक, द्वितीयक, एवं प्राथमिक सूचना स्त्रोतों का अवलोकन किया जायगा, इसका वर्णन भी किया है।

पाठ्यग्रंथ सूची

1 Choudhary, G.G. and Choudhary, Sudatta (2001). Searching CD-ROM and online information sources. London. Library Association Publishing.

2 Katz, William A. (1982). Introduction to reference work. Ed 4. New York, McGraw Hill. 2 vols.

3 Krishan, Kumar (1978). Reference service. Ed 2. New Delhi, Vikas Publishing House.

4 Psytherch, Roy (1987). Sources of information in librarianship and information science. Ed 2. England Gower Publishing Company, pp. 9-20.

5 Sen, B.K. (1994). Literature searches and bibliographies. In MLIS-04. Block-02 Unit 5. New Delhi : Indira Gandhi National Open University.

6 Taylor, R.S. (1962). Process of asking questions. American Documentation. 13(4): 391 - 396.

सूचना खोज प्रवृति एवं इनके आदर्शों पर सूचना प्रोद्योगिकी का प्रभाव
(Impact of Information Technology on Information Seeking Behaviour and its Models)

टी०डी० तिलवानी

वरिष्ठ सहायक आचार्य एवं विभागाध्यक्ष, ग्रन्थालय एवं सूचना विज्ञान विभाग, मोहनलाल सुखाड़िया विश्वविद्यालय, उदयपुर,

सार (Abstract)

प्रस्तुत लेख में सूचना खोज प्रवृति की अवधारणा को परिभाषित करते हुए इसके विभिन्न सामान्य घटकों का उल्लेख किया गया है। ग्रन्थालय विज्ञानियों द्वारा प्रस्तुत आई०एस०बी० के विभिन्न आदर्शों (मॉडलो) की चर्चा की गयी है। साथ ही आधुनिक सूचना युग में सूचना प्रोद्योगिकी के आगमन एवं इसके आई०एस०बी० पर पड़ने वाले प्रभाव पर भी प्रकाश डाला गया है। अन्त में ग्रन्थालय एवं सूचना तंत्र द्वारा उपयोगकर्ताओं का गहन अध्ययन करके उनकी सूचना आवश्कताओं, सूचना के प्रति व्यवहार तथा प्राथमिकताओं आदि का सही सही आकलन करके योजनाबद्ध तरीके से सूचना सेवाओं को अभिकल्पित करने का सुझाव दिया गया है।

1. परिचय (Introduction)

सूचना किसी राष्ट्र का एक महत्त्वपूर्ण संसाधन (Resources) हैं। व्यक्तिगत, प्रबंधकीय अथवा शासकीय स्तर पर महत्त्वपूर्ण निर्णय लेने हेतु इसे एक अपरिहार्य सामग्री माना गया है। भारत जैसे किसी भी विकासशील देश के सामाजिक, आर्थिक एवं सांस्कृतिक विकास के

लिये यह वास्तव में एक आवश्यक तत्व है। यह एक सर्वस्वीकृत तथ्य है कि जो देश सूचना के क्षेत्र में अधिक सम्पन्न है वही देश सामाजिक एवं आर्थिक क्षेत्र में भी सर्वसम्पन्न है।[1]

औद्योगिक क्रान्ति के बाद आज विश्व सूचना क्रान्ति (Information Technology) की ओर बढ़ रहा है। विभिन्न क्षेत्रों के बौद्धिक क्रियाकलापों में दिन प्रति दिन सूचना पर निर्भरता बढ़ती जा रही है। प्रौद्योगिक उन्नति (Technological Advances) ने सूचना को ऊर्जा एवं शक्ति का एक नया आधारभूत स्त्रोत बना दिया है। सूचना एक शक्ति है जो किसी देश के विकास एवं प्रगति में आवश्यक भूमिका का निर्वहन करती है। इसलिये यह आवश्यक है कि सभी प्रकार की सूचनाओं का अर्जन करके उन्हें व्यवस्थित कर सही उपयोगकर्ताओं तक पहुंचाया जाय जिससे उनका अधिकतम उपयोग हो सके। ऐसा करने के लिये उपयोगकर्ताओं की सूचना सम्बन्धी आवश्यकताओं का सही सही आंकलन करना होगा। क्योंकि सूचना सम्बन्धी क्रियाकलापों के लिये यही एक प्राथमिक आधार है। पाठकों की सूचना आवश्यकताओं का पूर्व निर्धारण करना किसी भी सूचना प्रणाली में, प्रभावशाली सूचना सेवा का प्रावधान करने के लिये नितान्त आवश्यक है। क्योंकि विभिन्न पाठकों की सूचना आवश्यकताएँ भिन्न–भिन्न हो सकती हैं, अतः सावधानी पूर्वक उनकी सूचना आवश्यकताओं का आंकलन करना जरूरी है। इसी प्रसंग में उपयोगकर्ताओं की सूचना प्रवृति (Information Behaviour) सूचना खोज प्रवृति (Information Seeking Behaviour-ISB) तथा सूचना आवश्यकताओं की प्रकृति एवं प्रकार का अध्ययन करना आवश्यक है। जिससे सूचनाओं के संग्रहण (Storage), संगठन (Organisation) एवं प्रसार (Dissemination) को प्रभावशाली कौशल द्वारा तुरन्त विकसित किया जा सके।

सूचना खोज प्रवृति (ISB) के विभिन्न आदर्शों की चर्चा करने से पहले इस अवधारणा का अर्थ एवं परिभाषा को जानना आवश्यक है। इनका उल्लेख आगामी बिन्दु में किया गया है।

2. सूचना खोज प्रवृति का अर्थ (Meaning of ISB)

विभिन्न लेखकों एवं अनुसंधानकर्ताओं ने अपने अध्ययन में सूचना खोज प्रवृति (Information Seeking Behaviour - ISB) पद का प्रयोग अन्य सम्बद्ध पदों के साथ पर्याय स्वरूप में किया है। जैसे – सूचना खोज प्रतिरूप (Information Seeking Pattern - ISP),

सूचना एकत्रण प्रवृति (Information Gathering Habit), इत्यादि। ये पद पाठकों द्वारा अपने उद्देश्यों की पूर्ति हेतु विभिन्न सूचना माध्यमों (Information Channels) से आवश्यक सूचना प्राप्त करने के प्रयासों पर बल देते हैं। इस प्रकार इन पदों को पूर्व एवं वर्तमान के अध्ययनों में एक दूसरे के स्थान पर प्रयुक्त किया गया है।

श्रीधर[2] के अनुसार जब अनुसंधानकर्ता को सूचना की आवश्यकता होती है तो सर्वप्रथम वह वांछित सूचना की खोज या अनुयोग (Seeking) करता है और इस अनुयोग या खोज से पहले वह सूचना एकत्रण (Information Gathering) करता है, और कई बार यही उपक्रम अनुयोग को प्रकट करता है। अतः सूचना खोज अथवा अनुयोग से अभिप्राय उपयोगकर्त्ता (User), सूचना (Information), एवं तंत्र (System) में आपसी सम्बन्ध स्थापित करना है ताकि बेहतर परिणाम प्राप्त हो सके।

चिंग–चिह चेन[3] के मतानुसार सूचना खोज प्रवृति (ISB) वे पथ हैं जिन पर चल कर उपयोगकर्ता अपनी आवश्यकता का समाधान करने का प्रयास करता है।

अतः सूचना खोज प्रवृति से तात्पर्य उन क्रियाओं एवं कौशल (Actions and Strategies) से हैं जिन के परिणामस्वरूप पृथक ज्ञान तत्वों (Discrete Knowledge Elements) का पता लग सके। इसका सम्बन्ध निम्नांकित तीन मूलभूत संसाधनों के एकीकृत उपयोग (Integrative Utilisation) से है –

– व्यक्ति (People)

– सूचना (Information)

– तंत्र (System)

ऐसी प्रवृत्ति जिससे उच्चतम सूचना संतुष्टि (Highest Information Satisfaction) की अनुभूति हो, को सर्वश्रेष्ठ प्रवृति कहा जा सकता है।

3. सूचना खोज प्रवृत्ति के आदर्श (Models for Information Seeking Behaviour)

विभिन्न अनुसंधानकर्ताओं ने समय–समय पर सूचना खोज प्रवृति (ISB) के लिए कई आदर्श (Models) प्रस्तुत किये हैं। किसी सूचना प्रणाली (Information System) के साथ पाठकों के परस्पर सम्बन्धों

का परीक्षण करने हेतु ये आदर्श बहुत सहायक होते हैं। कुछ महत्वपूर्ण एवं प्रभावकारी आदर्शों का उल्लेख निम्न प्रकार है –

3.1 मार्कयोनिनी एवं श्नाइडरमेन का सूचना खोज आदर्श (Marchionini and Shneiderman's Model for Information Seeking)

मार्कयोनिनी एवं श्नाइडरमेन[4] (Marchionini and Shneiderman) ने सूचना खोज की रूपरेखा (Framework) के अन्तर्गत निम्नांकित पांच समीक्षात्मक घटकों (Critical Components) एवं उनके अभिलक्षणों (Characteristics) की पहचान की है –

– उपयोग (Use)

– सैटिंग्स (Settings)

– टास्क डोमेन (Task Domain)

– खोज प्रणाली (Search System)

– निष्कर्ष (Outcome)

इस फ्रेमवर्क में डिजाइनरों ने प्रमुख रूप से चर राशि (Variables) पर बल दिया है जो कि किसी तंत्र (System) की उपादेयता (Utility) एवं उपयोगिता (Usability) को प्रभावित करता है। उन्होंने इन पांचों घटकों के संयोजन से ही इस आदर्श का सृजन किया है। उनके अनुसार उपयोगकर्ता अपने मानसिक आदर्शों (Mental Models) का विकास हाइपरमिडिया तंत्रों (Hypermedia Systems) से विभिन्न कारकों (Factors) जैसे प्रशिक्षण, कंप्यूटर अनुभव, एवं नियमावलियों के अध्ययन के आधार पर करता है। इस आदर्श की गति (Speed) एवं शुद्धता (Accuracy) चर राशियों जैसे–कंप्यूटर पूर्वानुभव, उपयोग की आवृति (Frequeny) एवं टास्क डोमेन की जटिलता (Complexity) के परस्पर संबंध पर निर्भर करती है।

3.2 मार्कयोनिनी का आदर्श (Marchionini's Model)

मार्कयोनिनी[5] के आदर्शानुसार सूचना खोज अथवा अनुयोग (IS) के समस्या के समाधान के रूप में लेना होगा। इसमें वांछित सूचना (Sought Information) एवं अन्वेषण प्रक्रिया (Search Process) जो कि क्रमशः समस्या (Problem) एवं समाधान पथ (Solution Path)

को प्रकट करते हैं, सरल या जटिल हो सकते हैं। सूचना खोज के लिये उन्होंने पांच प्रक्रियाओं की पहचान की है। ये निम्नलिखित है।

- समस्या की परिभाषा (Defining Problem)
- अन्वेषण हेतु संसाधनों का चयन (Selecting the Resources for Search)
- समस्या की सुस्पष्टता अन्वेषण कौशल के रूप में (Artification of Problem in Terms of Search Strategy)
- सुस्पष्ट समस्या के परिणामों का परीक्षण (Examining the Results of Articultaed Problem), तथा
- उपयोगी स्वरूप में अभीष्ट सूचना का निष्कर्ष (Extracting Desired Information in Useful; Form)

3.3 श्शू चिंग येंग आदर्श (Shu Ching Yang Model)

श्शू चिंग येंग[6] ने अपने आलेख में सूचना खोज के आदर्श को निम्नांकित पांच प्रक्रियाओं द्वारा प्रदर्शित किया है।

- सूचना के स्त्रोतों का चयन (Selecting Sources of Information)
- अन्वेषण निष्पादन (Executive the Search)
- समस्या की व्याख्या करना (Interpreting the Problem)
- प्रासंगिकता हेतु निर्णय (Judging the Relevance), एवं
- कायम रखना अथवा अस्वीकार करना (Retaining or Rejecting)

आई०एस० के आदर्श में इन प्रक्रियाओं को चित्र 1 में दर्शाया गया है।

3.4 चिंग चिह चेन का सूचना खोज प्रतिरूप के लिये आदर्श (Ching- Chih Chen's Model; of Information Seeking Pattern)

आई०एस०पी० हेतु चिग चिह चेन[7] ने एक बहुत ही उपयोगी मॉडल प्रस्तुत किया है। इनके मतानुसार आई०एस०पी० वे पथ है जिन पर चलकर उपयोगकर्ता अपनी आवश्यकता का समाधान करने का

प्रयास करता है। इस मॉडल को निम्नांकित छः चरणों में विभाजित किया गया है।

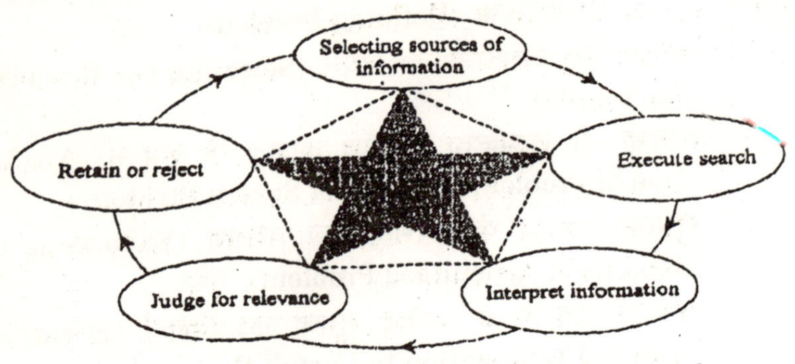

Fig. 1. Shu Ching Yang Infrmation Seeking Model

- उपयोगकर्ता की पृष्ठभूमि एवं अभिलक्षण (Background and Characteristics of a user)
- सूचना आवश्यकता की प्रकृति एवं प्रकार (Nature & Type of Information Need)
- सूचना प्रदाता के प्रकार एवं उपलब्धता (Type and Availabilityu of Information Providers)
- सूचना प्रदाता में किसी मांग का जवाब देने का सामर्थ्य (Information Providers Capability of responding to a Requent)
- सूचना प्रदाता एवं सूचना खोजकर्ता के मध्य किसी अवरोध का होना (Existence of Any Barrier between Information Provider and Information Seeker)
- सूचना प्रदाता द्वारा प्रत्युतर में दी गयी सूचना से उपयोगकर्ता की संतुष्टि की सीमा (Degree of Satisfaction perceived by Users with the Response of Information Providers)

इस फ्रेमवर्क में उपयोगकर्ता की पृष्ठभूमि एवं लक्षणों, सूचना आवश्यकताओं की प्रकृति एवं प्रकार, सूचना प्रदाता की सक्षमता, आई०एस०पी० के अवरोध (Barriers), उपभोक्ताओं की संतुष्टि की सीमा सम्बन्धी पहलुओं पर विशेष बल दिया गया है।

3.5 बेटस मॉडल (Bates Model)

बेटस[8] द्वारा प्रस्तावित सूचना खोज का बेरीपिकिंग आदर्श (Baerrypicking Model) सूचना पुनः प्राप्ति के उत्कृष्ट आदर्श से विषमता लिये है। इसकी संरचना के अन्तर्गत निम्नांकित चार बिन्दुओं का समावेश है –

– पुनरावृति समस्या की विकसित प्रकृति (Iterative, Evolving Nature of Problem)

– गतिशील, संशोधित अन्वेषण प्रश्न (Dynamic, Modified Search Query)

– बेरीपिकिंग अन्वेषण व्यवहार (Berrypicking Search Pattern) एवं

– बहुसंसाधनों से अन्वेषण कौशल (Search Strategy drawn from Multiple Resources)

यह एक शक्तिशाली मॉडल इस संदर्भ में है कि इसका उपयोग स्थिर एवं एकांकी क्वेरी की अपेक्षा गतिशील एवं संशोधित अन्वेषण के लिये किया जा सकता है। तथापि एक बार समस्या के निर्धारण की अपेक्षा यह मॉडल उसे बार बार विकसित करने का अवसर प्रदान करता है। यहां अन्वेषण से तात्पर्य यह है कि प्रत्येक उपयोगकर्ता के लिये ग्रंथावली अथवा सूचना अधिकारी आवश्यक सूचना या प्रलेख की खोज करके उन्हें सामग्री प्रदान करता है।

उपयोगकर्ता द्वारा उक्त सामग्री के उपयोग करने एवं पुनः अन्य सूचना की आवश्यकता होने पर खोज की इस प्रक्रिया को दोहराया जाता है। सूचना की प्रकृति बैरीपिकिंग पैटर्न (Berrypicking Pattern) पर आधारित होती है, जिससे सूचना की पुनः प्राप्ति एक सैट की अपेक्षा बिटस या टुकड़ों के रूप में एकत्रित की जाती है। इस फ्रेमवर्क में अन्वेषण की विकसित पुनरावृति एवं बहुसंसाधनों के उपयोग पर भी विशेष जोर दिया गया है।

3.6 गिरजा कुमार का आई०एस०बी० मॉडल (Girija Kumar's Model of ISB)

गिरजा कुमार[9] द्वारा प्रदत इस मॉडल का मुख्य सरोकार इस बात से है कि (1) किसे किस प्रकार की सूचना क्यों आवश्यकता है (2)

कैसे सूचना की प्राप्ति, उसका मूल्यांकन एवं उपयोग किया जाए (3) कैसे यूजर की सूचना का पता लगाया जाए एवं उन्हें संतुष्ट किया जाय। उनके अनुसार आई०एस०बी० के अन्तर्गत निम्नांकित प्रक्रियाएं होती है –

– उद्देश्य की पहचान (Indentifying Objective)
– आवश्यकता को परिभाषित करना (Defining Need)
– सूचना प्रणाली अभिगम (Accessing Information System)
– सूचना स्रोतों का गठन करना (Establishing Sources of Information)
– सूचना संप्राप्ति (Information Acquisition)
– सूचना उपयोग (Use of Information)
– संतोष / असंतोष (Satisfaction/Dissatisfaction)

इन चरणों (Stages) को चित्र 2 में प्रदर्शित किया गया है।

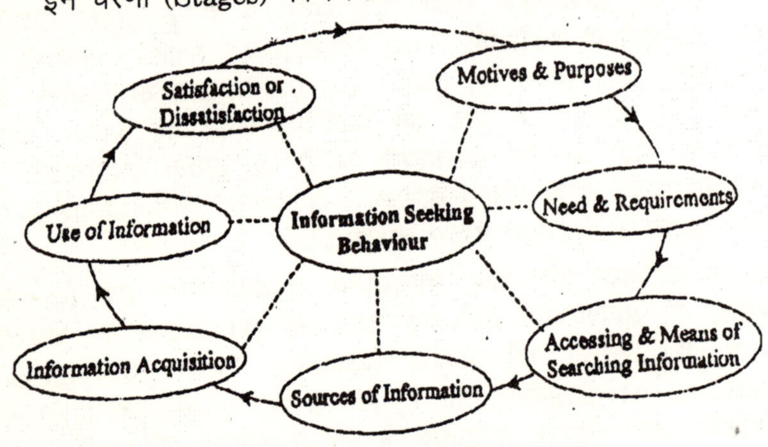

Fig. 2. Girija Kumar's Models of ISB.

इस धारणा के अनुसार उपयोक्ता को किन्हीं उद्देश्यों अथवा कार्यो की पूर्ति हेतु ही सूचना की आवश्यकता होती है। इन आवश्यकताओं को संतुष्ट करने के लिये उपयोक्ता कई रास्ते एवं अभिगमों को अपनाकर सूचना स्रोतों का अन्वेषण अथवा खोज करता है। जैसा कि इस मॉडल के तीसरे एवं चौथे चरण में बतलाया गया है। तदुपरांत वे आवश्यक सूचनाओं का अधिग्रहण (Acquisition) नियमित अथवा अस्थायी रूप से इन स्रोतों से करने की कोशिश करता है। सूचना

अधिग्रहण की इस प्रक्रिया के दौरान वह विभिन्न सूचना स्रोतों का उपयोग करता है। साथ ही इनका मिलान वह अपने पूर्वनिर्धारित उद्देश्यों से भी करता है। इस प्रकार वह अपने उद्देश्यों एवं आवश्यकताओं के अनुरूप संतोष अथवा असंतोष की अनुभूति करता है।

3.7 एलिस का आई०एस०पी० मॉडल (Ellis Model of ISP)

सामाजिक विज्ञानियों के सूचना खोज व्यवहार (ISP) से एलिस[10] ने छह सजातीय विशेषताओं को प्रकट किया है। जिन्हें उपयोक्ता के प्रवृति मॉडल हेतु सूचना पुनः प्राप्ति पद्धति (Information Retrieval Systme) के अभिकल्पन (Design) के लिये प्रयोग किया जा सकता है।[11]

ये छः प्रमुख विशेषताएँ अथवा प्रक्रियाएँ निम्न प्रकार है –

– प्रारम्भ (Starting)

– श्रंखलाबद्ध करना (Chaining)

– अवलोकन (Browsing)

– अन्तर बताना (Differentiating)

– परिवीषण करना (Monitoring)

– सारकरण (Extracting)

सामाजिक विज्ञानियों की सूचना प्रवृति को इस मॉडल द्वारा टेस्ट करने के बाद, एलिस ने इस मॉडल को भौतिक विज्ञान एवं रसायन विज्ञान से संबद्ध विज्ञानियों पर प्रयोग किया। इस प्रशिक्षण में उन्होंने यह पाया कि मूल आदर्श (Original Model) में जो कि सामाजिक विज्ञानियों के लिये प्रस्तावित (Proposed) है, उसमें बहुत अल्प संशोधन के उपरान्त इसे अन्य क्षेत्रों जैसे फिजिक्स एवं केमिस्ट्री से जुड़े लोगों की सूचना प्रवृति का भी अध्ययन करने हेतु लागू किया जा सकता है।

3.8 विल्सन का सूचना खोज प्रवृति मॉडल (Wilson's Model of Information Seeking Behaviour)

विल्सन[12] द्वारा विकसित सूचना प्रवृति के सामान्य मॉडल से सूचना खोज प्रवृति को परिभाषित किया जा सकता है। उनके अनुसार

इस मॉडल में कम से कम निम्नांकित तीन तत्व का समावेष आवश्यक है।

– "सूचना आवश्यकता एवं इसके कारक (Information Need and its drivers)
– सूचना बोध से संबद्ध व्यक्तिगत प्रत्युत्तर को प्रभावित करने वाले कारक (Factors that affect the Individuals Response to the Perception of Need)
– प्रत्युत्तर में समाहित क्रियाएं या प्रतिक्रियाएं (Processes or Actions involved in that Response)"[13]

इस फ्रेमवर्क में विल्सन ने स्पष्ट रूप से यह कहा है कि जब यूजर सूचना आवश्यकता का अनुभव करे उस समय उसकी सेवक भाव से उचित सहायता की जाय। इसे उपयोक्ता की सोच के संदर्भ में समझना चाहिए। तथा उसे उचित प्रत्युत्तर देने के हर संभव प्रयास उपयोक्ता को सार गर्भित आवश्यकताओं से मिलान करते हुए किये जाने चाहिये।

3.9 गुथराई एवं ड्रेहर का सूचना खोज आदर्श (Guthrie and Dreher's Model of IS)

गुथराई एवं ड्रेहर[14] द्वारा प्रस्तावित बोध प्रक्रिया आदर्श (Cognitive Processing Model) का संबन्ध खोजकर्ता द्वारा प्रलेखों से सूचना प्राप्ति के लेखे से है। इस मॉडल के निम्नांकित पांच घटक है।

– उद्देश्य तय करना (Goal Formation)
– श्रेणी करना (Category Selection)
– सूचना सार (Information Extraction)
– एकत्रीकरण (Integration)
– पुनरावृति (Recycling)

कोगनिशन प्रक्रिया[15] का सम्बन्ध मानसिक प्रक्रिया द्वारा प्राप्त उस ज्ञान से है जिसका सरोकार ज्ञान बोध, अन्तर्ज्ञान एवं तर्कशक्ति जैसे तत्वों से है। इस फ्रेमवर्क के घटक स्वतः स्पष्टीकृत है अतः इनकी विवेचना की आवश्यकता नहीं है।

3.10 टेलर का सूचना खोज प्रवृति आदर्श (Taylor's Model of ISB)

टेलर[16] द्वारा प्रतिपादित सूचना प्रवृति की परिभाषा के अनुसार यह सूचना उपयोग परिवेश (Information Use Environment) के कुछ तत्वों का उत्पाद (Product) है। इस मॉडल के तत्व इस प्रकार है।

- परिवेश में कार्यरत व्यक्ति (The peole Operates in an Environment)
- समस्याओं के प्रकार एवं उनकी संरचना (The Kinds and Structure of the Problems)
- विशिष्ट परिवेश में प्रतिबन्ध एवं अवसर (The Constraints and Opportunities of a Typical Environment)
- समस्याओं के क्या समाधान अथवा प्रस्ताव हैं तथा सूचना को उसके संदर्भ में कैसे उपयोगी एवं मूल्यवान बनाया जाय (What constituties a Solution of Resolution of Problem and What Makes an Information Useful and Valuable in their Contexts)

उनके मतानुसार विभिन्न व्यक्तियों के समूहों की सूचना प्रवृतियां भिन्न–भिन्न होती है।

3.11 कूलथायू का सूचना खोज आदर्श (Kuhlthau's Model of Information Seeking)

कुलथायू[17] का प्रस्तावित सूचना खोज का आदर्श ज्ञानोपार्जन के सिद्धान्तों (Learning Theories) के रचनात्मक फ्रेमवर्क (Constructive Framework) पर आधारित है। उनके अनुसार सूचना अन्वेषण ज्ञानोपार्जन की एक जटिल प्रक्रिया है, जो क्रमबद्ध चरणों की श्रृंखला पर आधारित है। प्रत्येक चरण में नियत कार्यों को सम्पन्न करते हुए इसे उचित प्रक्रिया से होकर अगली तर्क संगत कड़ी तक पहुचाया जाता है।

उनके द्वारा सूचना खोज को निम्न छः कड़िया द्वारा प्रदर्शित किया जा सकता है।

- प्रारंभ (Initiation)
- चयन (Selection)

– अन्वेषण (Exploration)

– निरूपण (Formumation)

– सकलन (Collection)

– प्रस्तुतीकरण (Presentation)

उनके अनुसार शुद्ध एव सम्पूर्ण ज्ञानोपार्जन प्रक्रिया में तीन अनुभवजनिक बातों का होना आवश्यक है। ये हैं –

(1) अन्वेषण की भौतिक क्रियाएं (Physical Actions of Seacrch)

(2) बुद्धि (Intellect)

(3) अन्वेषण का प्रभाव या अनुभव (Effect or Feeling of Search)

सूचना खोज प्रक्रिया के अन्तर्गत खोजकर्ता द्वारा विभिन्न चरणों पर सूचनाओं का संचय किया जाता है। लेकिन पांचवां चरण सर्वाधिक प्रभावकारी एवं दक्ष (Effective and Efficient) माना जा सकता है। क्योंकि यहां सूचना खोजकर्ता सूचनाओं के संकलन हेतु सूचना पुनः प्राप्ति पद्धति (Information Retrieval System) के अन्तर्गत परस्पर सम्पर्क में आता है।

उपरोक्त वर्णित चयनित मॉडल सूचना खोज की प्रवृति हेतु अत्यन्त उपयोगी माने गये हैं, क्योंकि प्रत्येक मॉडल में मुख्यतया सूचना, खोज की गतिशील प्रकृति के अलग–अलग पहलुओं पर विशेष जोर दिया गया है। ये मॉडल विश्लेषण के विभिन्न स्तरों पर उपयोगकर्ता द्वारा सूचना प्रणाली के साथ परस्पर सम्पर्क का परीक्षण करने में सहायक सिद्ध होते हैं।

4. सूचना प्रोद्योगिकी का आगमन (Emergence of Information Technology)

आधुनिक समय में प्रौद्योगिकी के क्षेत्र में हुए विभिन्न नवीन विकासों के फलस्वरूप किसी भी कार्य का निष्पादन करने में लगने वाले समय, श्रम एवं सूचनाएं व साधन प्रभावित होने से अछूते नहीं रहे हैं। विभिन्न प्रकार की प्रोद्योगिकीयों जैसे – कम्प्यूटर प्रोद्योगिकी, सूक्ष्म इलेक्ट्रोनिक्स, दूर संचार प्रोद्योगिकी, सी०डी० रोम तकनीक ने ग्रंथालयों के सूचना स्त्रोतों के त्वरित उपयोग को स्थानीय, क्षेत्रीय, राष्ट्रीय एवं अन्तर्राष्ट्रीय स्तर पर सरलतम बना दिया है। सूचना से सम्बन्धित

प्रक्रियाओं में प्रयुक्त होने वाली विभिन्न प्रोद्योगिकियों (Information Technology-IT) जिन्हें सूचना प्रोद्योगिकी कहा जाता है के प्रादुर्भाव एवं उपयोग ने आज सूचना के चयन, संकलन, संग्रहण, प्रक्रियाकरण एवं प्रकीर्णन की विधियों एवं साधनों को बिल्कुल परिवर्तित कर दिया है। साथ ही कंप्यूटर नेटवर्किंग के क्षेत्र में हुए विकासों ने भी इस कार्य में अपनी महत्वपूर्ण भूमिका का निर्वाह करते हुए विश्व के किसी भी स्थान से प्रलेखों में निहित सूचना के सम्प्रेषण में लगने वाले समय को अत्यन्त ही कम यहाँ तक कि नगण्य कर दिया है। सूचना प्रोद्योगिकी की इन्ही अपार विशेषताओं के कारण इनका उपयोग ग्रंथालयों में सूचना सेवाओ को प्रदान करने हेतु किया जा रहा है।

आज सूचना और संचार प्रौद्योगिकी (Information and Communication Technologyu-ICT) ने समूचे विश्व को अपने प्रभाव में ले लिया है। वृहद् रूप से आई०टी० का सम्बन्ध सूचना प्रणाली (Information System), डाटा स्टोरेज, डाटाबेस, विश्लेषण, पुनःप्राप्ति एवं बौद्धिक निर्णय क्षमता (Capability of Intellectual Decision) से हो गया है। 20वीं सदी में सूचना प्रोद्योगिकी ने जन्म लेकर 21वीं शताब्दी में इस क्षेत्र में अभूतपूर्व नव विचारों से ओतप्रोत हाईस्पीड गतिविधियां प्रत्येक राष्ट्र की प्राथमिकता बन चुकी है।

सूचना प्रोद्योगिकी के निरन्तर विकास ने मानव जीवन के प्रत्येक क्षेत्र में एक प्रकार की क्रान्ति का संचार किया है। आज प्रत्येक क्षेत्र में कंप्यूटर का उपयोग बढ़ने से परम्परागत पद्धतियों का उपयोग कम हो गया है। अतः वर्तमान में ग्रंथालय भी सूचना तकनीकी के अनुप्रयोग से अछूता नहीं है। आई०सी०टी० के तीव्र गति से उद्भव एवं विकास के कारण आज परम्परागत ग्रंथालय डिजिटल स्वरूप में परिवर्तित होते जा रहे हैं।। यह सब सूचना संचार (Infomation Communication) की विभिन्न तकनीकों जैसे – टेलीफोन, आप्टीकल फाइबर, सेटेलाइट आदि तथा आई०टी० की प्रणालियों जैसे सी०डी० की प्रणालियों जैसे सी०डी० रोग, डी०वी०डी० वर्ल्ड वाइड वेब आदि के विकास से ही सम्भव हो सका है।[18]

इस प्रकार प्रोद्योगिकी में नवप्रवर्तनों के फलस्वरूप आई०टी० व सी०टी० जैसे अन्तर्विषयी क्षेत्रों का आगमन हुआ है। पिछले चार दशकों में प्रोद्योगिक क्रान्ति ने सूचना के अधिग्रहण, संग्रहण, प्रक्रियाकरण, पुनःप्राप्ति एवं प्रसार की प्रविधियों पर बहुत गहरा असर किया है।

वर्तमान समाज को आकारबद्ध एवं विकसित करने तथा भविष्य के लिये नीतियों का निर्धारण करने हेतु आई०सी०टी० को एक प्रमुख कड़ी के रूप में माना जा रहा है।

5. सूचना खोज प्रवृति पर सूचना प्रसार प्रोद्योगिकी का प्रभाव (Impact of Information Communication Technology on Information Seeking Behaviour)

पूर्व मे की गयी चर्चानुसार सामान्यतया आई०एस०बी० के निम्न लिखित प्रमुख तीन घटक है – उपयोक्ता (User), सूचना (Information) एवं तंत्र (System)। आई०टी० ने आज इन तीनों तत्वों को प्रभावित किया है। इसके फलस्वरूप उपयोक्ता की सेच एवं सूचना आवश्यकता, सूचना की विविधता वच उसके अनेक स्वरूप, तथा तंत्र में निहित विभिन्न पद्धतियों एवं प्रक्रियाओं पर इसका उल्लेखनीय प्रभाव पड़ा है। इसे निम्नांकित बिन्दुओं में परिलक्षित किया गया है।

5.1 उपयोक्ता पर आई०टी० का प्रभाव (Impact of IT on User)

सूचना प्रसार प्रणाली (Information Communication System) में उपयोक्ता एक बहुत ही महत्वपूर्ण कड़ी हैं लेकिन इस कडी के अध्ययन पर अब तक अधिक ध्यान नहीं दिया है। जबकि नियमित उपयोक्ता की सूचना आवश्यकताओं को ध्यान में रखकर ही सूचना तंत्र (Information System) को अभिकल्पित (Design) किया जाना चाहिए। यही वे उपयोक्ता है जिन्हें निश्चित आवृति पर अधिक मात्रा में सूचना की आवश्यकता होती है। ऐसे यूजर की सूचना आवश्यकता एवं उपयोग को निम्नलिखित तीन तत्व प्रभावित करते हैं।

– उपयोक्ता के अभिलक्षण (Characteristics of User)

– उपयोक्ता के प्रकार (Types of user)

– सूचना खोज के उद्देश्य (Purpose or Motive of IS)

वर्तमान में सूचना विस्फोट के फलस्वरूप प्रकाशित सामग्री में आई असीमित वृद्धि ने उपयोक्ता द्वारा किसी अभीष्ट सूचना की खोज संबंधी कार्य को अत्यन्त दुष्कर बना दिया है। आई०टी० के प्रादुर्भाव से उपयोक्ता अपनी सूचना आवश्यकताओं को इन्टरनेट, डब्ल्यू डब्ल्यू डब्ल्यू, सी०डी० रोम, डिजिटल लाइब्रेरी आदि साधनों से तुरन्त खोज

सकता है। ग्रंथालय एवं सूचना केन्द्रों में भी आई०टी० के आगमन ने उपयोक्ता की सोच एवं प्रवृति को अत्यन्त प्रभावित किया है। इसके फलस्वरूप उपयोक्ता की निश्चित आवृति पर समुचित मात्रा में विविध प्रकार की एवं आवश्यकता उन्मुख (Pinpointed) सूचनाओं में उल्लेखनीय वृद्धि हुई है।

5.2 सूचना पर आई०टी० का प्रभाव (Impact of IT on Information)

वर्तमान युग सूचना क्रान्ति ;प्दवितउंजपवद त्मअवसनजपवदद्ध का युग कहा जाता हैं। किसी भी संगठन की सफलता उसकी सूचना संग्रहण की क्षमता एवं सूचनाओं को प्रोसेस करने की क्षमता पर निर्भर करती है। आज संसार के सभी क्षेत्रों में तीव्रता से बदलाव आता जा रहा हैं। अपना अस्तित्व बनाये रखने के लिये हर प्रतियोगी को प्रतिस्पर्धात्मक बने रहने की आवश्यकता है। तथा प्रतिस्पर्धा में बने रहने के लिये प्रतियोगी को समाज की सभी घटनाओं एवं तथ्यों से संबद्ध सूचनाओं से अवगत रहना आवश्यक है। इसी सूचना के आधार पर उपयोगकर्ता द्वारा महत्वपूर्ण निर्णय लिये जाते हैं।

सूचना समाज की संरचना में महत्वपूर्ण भूमिका निभाती है। इनका हमारे दैनिक जीवन में बड़ा महत्वपूर्ण स्थान हैं, क्योंकि ये ज्ञान को बढ़ाती है। किसी व्यक्ति के पास जितनी अधिक सूचनाएं होंगी वह उतना ही सहज एवं शक्तिशाली होगा। जिससे वह नई योजनाओं को सही समय पर क्रियान्वित कर सकता है। आज सूचना प्रोद्योगिकी, कंप्यूटर एवं संचार प्रणाली ने सूचना को बहुत अधिक प्रभावशाली बना दिया है। इस प्रोद्योगिकी का प्रयोग करके सूचना का मूल्य, उसकी गुणवता, शुद्धता, सुलभता एवं निर्णय क्षमता को सुनिश्चित किया जा सकता है।

5.3 सिस्टम पर आई०टी० का प्रभाव (Impact of IT on System)

सिस्टम से यहां अभिप्राय सूचना तंत्र या प्रणाली से है। यह सूचना के संरक्षण (Preservation) एवे संप्रेषण (Transmission) दोनों कार्यो को सम्पादित करता हैं। किसी भी सूचना तंत्र के दो भाग– इनपुट एवं आउटपुट के रूप में होते हैं। इनपुट भाग मे नये प्रलेख एवं सूचनाओं का लगातार प्रवाह बना रहात हैं, साथ ही सूचना के विश्लेषण,

वर्गीकरण के पश्चात् उनकी अनुक्रमणिका तैयार की जाती हैं। यह अनुक्रमणिका यूजर के विभिन्न अभिगमों (Approaches) को संतुष्ट करती हैं। इसे एक प्रभावशाली पुनःप्राप्ति के साधन के रूप में निर्मित किया जाता है। आउटपुट भाग पर उपयोक्ता को उसकी अभीष्ट सूचनाएं उपलब्ध करायी जाती हैं। इसके लिये उसे इंडेक्स की सहायता से अभीष्ट सूचना पर निर्दिष्ट किया जाता है। सूचना अन्वेषण प्रणाली को चित्र–3 द्वारा प्रदर्शित किया गया हैं[19]

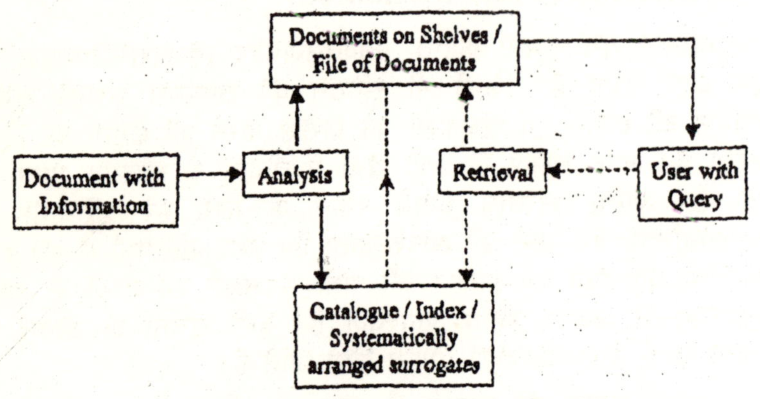

चित्र–3 सूचना अन्वेषण प्रणाली

आज ग्रंथालय एवं सूचना केन्द्र जो कि सूचना तंत्र के ही प्रतिरूप कहे जा सकते हैं। सूचना प्रोद्योगिकी को अपनाने के बाद एक क्रान्तिकारी बदलाव की ओर अग्रसर हो रहे हैं। ये हमारी शिक्षा एवं अनुसंधान प्रणाली के अभिन्न अंग कहे जा सकते हैं। इनका प्रमुख उद्देश्य सूचनाओं का अधिग्रहण, संग्रहण, प्रक्रियाकरण पुनः प्राप्ति एवं उसका प्रसार अपने नियमित उपयोगकर्ताओं को उनकी आवश्यकतानुरूप यथाशीघ्र करना हैं। तथापि सूचना प्रौद्योगिकी एवं कंप्यूटर के चलन ने सूचना तंत्र की विभिन्न पद्धतियाँ एवं प्रक्रियाओं को इस कदर प्रभावित किया है कि मानव की सीमित कार्य क्षमता को इस प्रोद्योगिकी ने असीमित कर दिया हैं।

इस प्रकार सूचना खोज प्रवृति के समस्त सामान्य घटकों अर्थात् उपयोगकर्ता, सूचना एवं सिस्टम पर सूचना प्रोद्योगिकी के प्रभाव को सहज ही महसूस किया जा सकता है। आज जरूरत इस बात की है कि इन तीनों तत्वों पर सूचना प्राद्योगिकी के परिवेश में गहराई से पुनः

विचार एवं खुली चर्चा की जाय ताकि उपयोगकर्ता के इस मनोवैज्ञानिक पक्ष अर्थात् सूचना खोज या अन्वेषण प्रवृति हेतु नये प्रतिमान प्रतिस्थापित किये जा सके। तथापि प्रत्येक उपयोक्ता को उसकी अभीष्ट सूचनाएँ सही समय पर वांछित स्वरूप में यथाशीघ्र देनें हेतु सुनिश्चित की जा सकें जिसे प्राप्त कर उसे पूर्ण संतुष्टि की अनुभूति हो सके।

6. सारांश (Conclusion)

यह एक सर्वविदित तथ्य है कि ग्रंथालय एवं सूचना तंत्र के अभिकल्पीयों (Designers) ने सेवाओं को अभिकल्पित अथवा उनका मूल्यांकन करते समय उनके नियमित एवं वास्तविक उपयोक्ता का अध्ययन शायद ही किया हो। यहां तक कि कभी कभी यह समझना कठिन हो जाता है कि कौन से उपयोक्ता ग्रुप है जिनको लक्ष्य बनाकर सेवाएं प्रारंभ की गयी है। भारतीय परिप्रेक्ष्य मे तो ग्रन्थालय एवं सूचना सेवाओं का परिवीक्षण (Monitoring) करते समय उपयोक्ता पक्ष की काफी उपेक्षा की गयी है। संकलन एवं सेवाएं उपयोक्ता की आवश्यकताओं के अनुरूप विकसित की जानी चाहिए। यह तभी संभव है जब हम वास्तव में उपयोक्ता की आवश्यकताओं, सूचना खोज प्रवृतियों, सूचना के प्रति उनका व्यवहार (Attitute) तथा प्राथमिकताओं (Priorities) का गहन अध्ययन कर उन्हें समझने का प्रयास करें। हमें उनको विश्वास में लेकर यह समझाना होगा कि ग्रंथालय अधिकारी उनकी आवश्यकताओं के साथ हैं। और हमारा प्रमुख ध्येय केवल, उन्हे उपलब्ध संसाधनों के साथ सर्वोत्तम देना है। अतः सेवाओं में निरंतर सुधार लाने के लिये उपयोक्ता व उनकी आवश्यकताओं को समझना नितांत आवश्यक है।

इस आलेख का अन्त टॉम विल्सन[20] के इस कथन से करना उचित होगा कि प्रभावी सूचना सेवाओं के उद्भव के लिये उपयोक्ता को समझना आवश्यक है। यदि हम उपयोक्ता की आवश्यकताओं तथा उन प्रक्रियाओं को जो इन आवश्यकताओं को संतुष्ट कर सकती हैं, को समझने में असफल रहे तो निश्चय ही ये सूचना सेवायें अस्थायी, अप्रयाप्त एवं असंतुष्ट करने वाली साबित होगी। जिसे उपयोक्ता द्वारा अंततः नकार दिया जायेगा। जब ऐसा होने लगे तो सूचना अधिकारी के

लिये बेहतर यह होगा कि वह नये कार्य की तलाश शुरू कर दे क्यों कि वर्तमान कार्य को वह लम्बे समय तक जारी नहीं रख पायेगा।

संदर्भ (References)

1. DEVARAJAN (G) : Users's Approach to Information in Libraries. New Delhi, Ess Ess publibication, 1989. P. 1.
2. SRIDHAR (M S) : Information Behaviour of Scientists and Engineers. ew Delhi, Concept. P. 40
3. CHING-CHIN CHEN: Information Seeking: Assessing and Anticipating User Nees. New York, Neel Schuman, 1982. P. 205.
4. SHU CHING YANG: Information Seeking as Problem-solving using a Quantitative Approach to uncover the Novice Learner's Information Seeking Process in a Perseus Hypertext System. *Library Information Science Research.* 19(1), 1997. P. 73.
5. Ibid P. 74
6. Ibid. P. 75-81
7. CHING-CHIN CHEN. Op. cit. 4, P. 205.
8. SHU-CHING YANG. Op. cit. 5, P. 73-4.
9. PRASAD (H.N.) Op. cit. 2, P. 39-40.
10. ELLIS (D.) : Behavioural Approach to Information Retrieval Design. *Jour. Doc.* 45(3), 1989, P. 171-2
11. KURUPPU (D.C.): Information Needs and Information Seeking Behaviour of Users in Organisations. *Information Study.* 5(1), 1999. P. 60.
12. WILSON (T.D.): Information Behaviour: An Interdisciplinary Perspective. *In:* International Conference on Research in Information Needs, Seeking and Use in different Context: Proceedings, Finland, 1996. Tylor Graham, 1997. P. 39.
13. ESKOLA (Eeva-Liisa): University Student's Infornation Seeking Behaviour in a changing Learning Enbitonmrnt. Information Research 4(2), 1998.P.5.
14. SHU CHING YANG. Op. Cit. 4, P. 73-4.

15. KEENAN (Stella) and JOHNSTON (Colin). Concise Dictionary of library and Information Science. Ed. 2. London, Bowker-Saur, 2000. P. 48.

16. TAYLOR (R.S.) : Information Use Environment. *In* Derwin (Brenda) and Voigt (Melvin J), Eds : Progress in Communication Scienceas. VIO. Norwood, N.J., Ablex, 1991. P. 221-2.

17. KUHLTHAU (Carol C.) : A Principle of Uncertainty for Information Seeking. *Journal Documentation,* 49, 1993. P. 339-55.

18. TILWANI (T.D.) and SHARMA (Arvind) : Digital Library : A New Era (Unpublished Paper).

19. PRASHER (R.S.) : Information and its Communication. New Delhi, Medallion Press, 1991. P. 33.

20. WILSON (TOM) : Information Seeking Behaviour : Designing Information Systems to meet our Clints Needs. *In* Conference of the Association of Carribean University Research and Institutional Libraries : Proceedings, San Juan, 1995. San Juan, ACURIL, 1995. P. 6.

राजस्थान सार्वजनिक ग्रन्थालय अधिनियम, 2006: आलोचनात्मक अध्ययन

Rajasthan Public Library Act, 2006 : Critical Study

एस०पी० सूद

सेवा निवृत एसोसियेट प्रोफेसर एव विभागाध्यक्ष, ग्रन्थालय एवं सूचना विज्ञान विभाग, राजस्थान विश्वविद्यालय, जयपुर

1. विषय प्रवेश (Introduction)

देश में सार्वजनिक ग्रन्थालयों की स्थापना एवं विकास राष्ट्र के व्यक्तियों को ज्ञान अर्जन कर उनके बौद्धिक, सामाजिक एवं आर्थिक विकास का एक प्रमुख साधन है। ग्रन्थालय सेवा द्वारा ही उनका सर्वांगीण विकास संभव है। ग्रन्थालय ज्ञान व सूचना प्रसारण का प्रमुख माध्यम है ऐसे सशक्त माध्यम की उचित व्यवस्था करना शासन की नैतिक जिम्मेदारी है और इस जिम्मेदारी का निर्वहन हेतु सार्वजनिक ग्रन्थालय अधिनियम का लागू किया जाना आवश्यक है।

2. ग्रन्थालय अधिनियम का अर्थ एवं परिभाषा (Meaning of Library Legislation and Definiition)

किसी भी संस्था अथवा कार्यप्रणाली को सुनियोजित ढंग से व्यवस्थित कर नियमबद्ध संचालित करने के लिए उसका आर्थिक आधार

सुदृढ़ होना, प्रशासन पक्ष सबल एवं नियमित होना एवं जनता में उसके प्रति रुचि होना आवश्यक है। यह तभी संभव है यदि उसके पीछे स्पष्ट एवं कानूनी आधार हो।

ग्रन्थालयों में संग्रहीत पाठ्य सामग्री की सुरक्षा एवं उसके उपयोग में वृद्धि, और उसकी सेवाओं को स्थायित्व प्रदान करने के लिए वैधानिक पृष्ठभूमि की आवश्यकता होती है। इसी की पूर्ति हेतु जो अधिनियम बनाया जाता है, उसे ही ग्रन्थालय अधिन्यिम कहते हैं। ग्रन्थालय अधिनियम सार्वजनिक ग्रन्थालयों की संरचना, स्थापना, अधिशासन, रख–रखाव, कार्मिक नियमों के निर्माण एवं संशोधन आदि से सम्बन्ध रखता है।

3. आवश्यकता एवं उद्देश्य (Need and Purpose)

विश्वविद्यालय ग्रन्थालयों, अभियांत्रिकी महाविद्यालय ग्रन्थालयों, चिकित्सा महाविद्यालय ग्रन्थालयों एवं अन्य विभागीय ग्रन्थालयों की तुलना में सार्वजनिक ग्रन्थालयों के लिए अधिनियम अति आवश्यक है क्योंकि अन्य ग्रंथालय सम्बन्धित संस्था के भाग होने के कारण उनके विकास का उतरदायित्व संस्था पर निर्भर करता है। वहीं सार्वजनिक ग्रन्थालयों हेतु इस प्रकार के तन्त्र का अभाव होता है। इस अभाव की पूर्ति सार्वजनिक ग्रन्थालय अधिनियम द्वारा ही सम्भव है। सार्वजनिक ग्रन्थालयों के चहुंमुखी विकास, उनकी कार्यप्रणाली को व्यवस्थित करने, उनके शक्ति स्रोत को उचित मार्ग में प्रवाहित करने, आर्थिक आवश्यकताओं की पूर्ति के लिए ऐसी अधिकारी सता की आवश्यकता होती है जो उचित निर्धारण करके ग्रन्थालय सेवा को व्यापक एवं सफल बना सके।

सार्वजनिक ग्रन्थालय द्वारा बिना भेदभाव – जाति, लिंग, आयु आदि के निःशुल्क सेवा प्रदान किये जाने के लिए सार्वजनिक ग्रन्थालय अधिनियम पारित किया जाना आवश्यक है। इसके अतिरिक्त इसके कुछ अन्य उद्देश्य निम्नलिखित हैं –

1. विश्वसनीय सूचना तथा स्वस्थ मनोरंजन सामग्री के संग्रह के प्रावधान हेतु।
2. ग्रन्थालय सामग्री के अधिकतम उपयोग हेतु समुचित व्यवस्था के प्रावधान हेतु।

3. अपाठकों को पाठक तथा पाठकों को सकारात्मक पाठक बनाने हेतु प्रेरित करने के लिए।
4. ग्रन्थालय सेवाओं के निःशुल्क प्रावधान हेतु निरन्तर वित्तीय अनुदान की व्यवस्था करने हेतु।

4. भारत में पारित सार्वजनिक ग्रन्थालय अधिनियम (Public Library Acts Passed in Indian States)

भारत में सार्वजनिक ग्रन्थालय आन्दोलन के प्रवर्तक एवं ग्रंथालय अधिनियम के प्रणेता डॉ० एस०आर० रंगनाथन, ने सर्वप्रथम 1930 में 'आदर्श ग्रन्थालय अधिनियम का प्रारूप' तैयार किया जिसे प्रथम अखिल एशिया शैक्षणिक सम्मेलन, वाराणसी ने स्वीकार किया गया। डॉ० रंगनाथन के प्रयत्नों से भारत में सर्वप्रथम सन् 1948 में तत्कालीन मद्रास राज्य में सार्वजनिक ग्रन्थालय अधिनियम पारित हुआ। इनके प्रयास स्वरूप ही 1956 में भारत सरकार ने के०पी० सिन्हा की अध्यक्षता में ग्रन्थालय परामर्शदात्री समिति का गठन किया जिसने अनुशंसा की कि केन्द्र व राज्यों में ग्रन्थालय अधिनियम बनने चाहिए।

आज तक भारत के निम्नलिखित 15 राज्यों में सार्वजनिक ग्रन्थालय अधिनियम पारित हो चुके हैं :

क्र०	वर्ष	राज्य	अधिनियम का नाम
1.	1948	तमिलनाडू	तमिलनाडू (मद्रास) सार्वजनिक ग्रन्थालय अधिनियम
2.	1960	आन्ध्र प्रदेश	आन्ध्र प्रदेश सार्वजनिक ग्रन्थालय अधिनियम
3.	1965	कर्नाटक	कर्नाटक (मैसूर) सार्वजनिक ग्रन्थालय अधिनियम
4.	1967	महाराष्ट्र	महाराष्ट्र सार्वजनिक ग्रन्थालय अधिनियम
5.	1979	प० बंगाल	प० बंगाल सार्वजनिक ग्रन्थालय अधिनियम
6.	1988	मणिपुर	मणिपुर सार्वजनिक ग्रन्थालय अधिनियम
7.	1989	केरल	केरल सार्वजनिक ग्रन्थालय अधिनियम
8.	1989	हरियाणा	हरियाणा सार्वजनिक ग्रन्थालय अधिनियम
9.	1993	मिजोरम	मिजोरम सार्वजनिक ग्रन्थालय अधिनियम
10.	1994	गोवा	गोवा सार्वजनिक ग्रन्थालय अधिनियम
11.	2002	गुजरात	गुजरात सार्वजनिक ग्रन्थालय अधिनियम

12.	2002	उड़ीसा	उड़ीसा सार्वजनिक ग्रन्थालय अधिनियम
13.	2005	उत्तराखण्ड	उत्तराखण्ड सार्वजनिक ग्रन्थालय अधिनियम
14.	2006	राजस्थान	राजस्थान सार्वजनिक ग्रन्थालय अधिनियम
15.	2006	उत्तर प्रदेश	उत्तर प्रदेश सार्वजनिक ग्रन्थालय अधिनियम

5. राजस्थान सार्वजनिक ग्रन्थालय आन्दोलन : ऐतिहासिक परिप्रेक्ष्य (Historical; Background of Rajasthan Public Library Act)

राजस्थान में ग्रंथालय अधिनियम की आवश्यकता का उल्लेख सर्वप्रथम डॉ० सम्पूर्णानन्द, तत्कालीन राज्यपाल राजस्थान द्वारा 13 अगस्त, 1962 को राजस्थान ग्रन्थालय संघ के उद्घाटन भाषण में किया गया।

इस दिशा में अगला प्रयास 10 मार्च, 1969 में राजस्थान ग्रंथालय संघ के अध्यक्ष प्रो० सतीश चन्द्र की अध्यक्षत में सम्पन्न कार्यकारिणी की बैठक में सार्वजनिक ग्रन्थालय अधिनियम पारित करने के उद्देश्य से ज्ञापन तैयार करने से हुआ। 4 अप्रैल, 1969 को राजस्थान ग्रंथालय सघ के प्रतिनिधि मण्डल जिसमे अध्यक्ष प्रो० सतीशचन्द्र, सचिव श्री एन०एन० गिडवाणी आदि ने तत्कालीन राजस्थान के मुख्यमंत्री श्री मोहनलाल सुखाड़िया से उनके निवास स्थान पर भेंट कर राजस्थान सार्वजनिक ग्रन्थालय अधिनियम पारित करने का अनुरोध किया। मुख्यमंत्री द्वारा निदेशक, प्राथमिक एवं माध्यमिक शिक्षा, बीकानेर को अधिनियम का प्रारूप तैयार कर सरकार को प्रेषित करने का आदेश दिया। 15 जनवरी, 1970 को सम्पन्न बैठक में ग्रंथालय अधिनियम पर विचार किया गया जिसमें राजस्थान ग्रन्थालय संघ की ओर से श्री एन०एन० गिडवाणी, श्री मोहनराव एवं राज्य ग्रन्थालयरी श्री सी०सी० भण्डारी ने भाग लिया।

फरवरी 1970 में राजस्थान विश्वविद्यालय द्वारा आयोजित गोष्ठी जिसमें राजस्थान के ग्रन्थालयियों द्वारा अधिनियम के प्रारूप पर विचार किया गया। यह प्रारूप मूल रूप से रंगनाथन के मॉडल पब्लिक एक्ट पर आधारित था।

वर्षों तक अधिनियम का प्रारूप शिक्षा विभाग एवं विधि विभाग के मध्य घूमता रहा। पुनः 1991 में प्रो० श्रीवास्तव की अध्यक्षता में गठित

समिति को इस अधिनियम के प्रारूप में संशोधन का कार्य सौंपा गया। समिति द्वारा 1993 के प्रारम्भ में संशोधित प्रारूप सरकार को प्रेषित किया गया।

पुनः 2002 में राजस्थान सरकार द्वारा डॉ० एस०पी० सूद, सेवा निवृत विभागाध्यक्ष की अध्यक्षता में समिति गठन कर इसके प्रारूप को संशोधित करने का कार्य सौंपा गया।

6. राजस्थान सार्वजनिक ग्रन्थालय अधिनियम, 2006 की मुख्य धाराएँ (Main Provisions of Rajasthan Public Library Act, 2006)

राजस्थान सार्वजनिक ग्रन्थालय अधिनियम, 2006 को राज्यपाल महोदय द्वारा 20 अप्रैल, 2006 को अनुमोदित किया गया तथा 24 अप्रैल, 2006 को लागू किया गया।

इस अधिनियम को कुल 8 अध्यायों में विभक्त किया गया है –

अध्याय 1 में इस अधिनियम के नाम का उल्लेख 'राजस्थान सार्वजनिक ग्रन्थालय अधिनियम, 2006' के रूप में किया गया है। इसका कार्यक्षेत्र सम्पूर्ण राजस्थान राज्य होगा।

इस अध्याय में इस अधिनियम से सम्बन्धित पदों जैसे – ग्रंथ, ग्रंथ जमा केन्द्र, ग्रन्थ सेवा केन्द्र, राज्य ग्रन्थालय परिषद का अध्यक्ष, राज्य ग्रन्थालय परिषद, निदेशक, जिला, खण्ड विस्तारी सेवा, ग्रन्थालय, ग्रन्थालय सेवा, स्थानीय प्राधिकारी, ग्रन्थालय सदस्य, विहित सार्वजनिक ग्रन्थालय, पंचायत समिति, सार्वजनिक ग्रन्थालय पद्धति, सार्वजनिक ग्रन्थालय संगम, नियम या विनिमय, वर्ष आदि को परिभाषित किया गया है।

अध्याय 2 में 'राज्य ग्रन्थालय परिषद्' के अन्तर्गत राज्य ग्रन्थालय परिषद के गठन का वर्णन किया गया है। इस परिषद के निम्नलिखित सदस्य होंगे –

(क) पदेन सदस्य –

(i) ग्रन्थालयों का प्रभारी मन्त्री – अध्यक्ष

(ii) ग्रन्थालयों के लिए उत्तरदायी शासन सचिव – उपाध्यक्ष

(iii) शासन सचिव, वित्त विभाग या उप सचिव से निम्न रैंक का उसका नामनिर्देशिति

(iv) निदेशक, महाविद्यालय शिक्षा

(v) निदेशक, प्रारम्भिक शिक्षा

(vi) निदेशक, माध्यमिक शिक्षा

(vii) निदेशक, पंचायती राज

(viii) निदेशक, स्थानीय स्वशासन

(ix) अध्यक्ष, माध्यमिक शिक्षा बोर्ड, राजस्थान

(x) सचिव, राजस्थान राज्य पाठ्य पुस्तक बोर्ड

(xi) ग्रन्थालयाध्यक्ष, राज्य केन्द्रीय ग्रन्थालय

(xii) निदेशक, सार्वजनिक ग्रन्थालय – सदस्य सचिव

(ख) नामनिर्देशित सदस्य –

(i) अध्यक्ष द्वारा ग्रन्थालय सेवाओं से सम्बन्धित विषयों में विशेषज्ञीय ज्ञान और रुचि रखने वाले व्यक्तियों में से नाम निर्देशित तीन सदस्य जिनमें से एक महिला होनी चाहिए।

(ii) जिला ग्रन्थालय का राज्य सरकार द्वारा नामनिर्देशित एक ग्रन्थालयाध्यक्ष

(iii) अध्यक्ष द्वारा नाम निर्देशित दो विख्यात विद्वान।

इस अध्याय में परिषद के मुख्यालय के रूप में जयपुर या अन्य स्थान जैसा कि राज्य सरकार राजपत्र में अधिसूचित करे, होगा।

इस अध्याय में परिषद के अध्यक्ष की शक्तियाँ, कर्त्तव्य और कार्यों का निम्नलिखित ब्यौरा दिया गया है –

(i) इस अधिनियम और नियमों के प्रशासन से सम्बन्धित समस्त विषयों के सम्बन्ध में उसे किये गये निर्देश पर या स्वप्रेरणा से राज्य सरकार को सलाह देना।

(ii) राज्य ग्रन्थालय विकास निधि में से व्यय का नियमों के अनुसार अनुमोदन करना।

(iii) ग्रन्थों के प्रयोग को बढ़ावा देने के लिये किये जाने वाले अद्युपायों के निर्देश देना और समुदाय में पढ़ने की आदत पैदा करना।

(iv) सार्वजनिक ग्रन्थालयों के कार्यकरण, प्रशासन और प्रगति पर धारा 22 के अधीन तैयार की गयी वार्षिक रिपोर्ट पर विचार करना और उस पर सुझाव देना और सिफारिशें करना।

(v) समस्त सार्वजनिक ग्रन्थालयों और सार्वजनिक ग्रन्थालय संगमों के कार्यकरण और प्रशासन का क्रमशः धारा 20 और 21 के अधीन की गयी रिपोर्टो और निरीक्षणों के आधार पर समय–समय पर पुनर्विलोकन करना और लोक शिक्षा और ग्रन्थालय सेवा के अधिक उपयोगी और प्रभावकारी उपकरण होने में आने वाली कठिनाईयों को दूर करने के अर्थोपायों का सुझाव देना।

(vi) सार्वजनिक ग्रन्थालयों के प्रशासन में सुधार के लिए किये जाने वाले अध्युपायों के सम्बन्ध में राज्य सरकार को सिफारिशें करना।

(vii) सार्वजनिक ग्रन्थालयों और सार्वजनिक ग्रन्थालय संगमों को सहायता अनुदान या अन्य वित्तीय सहायता के प्रयोजन के लिए पात्रता हेतु मानदण्ड के रूप में सम्पादन के मानकों और स्तरमानों का सुझाव देना।

(viii) सहायता अनुदान की मात्रा नियत करने के फार्मूले का सुझाव देना।

(ix) सहायता अनुदान से भिन्न वित्तीय सहायता के लिए उद्देश्यों और प्रयोजनों और ऐसी सहायता के लिए पूरे किये जाने वाले निबन्धनों और शर्तों के विषय में राज्य सरकार को सलाह देना।

(x) ग्रन्थालयों के लिए वार्षिक विकास योजना के लिए सुझाव देना और सिफारिशें करना।

(xi) ग्रन्थालय संगोष्ठी, सभाओं और सम्मेलनों का आयोजन और संचालन करना।

(xii) ग्रन्थालय सेवा के क्षेत्र में, राज्य सरकार द्वारा समय–समय पर जारी किये गये मार्गदर्शक सिद्धान्तों के अनुसार समेकित कार्यक्रम तैयार करना।

(xiii) राज्य में दक्ष ग्रन्थालय सेवा के आयोजन और प्रोन्नति के लिए सुझाव देना।

(xiv) आर्थिक संसाधन **जुटाने और** ग्रन्थालय सेवा की प्रोन्नति के लिए सुझाव देना।

(xv) राज्य में ग्रन्थालय **सेवा** में सुधार के लिए दीर्घकालिक और अल्पकालिक योजनाएँ तैयार करना।

(xvi) ऐसी शक्तियों का प्रयोग और ऐसे कृत्यों का पालन करना जो इस अधिनियम या तदधीन बनाये गये नियमों के द्वारा या अधीन उसे प्रदत्त या न्यस्त की गई है।

इस अध्याय में परिषद के सदस्यों की पदावधि, बैठकों, समितियों का गठन, परिषद के सदस्यों के भतों आदि का भी उल्लेख किया गया है।

अध्याय 3 'सार्वजनिक ग्रन्थालयों का निदेशक' के अन्तर्गत भाषा और ग्रन्थालयों के विद्यमान निदेशक को सार्वजनिक ग्रन्थालयों का निदेशक घोषित किया गया है। निदेशक के कार्यों का निम्नलिखित ब्यौरा दिया गया है –

(क) सार्वजनिक ग्रन्थालयों से सम्बन्धित समस्त विषयों का पर्यवेक्षण करेगा;

(ख) सार्वजनिक ग्रन्थालयों की स्थापना और विकास को प्रोन्नत करेगा;

(ग) सार्वजनिक ग्रन्थालयों की योजना, रख–रखाव, प्रोन्नत और विकास और सार्वजनिक ग्रन्थालय पद्धति के संगठन के लिए उतरदायी होगा;

(घ) ग्रन्थालय सेवा और ग्रन्थालय और सूचना विज्ञान में प्रशिक्षण पाठ्यक्रमों का संचालन करने वाली संस्था या सेवा को मान्यता देगा और सार्वजनिक ग्रन्थालयों के कर्मचारियों और अन्य व्यक्तियों के प्रशिक्षण के लिए कार्यक्रमों का आयोजन करेगा;

(ङ) मान्यता प्राप्त ग्रन्थालयों का रजिस्टर रखेगा और ऐसे ग्रन्थालयों के नाम और पतों का प्रकाशन करेगा;

(च) राज्य ग्रन्थालय विकास निधि के लेखाओं का प्रबन्ध और संधारण करेगा और उसका उचित उपयोग सुनिश्चित करेगा;

(छ) सार्वजनिक ग्रन्थालयों में शिक्षाप्रद पुराने और दुष्प्राप्य ग्रन्थों, पाण्डुलिपियों और अन्य दस्तावेजों के संग्रहण और संरक्षण के लिए व्यवस्था करेगा;

(ज) सार्वजनिक ग्रन्थालयों और सार्वजनिक ग्रन्थालय संगमों का निरीक्षण करेगा और उन्हें सलाहकार सेवा देगा;

(झ) परिषद् की ऐसी सिफारिशों का कार्यान्वयन करेगा जो राज्य सरकार द्वारा अनुमोदित हों;

(ञ) सार्वजनिक ग्रन्थालयों, सार्वजनिक ग्रन्थालय संगमों और मान्यता प्राप्त प्रशिक्षण संस्थाओं को सहायता अनुदान और अन्य वित्तीय सहायता के लिए स्कीमों और नियमों तथा विनियमों का प्रशासन करेगा और इस निमित्त समय–समय पर बनायी गयी स्कीमों, नियमों और मार्गदर्शक सिद्धान्तों के अनुसार ऐसे सहायता अनुदान और अन्य वित्तीय सहायता मंजूर और संवितरित करेगा;

(ट) धारा 22 के अधीन यथाअपेक्षिति रिपोर्ट तैयार और प्रस्तुत करेगा;

(ठ) ऐसी अन्य शक्तियों का प्रयोग और ऐसे अन्य कृत्यों और कर्त्तव्यों का पालन करेगा जो इस अधिनियम और नियमों के द्वारा या अधीन उसे प्रदत्त या उस पर अधिरोपित किये जावे।

अध्याय 4 'सार्वजनिक ग्रन्थालय पद्धति' में सार्वजनिक ग्रन्थालय की स्थापना एवं प्रबन्ध, ग्रन्थालय सलाहकार समितियों के गठन, उनके संविधान एवं कार्यो का उल्लेख किया गया है।

अध्याय 5 'सार्वजनिक ग्रन्थालयों के लिये वित' में सार्वजनिक ग्रन्थालयों के बजट, राज्य ग्रन्थालय विकास निधि और उसके धन का उपयोग आदि का वर्णन किया गया है।

अध्याय 6 'सार्वजनिक ग्रन्थालयों और सार्वजनिक ग्रन्थालय संगमों को मान्यता' में प्रदेश में राजस्थान सोसाइटी रजिस्ट्रीकरण अधिनियम, 1958 या राजस्थान लोक न्यास अधिनियम, 1959 के अधीन स्वैच्छिक एजेन्सी द्वारा संचालित सार्वजनिक ग्रन्थालय संगमों को मान्यता, अनुदान एवं अन्य वित्तीय सहायता आदि का उल्लेख किया गया है।

अध्याय 7 'रिपोर्ट और निरीक्षण' के अन्तर्गत सार्वजनिक ग्रन्थालयों के प्रभारियों द्वारा निदेशक को वार्षिक प्रतिवेदन और विवरणियों प्रस्तुत करने का उल्लेख किया गया है। इस अध्याय में सार्वजनिक ग्रन्थालयों और सार्वजनिक ग्रन्थालय संगमों के निरीक्षण के अधिकार का भी वर्णन किया गया है।

अध्याय 8 'प्रकीर्ण' में राज्य ग्रन्थालय परिषद् के सदस्यों के लोकसेवक होने, सद्भावपूर्ण की गई कार्यवाई के लिए संरक्षण नियम बनाने की शक्ति, विनियम बनाने की शक्ति का वर्णन किया गया है।

इस अधिनियम की मुख्य–मुख्य विशेषताएँ निम्नलिखित हैं –

1. राज्य ग्रन्थालय परिषद का गठन प्रस्तावित किया गया जिसके अध्यक्ष ग्रन्थालयों के प्रभारी मंत्री होगे, ग्रन्थालयों के लिए उतरदायी सचिव, उपाध्यक्ष एवं निदेशक सार्वजनिक ग्रन्थालय सदस्य सचिव होंगे। इनके अतिरिक्त वित्त विभाग के सचिव, निदेशक, महाविद्यालय शिक्षा, प्रारंभिक शिक्षा, माध्यमिक शिक्षा, पंचायती राज्य, स्थानीय स्वशासन, अध्यक्ष माध्यमिक शिक्षा बोर्ड, सचिव, राजस्थान राज्य पाठ्यग्रन्थ बोर्ड एवं ग्रन्थालयी, राज्य केन्द्रीय ग्रन्थालय के अतिरिक्त 2 विधानसभा सदस्य, 2 विख्यात विद्वानों, 3 विषय विशेषज्ञों, जिनमें एक महिला एवं एक जिला ग्रन्थालयी को भी नाम निर्देशित सदस्य बनाया जायेगा।

2. सार्वजनिक ग्रन्थालय के निदेशक का कार्य वर्तमान में भाषा एवं ग्रन्थालयों के विद्यमान निदेशक को सौंपा गया है। जो सार्वजनिक ग्रन्थालयों से संबंधित समस्त विषयों का पर्यवेक्षक, ग्रन्थालयों की स्थापना एवं विकास, सार्वजनिक ग्रन्थालय पद्धति के संगठन के लिए जिम्मेदार होगा। साथ ही मान्यता प्राप्त ग्रन्थालयों का रजिस्टर रखेगा और अनुदान प्रदान करेगा। सार्वजनिक ग्रन्थालयों के शिक्षाप्रद पुराने एवं दुष्प्राप्य ग्रन्थों, पाण्डुलिपियों और अन्य प्रलेखों के संग्रहण एवं संरक्षण की व्यवस्था करेगा।

3. राज्य में सार्वजनिक ग्रन्थालयों की जाँच संग्रहालय के लिए राज्य केन्द्रीय ग्रन्थालय, मण्डल स्तरों पर मण्डल ग्रन्थालय, सभी जिलों के लिए जिला ग्रन्थालय, पंचायत समिति के लिए

पंचायत समिति ग्रन्थालय तथा आवश्यकतानुसार ग्रामीण ग्रन्थालय आदि स्थापित किये जाएगें।

4. राज्य केन्द्रीय ग्रन्थालय, मण्डल ग्रन्थालय एवं जिला ग्रन्थालयों के लिए ग्रन्थालय सलाहकार समितियों के गठन का प्रावधान किया गया है।
5. किसी भी प्रकार की ग्रन्थालय अधिकर (Library Cess) के स्थान पर योजना एवं गैर–योजना व्यय के लिए प्रतिवर्ष वार्षिक बजट तैयार किया जायेगा जिनमें विद्यालय ग्रन्थालयों के अतिरिक्त नवीन ग्रन्थालयों की स्थापना, अनुदानित संस्थाओं के लिए वित आदि का प्रावधान सम्मिलित होगा।
6. राज्य ग्रन्थालय विकास निधि की स्थापना जिसमें सरकार से प्राप्त अनुदान, केन्द्रीय संरक्षण से प्राप्त अंशदान, जनता या अन्य किसी भी एजेन्सी द्वारा किये जाने वाला अनुदान सम्मिलित होगा।
7. स्वैच्छिक एजेन्सी द्वारा संचालन व सार्वजनिक ग्रन्थालयों की मान्यता एवं अनुदान का प्रावधान।
8. सार्वजनिक ग्रन्थालयों से सम्बन्धित ग्रन्थालय संघ एवं संगमों को मान्यता एवं अनुदान का प्रावधान।

7. राजस्थान सार्वजनिक ग्रन्थालय अधिनियम, 2006 का आलोचनात्मक अध्ययन (Critical Study of Rajathan Public Library Act, 2006)

1. अधिनियम पारित हुए 15 राज्यों में मात्र पश्चिम बंगाल ही एक मात्र ऐसा राज्य हैं जहाँ अलग से ग्रन्थालय मन्त्री की नियुक्ति का प्रावधान है। अलग से नियुक्त मंत्री ग्रन्थालयों के निर्धारण कर पूर्णतया जिम्मेदार होता है। अच्छा होता कि राजस्थान में भी अलग से ग्रन्थालय मंत्री की नियुक्ति का प्रावधान किया जाये।
2. राज्य ग्रन्थालय परिषद् में 20 सदस्यों के मनोनयन का प्रावधान किया गया है जिसका अध्यक्ष ग्रन्थालयों का प्रभारी मंत्री एवं निदेशक सार्वजनिक ग्रन्थालय सदस्य सचिव होगा। इसमें ग्रन्थालयों से सम्बन्धित पात्र ही सदस्य – 1. ग्रन्थालयी,

राज्य केन्द्रीय ग्रन्थालय एवं जिला ग्रन्थालयी ही सदस्य होंगे शेष सभी सदस्य विभिन्न विभागों के अधिकारी होंगे।

3. राज्य में राज्य ग्रन्थालय विकास निधि के गठन की तो बात की गई है परन्तु इस निधि के आय के स्रोतों का स्पष्ट उल्लेख नहीं किया गया है। चूँकि अधिनियम में किसी प्रकार के ग्रन्थालय उपकर का प्रावधान नहीं किया गया है और न ही शिक्षा के बजट का कुछ प्रतिशत ग्रन्थालयों के विकास हेतु प्रस्तावित किया गया है।

4. सार्वजनिक ग्रन्थालय के निदेशक का पद वर्तमान में भाषा एवं ग्रन्थालय विभाग के निदेशक के अन्तर्गत होगा। सार्वजनिक ग्रन्थालयों के सम्पूर्ण विकास के लिए जहाँ सभी राज्यों में पूर्णकालिक ग्रन्थालय निदेशक के पद का प्रावधान है वहीं राजस्थान सार्वजनिक ग्रन्थालय अधिनियम में विभाग का निदेशक भाषा एवं ग्रन्थालय दोनों विभागों का प्रभारी होगा। राज्य में अभी राजस्थान प्रशासनिक सेवा के सदस्य को विभाग का निदेशक नियुक्त किया जाता है। उसके अधीन कम से कम एक उपनिदेशक ग्रन्थालय सेवाओं से जुड़ा व्यक्ति होना चाहिए।

5. अध्याय 4 सार्वजनिक ग्रन्थालय पद्धति के अन्तर्गत धारा 13 सार्वजनिक ग्रन्थालयों की सहायता और प्रबन्ध में राज्य सरकार राज्य के लिये राज्य केन्द्रीय ग्रन्थालय, मण्डल के लिए मण्डल ग्रन्थालय, जिले के लिऐ जिला ग्रन्थालय, पंचायत समिति के लिए पंचायत समिति ग्रन्थालय और ऐसे अन्य ग्रामीण ग्रन्थालय स्थापित करेगा का उल्लेख है। वहीं बड़े शहरों में ब्रांच ग्रन्थालय, मुहल्ला ग्रन्थालय, चल ग्रन्थालय आदि के बारे में कोई उल्लेख नहीं किया गया है। क्या जयपुर जैसे बड़े शहर में जहां मात्र एक केन्द्रीय ग्रन्थ एवं एक मण्डल ग्रन्थालय है, जयपुर की 20–25 लाख आबादी एवं 50 किमी क्षेत्रफल की ग्रन्थीय आवश्यकताओं की पूर्ति करने के सक्षम होगा? वहीं कोटा, उदयपुर, अजमेर, बीकानेर, जोधपुर आदि शहरों में मात्र एक मण्डल ग्रन्थालय शहरी आवश्यकताओं की पूर्ति कर पायेगा?

अध्याय 5 सार्वजनिक ग्रन्थालयों के लिये वित धारा 15 में निदेशक सार्वजनिक ग्रन्थालय निदेशालय प्रतिवर्ष बजट तैयार करने का प्रावधान प्रस्तावित करता है।

8. राजस्थान में सार्वजनिक ग्रन्थालय अधिनियम पारित होने के बाद का ग्रन्थ सार्वजनिक ग्रन्थालय परिदृश्य (Public Library Scene after the Enactment of Public Library Act in Rajasthan)

राजस्थान में सार्वजनिक ग्रन्थालय अधिनियम, 2006 पारित होने के पश्चात् भी सार्वजनिक ग्रन्थालयों की स्थिति में विशेष अन्तर नहीं आया है। राजस्थान में निम्नलिखित सार्वजनिक ग्रन्थालय कार्यरत हैं –

जयपुर में सर्वपल्ली राधाकृष्णन राज्य केन्द्रीय ग्रन्थालय कार्यरत हैं जिसमें 68,910 ग्रन्थों का संग्रह एवं 200 पत्रिकाएँ मँगाई जाती हैं। ये ग्रन्थालय निम्नलिखित सेवाएँ प्रदान करता है –

1. ग्रन्थ आदान–प्रदान सेवा
2. वाचनालय सेवा
3. सन्दर्भ एवं निर्देशन सेवा
4. रिप्रोग्राफिक सेवा
5. बाल कक्ष सेवा
6. श्रव्य–दृश्य ग्रन्थालय सेवा
7. ग्रन्थालयकर्मियों के लिये समय–समय पर पुनश्चर्या कार्यक्रम एवं सम्मेलनों का आयोजन

राजस्थान के प्रत्येक मण्डल – जयपुर, अजमेर, जोधपुर, उदयपुर, कोटा एवं बीकानेर में मण्डल ग्रन्थालय (Divisional Library) कार्यरत हैं। इन सभी ग्रन्थालयों द्वारा पाठकों के लिए निम्नलिखित सेवाओं का प्रावधान है –

1. ग्रन्थ आदान–प्रदान सेवा
2. वाचनालय सेवा
3. रिप्रोग्राफिक सेवा (सिर्फ जयपुर के महाराजा मण्डल ग्रन्थालय द्वारा ही प्रदान की जाती है।)

4. बाल कक्ष सेवा
5. सन्दर्भ सेवा

राजस्थान के सभी 31 जिलों में जिला पुस्तकालय स्थापित हैं। इन ग्रन्थालयों द्वारा ग्रन्थ आदान–प्रदान सेवा, वाचनालय सेवा, सन्दर्भ सेवा एवं बाल कक्ष सेवाएँ ही प्रदान की जा रही हैं।

राज्य की 237 पंचायतों में अधिनियम पारित होने के पूर्व अंशकालीन ग्रन्थालय कार्यरत थे, अब उन्हें पूर्णकालीन बना दिया गया है। यह ग्रन्थालय ग्रन्थ आदान–प्रदान एवं वाचनालय सेवाएँ ही प्रदान कर रहे हैं।

8.1 वित्त प्रावधान (Finance)

अधिनियम पारित होने के पूर्व ही सार्वजनिक ग्रन्थालयों के लिए जो वित उपलब्ध हो रहा था उसमें कोई विशेष परिवर्तन नहीं हुआ है। क्योंकि अधिनियम में इस हेतु किसी ग्रन्थालय कर (Library Cess) का प्रावधान नहीं किया गया है और न ही शिक्ष के बजट का कुछ प्रतिशत इस हेतु प्रावधान रखा गया है। शासन द्वारा सामान्य वित के अतिरिक्त 11वें बित आयोग से प्राप्त 7.40 करोड़ रुपये से प्राप्त ब्याज एवं राजस्थान पाठ्य पुस्तक मण्डल से प्राप्त उपकर (Levy) तथा राजा राममोहन राय ग्रन्थालय प्रतिष्ठान द्वारा प्रदत्त पाठ्य सामग्री तथा मैचिंग ग्रान्ट ही इन ग्रन्थालयों के वित के प्रमुख साधन है। 12वें वित आयोग द्वारा भी राज्य के 12–13 हेरिटेज ग्रन्थालयों (Heritage Libraries) के विकास हेतु दो करोड़ रुपये की धनराशि प्राप्त हुई है।

8.2 भवन (Building)

अधिकतर ग्रन्थालयों के स्वयं के भवन है बाकी भवनों का निर्माण कार्य चल रहा है। 100 पंचायत समिति ग्रन्थालयों के भवन का निर्माण कार्य पूर्ण हो चुका हैं। इसी काल में अजमेर मण्डल ग्रन्थालय भवन का निर्माण कार्य पूर्ण हुआ है।

8.3 कम्प्यूटरीकरण (Computerization)

राधाकृष्णन राज्य ग्रन्थालय, मण्डल ग्रन्थालयों एवं जिला ग्रन्थालयों में कम्प्यूटरीकरण का कार्य प्रगति पर है। महाराजा मण्डल ग्रन्थालय

जयपुर की वेबसाइट (Website) बनकर कार्य कर रही है। इस हेतु सभी ग्रन्थालयों को एक–एक कम्प्यूटर प्रदान किया गया है तथा राज कोम द्वारा विकसित ई–पुस्तकालय सॉफ्टवेयर प्रदान किया गया है।

Contributors

Anju Vyas (Mrs.) M.A. (Ancient History), MLIS (BHU) is working as Librarian, Centre for Women's Development Studies, New Delhi since last more than 25 years. Prior to that she worked with U.P. State Archives and National Institute of Science, Technology and Development Studies (NISTADS). She jointly organised international conference on Empowering Women through Information and Knowledge: from Oral Traditions to ICT, May 30 - June 2, 2003 at SNDT Women's University. She is Moderator of BOL and has organised many workshops across the country. Mrs. Vyas has to her credit a number of articles in various journals, chapters in books and has presented papers in national and international seminars. She was awarded Commonwelath Scholarship at U.K. during 1978-80 and Dr. C.D. Sharma Memorial Award in 2002 for Advancement and Promotion of Library Movement.

B. Seenaiah has been working as Library Assistant at NALSAR, University of Law, Hyderabad since 2001. He holds M.A. degree in Sociology from Osmania University (2000) and M.L.I. Sc. from Dr. B.R. Ambedkar Open University (2005), Hyderabad.

B.L. Gajja (Dr.) M.A. (Economics), Ph.D. (Dairy Economics) is presently working as Principal Scientist, Central Arid Zone Research Institue, Jodhpur - 342 003 (Raj.) Total Publications - 170, Research Papers 107, Chapters in Books 14, Ph.D Student - 3, Area of Specilization- Environmntal Economics, Impat Assessment of Production Technologies, Information Communication Technology, Natural Resource Management.

C. Lal retired as Librarian from Agra Collge, Agra is an eminent library professional. He participated in several seminars/ conferences/workshops and contributed many articles on latest themes. His area of interest is library softwares and e-resources.

D.V. Kothari, M.A., M.Lib. & Inf. Sc. Ex.-Sr. Tech. Officer, Central Arid Zone Research Institute, Jodhpur (Rajasthan) and presently working as HoD, Jodhpur National University, Jodhpur. He is Life Member of ILA, IASLIC, RLA and Pustakalaya Parishad, Jodhpur (Raj.). He attended one International, three national and three state level conferences. He has edited/compiled six books.

Dayal Singh Bhati, M.A., MLIS is working as Librarian in Army Public School, Jodhpur - 342 001. He is on the way to complete his M.Phil. degree soon. Shri Singh actively participates in National Level Conferences. His area of interest is digitization of library resources. He is Life Member of ILA, IASLIC, Pustakalaya Parishad and SALIS.

Deep Singh is an eminent professional working as Librarian in India's Premier Engineering Institute, Malviya National Institute of Technology (MNIT), Jaipur. He is a life member of ILA, IASLIC, RLA and many other professional organizations. He has contributed several research papers and has conducted case studies. He has worked on many prestigious projects and has chaired many sessions in national and regional seminars.

Geeta G. Gadhavi (Mrs.) is a Asst. Professor and Co-ordinator at Dept. of Library & Information Science, Gujarat University, Ahmedabad. She is having 13 years teaching experience. Her area of interest is IT applications in Libraries, Research in LIS and Management. She has guided 30 students for MLISc projects and more then 70 Information Products on various topics. She has attended many seminars and conferences of National and local level and contributed Five National and one International conference paper. Her contribution for the development of LIS syllabus is noteworthy. She has successfully organised one national level conference and one refresher course. She is a Life member of Gujarat Granthalay Seva Sangh, IATLIS, ILA and ADINET.

Jagdish Arora (Dr.) joined as the Director of Information and Library Network (INFLIBNET) Centre in August, 2007. Prior to his present assignment, Dr. Arora has worked as the Librarian and Deputy Librarian at the Indian Institute of

Technology Delhi from Sept. 2003 to August 2007 and from March 1991 to June 2002 respectively. He was also the National Coordinator of the INDEST-AICTE Consortium. Dr. Arora is recipient of Fulbright Professional Fellowship in Library and Information Science (1997 – 98), SIS Fellow (1999), Young Librarian of the Year (2001, SATKAL), Librarian of the Year (IASLIC, 1999) and ILA-Kuala Best Librarian Award, 2004. Dr. Arora was the Principal Investigator for several projects sponsored by agencies like AICTE, Deptt. of Biotechnology (DBT), Ministry of Information Technology (MIT), Ministry of Human Resource Development (MHRD), the National Highway Authority of India and University Grants Commission. Dr. Arora has more than 60 research articles to his credit.

K. Kumar (Dr.) M.A., MLIS is presently working as Librarian, Govt. College, Chhara, Aligarh (U.P.). His area of interest is networking and he has designed one model for networking.

Kadire Krishna is at present working as Asstt. Librarian at NALSAR University of Law, Hyderabad. He is B.A., B.L.I.Sc. & M.L.I.Sc. from Osmania Unviersity, Hyderabad. He was with American Studies Research Centre (ASRC) for a long period from (1965 to 1996) as a Library Asstt. and later as an Asstt. Librarian. Since 2006 he has been working at NALSAR Library, University of Law. He attended conferences organized by ILA, IASLIC, ASRC and local professional bodies.

Kamal Kant Gupta, MLIS is working as Librarian, University Rajasthan College, Jaipur since 2005. He actively participated in CALIBER (2002) and NACLIN (2002) and presented papers. His area of interest is E-Libraries and digitization. He has also worked with Index India (1993-98).

Kundan Mal Gawaria (Dr.) M.Com. (Business Administration), M.Tech. (IT), Ph.D. (Economics), is presently working as Technical Officer, Central Arid Zone Research Institute, Jodhpur.

M. Ishwara Bhat (Dr.) is the Librarian at Birla Institute of Technology and Science, Pilani, Rajasthan since 2002. He is also a Faculty Member attached to Humanities Studies Group of the Institue. Prior to joining BITS Pilani, Dr. Bhat was with the British Council for 18 years.

M.R. Rawtani (Dr.) is an Associate Professor and Head in the Dept. of Library and Information Science, University of Rajasthan, Jaipur. He obtained his M.A.; LLB; M.Lib.Sc. & Doc. (Gold Medalist) and Ph.D. from Rajasthan University, Jaipur. He served as Asstt. Librarian in National Institute of Ayurveda (1980-83), Jaipur. Before joining the present post. He is a member of Indian Library Association, IASLIC, IATLIS and Rajasthan Library Association. He has contributed twenty articles and three books. Hc is supervising many research scholars for the doctoral programme of the University of Rajasthan.

Madan Singh Rana B.Sc. (Hons.) Chemistry; M.A. (Sociology); M.Lib. & Inf. Sc. is presently working as University Librarian, Banasthali Vidyapeeth, Banasthali, Tonk (Raj.). Prior to this he worked as Librarian in Wildlife Institute of India, Dehradun 248 001. He remained Council Member ILA; President UPLA-Doon branch, 1998-99. He participated in three international, eight national and one state level conference. He has published three books, 10 articles and completed five projects. He has three foreign visits at his credit and was also rewarded by ILA- Kaula Best Librarian Award.

Mihir Ranjan Panda is B.Com., M.L.I.Sc. At present he is working as Library Assistant at Indian Institute of Management, Bangalore. Prior to this he worked as Library Assistant at NALSAR University of Law, Hyderabad for four years (2005-09). He began his career as Technical Assistant with VTLS Software Company, Delhi prior to joining NALSAR University of Law.

Monika Sharma (Mrs.) is working as Librarian, UIET, Panjab Universtiy, Chandigarh (India).

Mukesh Gehlot, M. Tech (IT) is working as Technical Officer (T-5) in Central Arid Zone Research Institute, CAZRI-ICAR, Jodhpur.

P. Radha (Mrs.) has been working as Asstt. Librarian at NALSAR, University of Law, Hyderabad since 2001. She did M.A. (Economics) in 2008 and M.L.I.Sc. in 2001 with a project work on "Storage Technology". She also did a Law Degree from Osmania University in 1998. She attended All India Library Conference in 2007. She did her one year Internship at Osmania University Centre for International Programmes - OUCIP.

P.S.G. Kuamr (Dr.) B.Sc. (Agri.); M.Lib. & Inf. Sc.; Ph.D. (Lib. & Inf. Sc.) worked as University Librarian & Head, Deptt. of Lib. & Inf. Sc., Nagpur University, Nagpur. Dr. Kumar remained president of ILA, IATLIS, LA SAARC, JOCLAI. He organised five national conferences and chaired 18 sessions in various conferences. He has at his credit 27 Books, 57 articles and 69 reviews. He had five professional foreign visits. He was rewarded with FID and IFLA awards.

Parvinder Kaur (Mrs.), M.A., MLIS is presently working in National Ayurvedic University Library, Jodhpur since last two years. She actively participates in `Pustakalya Parishads' activities and seminars.

Pawan Kumar Gupta (Dr.), M.Sc. (Botany) MLLS (Delhi), Ph.D. is presently working as Hony. Director, since 1982 in Rajasthan University Library, Jaipur. Dr. Gupta also worked as Chief Librarian, National Forest Library Since March to Oct. 1997. He is life member of ILA, IASLIC, RLA, Jaipur Library Society, and JALLS. Professionally he worked as Vice-president (West) ILA, President RLA, and President IPLA Rajasthan Chapter. Dr. Gupta was honoured with `Dr. C.D. Sharma Memorial Award for promotion of Library and Information Science in the year 1996 and Best Librarian award by Rajasthan Patrika in 2003. Dr. Pawan Participated in One International, 30 National and 25 State level conferences. He has at his credit of organizing 4 National, 15 State level conference. He authored/ edited 8 Books, 35 articles and completed two projects. Dr. Gupta has two foreign visits (USA & UK).

Prabha Sharma (Dr.) is Working as Deputy Librarian at Rajasthan University Library, Jaipur. Earlier she was working as Assistant Librarian in prestigious Maharani's College (a constituent college of University of Rajasthan) Jaipur. She is actively involved in professional associations. At present she is President of the Jaipur Library & Information Society (JALIS). She is a regular contributor to L&IS literature. She was rewarded with the prestigeous Rajasthan Patrika award for active library services.

a teacher of LIS at Department of L&IS, University of Rajasthan for over two decades and superannuated as Associate Professor from this Department. She has been actively involved in professional activities as author of books in LIS, as contributor of periodical articles etc, Her book on 'Reference Service' in Hindi language has been very popular.

Vimal Kishore Purohit, MCA is working as Technical Officer (T-6) in Central Arid Zone Research Institute, CAZRI-ICAR, Jodhpur.

Vinod, D. MLISc., M.Phil, PGDLAN is currently working as Asstt. Librarian, National Law University, Jodhpur. He has participated in various national and international conferences and seminars. He has been associated with a number of libraries like Indian Institute of Technology, Kharagpur. His areas of research is in law librarianship and e-libraries